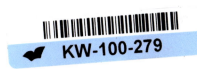

The Transformation of the Social Right to Healthcare

This pathbreaking book investigates welfare state change in the area of healthcare – a field widely neglected by comparative welfare state research. While some work on healthcare expenditure exists, healthcare rights have not been systematically studied since social rights have exclusively focused on entitlement to cash benefits. Addressing this research gap, Böhm analyses in what way the social right to healthcare has been modified in the course of general welfare state transformation since the late 1970s. Taking England and Germany as examples, she assesses how healthcare reforms conducted under the conditions of constrained budgets, demographic ageing, and rapid medical progress, have altered access to and generosity of public healthcare systems over the past 35 years. The book's findings significantly increase our understanding of social rights and reveals fundamental differences of approach: while Germany provides absolute and enforceable rights to healthcare for each (entitled) individual, English social healthcare rights are directed towards the population as a whole and contingent upon the availability of resources, i.e. they are not absolute and not enforceable. This distinction between individual and collective social rights will be an important contribution to the theory of social rights given its applicability to other types of social rights and its usefulness in tracing changes in social rights over time.

Katharina Böhm, is Junior Professor for health policy and politics at the Ruhr University Bochum, Germany. She has published on various health policy issues, including priority setting and rationing, Europeanization of health policy and German health policy reforms.

Social Welfare Around the World
Series editor: Bent Greve
Roskilde University, Denmark

This series publishes high quality research monographs and edited books focusing on development, change in provision and/or delivery of welfare – with a primary focus on developed welfare states. The books provide overviews of themes such as pensions, social services, unemployment or housing, as well as in-depth analysis of change and impact on a micro level. The impact and influence of supranational institutions on welfare state developments are studied as are the methodologies used to analyse the ongoing transformations of welfare states.

Forthcoming titles:

The Transformation of the Social Right to Healthcare
Evidence from England and Germany
Katharina Böhm

Welfare State Transformation in the Yugoslav Successor States
From social to unequal
Marija Stambolieva

The Transformation of the Social Right to Healthcare

Evidence from England and Germany

Katharina Böhm

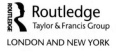

Routledge
Taylor & Francis Group

LONDON AND NEW YORK

First published 2017
by Routledge
2 Park Square, Milton Park, Abingdon, Oxon OX14 4RN

and by Routledge
711 Third Avenue, New York, NY 10017

*Routledge is an imprint of the Taylor & Francis Group,
an informa business*

© 2017 Katharina Böhm

British Library Cataloguing in Publication Data
A catalogue record for this book is available from the British Library

Library of Congress Cataloging-in-Publication Data
Names: Böhm, Katharina, author.
Title: The transformation of the social right to healthcare : evidence from
　　England and Germany / by Katharina Böhm.
Description: Farnham, Surrey, UK, England ; Burlington, VT : Ashgate,
　　2017. | Series: Social welfare around the world | Includes bibliographical
　　references and index.
Identifiers: LCCN 2015045904 (print) | LCCN 2016015764 (ebook) |
　　ISBN 9781472479143 (hardback : alk. paper) | ISBN 9781315552071 (ebook)
Subjects: LCSH: Social medicine—England. | Social medicine—Germany. |
　　Right to health—England. | Right to health—Germany. | Medical care—
　　England. | Medical care—Germany. | Health—Social aspects—England. |
　　Health—Social aspects—Germany.
Classification: LCC RA418 .B63 2017 (print) | LCC RA418 (ebook) |
　　DDC 362.10942—dc23
LC record available at https://lccn.loc.gov/2015045904

ISBN: 978-1-4724-7914-3 (hbk)
ISBN: 978-1-315-55207-1 (ebk)

Typeset in Times New Roman
by Apex CoVantage, LLC

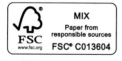

Printed and bound by CPI Group (UK) Ltd, Croydon, CR0 4YY

To Daniel

Contents

Illustrations

Figures

Tables

Acknowledgements

This book is a revised version of my doctoral thesis which I wrote between 2009 and 2014. During this time, I received various help and support from many people without whom I would not have been able to realise this project.

My lasting gratitude goes to *Claudia Landwehr*, my main supervisor and boss of the research project 'Decision-making processes and distributive effects', which I worked for during the last six years at Goethe University Frankfurt and Gutenberg University Mainz. It is almost impossible to specify what I learned and received from her. Claudia introduced me to the academic world and helped me to acquire all the knowledge and research skills essential for a political scientist. I most appreciate that she gave me all the leeway I needed, but was always there if I required advice.

Thomas Gerlinger sparked my interest in the topics of health policy and politics when I was a student at Goethe University and taught me all the fundamentals about this policy area. Having served as supervisor for my Diploma thesis, Thomas encouraged me to take up a PhD, which I would never have thought of as a possible career without him. With his immense knowledge about German and European health policies and politics, Thomas was a great support as second supervisor of my PhD. I am very grateful for all the inspiring discussions we had during the time of writing.

A third important academic mentor for me was *Julien Le Grand*, my supervisor during my visiting scholarship at the Social Policy Department of the London School of Economics and Political Science in 2011. I very much enjoyed our meetings, during which I learned a lot about the huge cultural and institutional differences between our two healthcare systems.

I also wish to thank all my colleagues and friends I worked with during the last six years, of which I can only name some here: my colleagues from the Department of Medical Sociology at Goethe University Frankfurt who provided me with helpful comments at the research seminars during the first phase of my dissertation; my colleagues at the Department of Political Science at Goethe University Frankfurt and Gutenberg University Mainz who contributed to a great working atmosphere and with whom I spent many inspiring lunch and coffee breaks; and last but not least, Dorothea Klinnert, Katharina Kieslich and Ralf Götze who read

xii *Acknowledgements*

earlier versions of my PhD manuscript and helped to improve the book with many useful comments.

I thank my parents for always endorsing me to cut my own way and for rendering my studies possible. With all my heart, I dedicate this book to my husband Daniel who lived with me through all the ups and downs of this project. Thank you for encouraging me in times of hopelessness and sharing the happy moments. Your endless love and support in everyday life gave me the strength to write this book.

Abbreviations

AHA	area health authority
BA	*Bundesagentur für Arbeit*, Federal Employment Agency
BAÄK	*Bundesausschuss der Ärzte und Krankenkassen*, Federal Committee of Physicians and Sickness Funds
BAZÄK	*Bundesausschuss der Zahnärzte und Krankenkassen*, Federal Committee of Dentists and Sickness Funds
BGBl.	*Bundesgesetzblatt,* Federal Law Gazette
BMG	*Bundesministerium für Gesundheit* (1991–2002, since 2005)
	Bundesministerium für Jugend, Familie und Gesundheit (1969–1986)
	Bundesministerium für Jugend, Familie, Frauen u. Gesundheit (1986–1991)
	Bundesministerium für Gesundheit und Soziale Sicherung (2002–2005)
	Federal Ministry of Health
BT–Drs.	*Bundestag–Drucksache*, Official Records of the Bundestag
CCG	clinical commissioning group
CDU	*Christlich Demokratische Union Deutschlands*, Christian Democratic Union of Germany
CSU	*Christlich Soziale Union Deutschlands*, Christian Social Union of Germany
DH	Department of Health
	Department of Health and Social Services (1968–1988)
DM	Deutsche Mark
dpts	dioptres
EC	European Community
ECJ	European Court of Justice
EEA	European Economic Area
EEC	European Economic Community
EU	European Union
EWCA	Court of Appeal of England and Wales
EWHC	High Court of Justice of England and Wales
f.	following page
ff.	following pages
FCC	Federal Constitutional Court

FDP	*Freie Demokratische Partei,* Free Democratic Party
FJC	Federal Joint Committee, *Gemeinsamer Bundesausschuss*
FSC	Federal Social Court
GDP	gross domestic product
GDS	General Dental Services
GMS	General Medical Services
GP	general practitioner
HIV	human immunodeficiency virus
HMSO	Her Majesty's Stationery Office
HSR	health system research
i.c.w	in conjunction with
IQWiG	*Institut für Qualität und Wirtschaftlichkeit im Gesundheitswesen*, Institute for Quality and Efficiency in healthcare
m.	million
MR	Master of the Rolls and Records of the Chancery of England
n.	note
NHS	National Health Service
NIC	national insurance contributions
NICE	National Institute for Clinical Excellence (1999–2005)
	National Institute for Health and Clinical Excellence (2005–2013)
	National Institute for Health and Care Excellence (since 1 April 2013)
No.	number
OECD	Organisation for Economic Co-operation and Development
OTC	over-the-counter
p.	page
pp.	pages
p	pence
para.	paragraph
PCT	primary care trust
PDS	*Partei des Demokratischen Sozialismus*, Party of Democratic Socialism
PMI	private medical insurance
PPC	Pre-payment certificate
PPI	Public Service Provision Index
QALY	Quality Adjusted Life Year
s.	section
sch.	schedule
SCIP	Social Citizenship Indicator Programme
SHI	statutory health insurance
SI	statutory instrument
SoS	Secretary of State for Health
	Secretary of State for Health and Social Services (1968–1988)
SPD	*Sozialdemokratische Partei Deutschlands*, Social Democratic Party of Germany
SPI	statutory pension insurance
TAC	Technology Appraisal Committee

UK   United Kingdom
WASG   *Arbeit und soziale Gerechtigkeit – Die Wahlalternative*, The Electoral
            Alternative for Labour and Social Justice
WSR   welfare state research

Law abbreviations

UK Law

NHS Act	National Health Service Act

German Law

AFG	*Arbeitsförderungsgesetz*	Employment Promotion Law
AMNOG	*Arzneimittelmarktneuord-nungsgesetz*	Act on the Reform of the Market for Medicinal Products
AssPflStatRG	*Gesetz zur Regelung des Assistenzpflegebedarfs in stationären Vorsorge- oder Rehabilitationseinrichtungen*	Act to Regulate the Additional Care Need in Stationary Prevention or Rehabilitation Hospitals
BeitrEntlG	*Beitragssatzentlastungsgesetz*	Health Insurance Contribution Rate Exoneration Act
BeitrSchuldG	*Gesetz zur Beseitigung sozialer Überforderung bei Beitragsschulden in der Krankenversicherung*	Act to Reduce the Excessive Burden of Contribution Debts in Health Insurance
BPflV	*Bundespflegesatzverordnung*	National Order on Hospital Rates
BSSichG	*Beitragssatzsicherungsgesetz*	Contribution Rate Stabilisation Act
GKV–FinG	*GKV–Finanzierungsgesetz*	Act for Sustainable and Socially Balanced Financing of SHI
1.GKV–NOG	*1. GKV–Neuordnungsgesetz*	First SHI Restructuring Act
2.GKV–NOG	*2. GKV–Neuordnungsgesetz*	Second SHI Restructuring Act

GKV–OrgWG	*Gesetz zur Weiterentwicklung der Organisationsstrukturen in der GKV*	Act on the Further Development of Organisational Structures in SHI
GKVRefG	*GKV–Gesundheitsreformgesetz 2000*	SHI Reform Act 2000
GKVSolG	*GKV–Solidaritätsstärkungsgesetz*	Act on the Promotion of Solidarity in SHI
GKV–VStG	*GKV–Versorgungsstrukturgesetz*	Act to Improve the Provision of SHI Services
GKV–WSG	*Gesetz zur Stärkung des Wettbewerbs in der gesetzlichen Krankenversicherung*	Act to Strengthen Competition in Statutory Health Insurance
GMG	*GKV–Modernisierungsgesetz*	SHI–Modernisation Act
GRG	*Gesundheitsreformgesetz*	Health Insurance Reform Act
GSG	*Gesundheitsstrukturgesetz*	Healthcare Structure Act
HBegleitG	*Haushaltsbegleitgesetz*	Accompanying Budget Law
KFRG	*Krebsfrüherkennungs- und -registergesetz*	Act on Cancer Screening and Clinical Cancer Registry
KOV–AnpG	*KOV–Anpassungsgesetz*	KOV–Adjustment Act
KSVG	*Künstlersozialversicherungsgesetz*	Law on Social Insurance for Artists
KVEG	*Kostendämpfungs–Ergänzungsgesetz*	Health Insurance Cost-Containment Amendment Act
KVKG	*Krankenversicherungs–Kostendämpfungsgesetz*	Health Insurance Cost-Containment Act
KVLG	*Gesetz über die Krankenversicherung der Landwirte*	Law on Health Insurance for Farmers
PsychThG/SGB5uaÄndG	*Gesetz über die Berufe des Psychologischen Psychotherapeuten und des Kinder- und Jugendlichenpsychotherapeuten, zur Änderung des SGB V und anderer Gesetze*	Act on the Professions of Psychological Psychotherapists and Children and Teenager Psychotherapists and SGB V and Other Laws Amendment Act
RKG	*Reichsknappschaftsgesetz*	Law on Social Insurance for Mineworkers
RVO	*Reichsversicherungsordnung*	Imperial Insurance Code
SFHG	*Schwangeren- und Familienhilfegesetz*	Help for Expectant Mothers and Families Act

SGB I	*Erstes Sozialgesetzbuch*	Social Code Book I
SGB III	*Drittes Sozialgesetzbuch*	Social Code Book III
SGBIIIÄndG	*SGB III Änderungsgesetz*	Social Code Book III Amendment Act
SGB V (1.–9.) SGBVÄndG	*Fünftes Sozialgesetzbuch (1.–9.) SGB V Änderungsgesetz*	Social Code Book V (1.–9.) SGB V Amendment Act
SVBG	*Gesetz über die Sozialversicherung Behinderter*	Law on Social Insurance of the Disabled

EU-Law

Treaties

TEEC	Treaty establishing the European Economic Community
TFEU	Treaties of the European Union
EC	Treaty establishing the European Community

Regulations

883/2004/EC	Regulation (EC) No 883/2004 of the European Parliament and of the Council of 29 April 2004 on the coordination of social security systems
1408/71/EEC	Council Regulation (EEC) No. 1408/71 of 14 June 1971 on the application of social security schemes to employed persons, to self-employed persons and to members of their families moving within the Community.

Introduction

Everyone gets ill. A common cold, a broken leg or the evil of cancer, we all face various diseases in the course of life. Some of them cause only minor discomfort, some badly impact on our wellbeing, and some even threaten our lives. When we are sick, we often have to rely on help: if we catch a cold, we are happy if someone brings tissues and a cup of hot tea to our bedside. In more severe cases, we require medical attention and general assistance with many necessities of life. But who will be the one to help us? Whose duty is it to help: that of our family, the community, the state? To what extent can we expect them to help? And to whom is help due?

The answers to these questions differ between societies depending upon their general understanding of the division of rights and responsibilities between the individual, the community and the state, and thus inevitably require normative decisions. Answers also vary over time because they depend on knowledge of disease and the existence of available treatments. Western welfare states have responded to the needs of those who are ill by granting a universal social right to healthcare, i.e. providing their citizens with more or less comprehensive entitlements to healthcare, which are then realised by the public healthcare system. Although these systems vary in organisation, funding and provision, as well as in degree of generosity, they coincide in the acknowledgement of society's duty toward its ill members and provide extensive public protections against the risks of illness. Yet decisions regarding the beneficiaries and concrete content of the social right to healthcare are determined through societal compromise and thus evolve uniquely in each welfare state.

To what degree social rights to healthcare differ between welfare states, and how they are amended over time, are questions not well studied because comparative welfare state research has not yet paid much attention to the area of healthcare. Addressing this research gap, this book pursues the question in what way the social right to healthcare has been modified in the course of general welfare state transformation since the late 1970s. Taking England and Germany as examples, it assesses how healthcare reforms conducted under the conditions of constrained budgets, demographic ageing and rapid medical progress, have altered access to and generosity of public healthcare systems over the last 35 years. The goal of this study is not to document the outcome of reforms, but to investigate changes in the legal definition of healthcare entitlement, in order to reveal shifts in the rights and responsibilities of the individual, the society and the state.

The study furthermore targets a second research question: it assesses the driving forces of reform thereby addressing the controversial scholarly debate about how welfare state transformation can best be explained. Amongst the most seminal contributions to this debate is Pierson's 'new politics' approach (Pierson 1996; 2001). Pierson claims that politics in times of austerity fundamentally differ from politics during welfare state expansion, and therefore, classical welfare state theories such as the power resource theory are not capable of explaining reform. Pierson's 'new politics' thesis has been tested for several welfare areas, but not yet satisfactorily for healthcare.[1] Using the findings of the first part of this study as the dependent variable, I test some of Pierson's assumptions for the case of social healthcare rights.

Since the late 1970s, Western welfare states have faced a variety of severe problems. Recurring recessions and generally low growth paired with neo-liberal reforms have squeezed social budgets. In addition, fundamental socio-economic changes, such as altered family structures and demographic shifts, have added pressure to social programmes and posed new challenges for traditional welfare state arrangements. Public healthcare systems have been particularly affected, because they not only suffered from restricted financial resources, but also faced snowballing increases in expenditures stemming from medical progress and rising demand. In response to these challenges, welfare states have conducted more or less comprehensive reforms of their healthcare systems. The content and course of reforms differed greatly between countries, but the most prevalent reform measures included privatisation of costs, introduction of capped budgets, privatisation of provision, as well as the introduction and expansion of market elements (Freeman and Moran 2000; Gerlinger 2009; Schmid, Cacace and Rothgang 2010; Starke and Obinger 2009).

Although much has been written about health reforms occurring over the last three decades, very little has been said about the impacts of austerity and societal changes on the social right to healthcare. Usually, social rights are the subject of comparative welfare state research (WSR), but so far, WSR has given little attention to the area of healthcare. Rather, the focus has mainly been on cash benefits (Hacker 2004; Moran 2000; Rothgang 2010). The most knowledge about healthcare reforms in advanced welfare states stems from the field of health system research (HSR). However, the two disciplines pose disparate research questions and apply differing analytical categories. HSR aims primarily to improve health services and health outcomes (WHO 2009). Therefore, it usually treats aspects of healthcare systems such as the financing, provision or organisation as the independent variable and assesses their effects on the performance of the system (Mills et al. 2008; similarly, Velasco-Garrido and Busse 2010). WSR, on the contrary, seeks to explain the formation of, changes to, and differences between welfare state arrangements (Clasen and Siegel 2007, pp. 3f.) by analysing power relations within society at large, and in politics in particular, by examining normative values guiding welfare policies, and by identifying the institutional characteristics of welfare states potentially impacting policy decisions, to name only some of its main fields of inquiry. Social programmes usually function as dependent variables in WSR studies.

Several health reform studies follow a WSR design (e.g. Giaimo and Manow 1999; Jensen 2011a; Jordan 2011), but so far none have taken the step of analysing health reforms with a social rights perspective. Social rights are – aside from expenditure data and institutional characteristics of welfare programmes – one of the most common indicators for measuring welfare state change (Clasen and Clegg 2007). They are the direct outcome of political conflict and struggle (Blank 2007, p. 7) and hence are better suited than expenditure studies to reveal the driving forces of reforms. However, as the social right to healthcare has not been studied yet, information about changes to this right must be gathered before the causes of welfare state reform can be analysed in a second step.

In the tradition of classical social rights studies such as Esping-Andersen (1990), Kangas and Palme (2007) and Korpi (2003), I define social rights as the legal entitlement to healthcare. Hence, the subject of this study is the legal healthcare entitlement regulation and reform which has occurred over the last three and a half decades. The framework for the analysis is based on the two 'constitutive dimensions of social rights, accessibility and generosity' (Kvist 2007, p. 201). The *access* dimension assesses who is generally entitled to receive benefits, i.e. the beneficiaries of the social programme. The *generosity* of healthcare entitlements is difficult to measure because healthcare benefits are services or benefits in kind, and thus unique to the individual patient. Based on a modified version of the framework developed by Busse, Schreyögg and Gericke (2007) for the inter-country comparison of healthcare entitlement, generosity in this study is understood as consisting of two elements: service coverage and cost coverage. *Service coverage* means the goods and services supplied by the public healthcare system, or more specifically, the goods and services to which eligible persons are entitled. In contrast, *cost coverage* captures the degree of treatment costs borne by the public system. This dichotomous assessment of generosity takes into account that not all goods and services covered by a public healthcare system are automatically reimbursed in full because co-payments and charges often apply.

In general, broad cuts in healthcare entitlement are not to be expected because public healthcare systems typically enjoy broad public support, making them highly immune to retrenchment efforts. This broad support is based on a high level of legitimacy due to universal or majority coverage of the population. Legitimacy is further strengthened by the fact that nearly everyone who benefits also contributes financially in some way or another (Giaimo 2001). Furthermore, in Western societies, 'neither violence nor hunger is any longer the primary security concern of the population, and so the risk of poor health has now emerged as the most imminent threat to the physical wellbeing of individuals' (Jensen 2008, p. 159), and all provisions reducing the risk of illness or restoring health are given high priority. Finally, cuts in health services may cause unnecessary death, or may result in avoidable pain and suffering. Thus, everyone has a vital interest in comprehensive public healthcare provision.

All of the above factors render cuts to public healthcare a delicate task for policy makers. Nevertheless, the two case studies in this book show that healthcare entitlement has been repeatedly subject to retrenchments. Thus, healthcare entitlement is well suited to test Pierson's 'new politics' thesis. The study examines the conditions under which retrenchment reforms are likely, and tests the relevance of partisanship and institutional factors for explaining retrenchment reforms, while using the findings for healthcare entitlement retrenchment as the dependent variable.

Of more relevance than retrenchment, however, are the qualitative transformations of the social right to healthcare that the study finds in both countries: in Germany, the social right to healthcare has become more universal, and the English collective right has become more individualistic. While the German universalisation can be seen as a process of catching up with the general standards of OECD public healthcare systems, the individualisation of the collective social right in England indicates an elemental shift within the tripartite relationship of individual, society and state. For this reason, the individualisation process in England is explored in more detail, its driving forces are evaluated and its likely impact on the future of healthcare entitlement in England in particular, and on social rights in Europe in general, is discussed.

Outline of the book

Chapter 1 develops and presents the theoretical framework of this book in six parts. Part I introduces the subject by providing an overview of the current WSR literature on welfare state transformation, as well as HSR literature on healthcare reform. Based on this literature review, part II identifies research gaps and presents the two research questions of this study: how has the social right to healthcare been changed over the last 35 years? And: how can these transformations be explained? Part III then discusses T. H. Marshall's seminal ideas on social citizenship, as well as other more recent scholarly work on social rights. From this, the definition of social rights that guides this study is derived: social rights are defined as legal entitlements to social benefits, and their content and goals are perceived as contested and historically contingent. Part IV addresses the first research question and develops the analytical framework for the empirical investigation of healthcare entitlement reform. For this purpose, the basic analytical categories of social rights studies – access and generosity – are adapted to the special character of healthcare. In a next step, specific research questions for each of the analytical categories are developed. Part V is dedicated to the second research question. As a lead-in to this section, Pierson's 'new politics' approach is described and some of its critiques are discussed. Then, some of Pierson's central hypotheses are selected for testing in Chapter 5. Next, taking into account further factors potentially explaining healthcare entitlement reforms, a causal model of healthcare entitlement reforms is developed to guide the empirical investigation in Chapter 5. Finally, part VI covers research design and methodology: it explains the case study selection, specifies the period of investigation and expounds on the methods.

Chapters 2 and *3* build the empirical core of this book. The two case studies describe healthcare entitlement reforms in England (Chapter 2) and Germany (Chapter 3) since the late 1970s. The chapters are similarly structured: following a brief overview of the national healthcare system, a detailed description of legal healthcare entitlement and its development since the late 1970s is given. In a third step, healthcare entitlement reforms of the last three and a half decades are analysed. The reforms are presented separately for each government which allows for testing (in Chapter 5) of the influence of partisan politics. In addition to in-depth descriptions of reforms, the sections provide basic information about the particular government, the specific economic situation and relevant health policy issues of the respective period. In the case of England, two additional sections follow: the first concerns the courts' special role in defining healthcare entitlement, and the second one examines the particular influence European Union (EU) law has had on healthcare entitlement in England. Unique to the German case is the joint self-administration's role in defining healthcare entitlement, which is additionally discussed in Chapter 3. Both case studies conclude with a summary and discussion of the main findings.

Chapter 4 answers the first research question. Summing up and comparing the case study findings, the extent and mode of retrenchment are evaluated for each of the analytical categories developed in Chapter 1. In part II, changes to the governance of healthcare entitlement are discussed. A particular focus of Chapter 4 lies on the qualitative transformations of the social right to healthcare that have taken place in England and Germany: part III considers the universalisation of healthcare rights in Germany, while part IV closely examines the individualisation of the collective social right to healthcare in England.

Chapter 5 strives to explain the core findings of the study, i.e. the retrenchment of healthcare entitlement during the 1980s and 1990s, and the individualisation of the social right to healthcare in England. To clarify the driving forces behind retrenchment reforms, part I first outlines the periods of retrenchment in both countries and then discusses the explanatory factors identified in Chapter 1. A comparison of the results for both countries reveals the continuing importance of partisan politics and standard political institutions in explaining welfare state change. Part II diagnoses the Europeanisation of healthcare entitlement and marketisation processes on the national level as the two central roots of the transformation of the collective social right to healthcare in England. Both processes are found to establish a consumer role for citizens which brings about more individualistic social rights.

The *Conclusion* highlights the main findings of the study, recognises its limitations and also discusses the future of the social right to healthcare in Europe.

Note

1   Two recent studies (Jordan 2011; Jensen 2011a) examined the relationship between ruling government party and public health expenditure. Aggregated spending data, however, is not a good measure for assessing the influence of partisanship on policy output. See Chapter 1.5 for a detailed discussion of the studies and the drawbacks of spending data.

1 The social right to healthcare and the transformation of the welfare state

The purpose of this first chapter is to provide the theoretical basis for the empirical analysis of the transformation of the social right to healthcare. In the first part, the general topic of this book – welfare state transformation in the area of healthcare – is introduced: the problems mature welfare states have been confronted with since the mid-1970s are delineated and the reforms which came in response are described. Special attention is paid to the challenges facing public healthcare systems and to healthcare reforms designed to overcome these challenges. Although the research on welfare state transformation and healthcare reform is vast, there remain several research gaps which are identified in the second part of the chapter. The research questions of this study are formulated to address these gaps. Basically, the study follows two research questions, of which one is descriptive and the other causal. Part four focuses on the descriptive research question. It develops an analytical framework for the empirical assessment of healthcare entitlement reforms and establishes more specific research questions. Part five is dedicated to the causal research question and discusses common welfare state theories explaining the (non)formation of retrenchment reforms. From this, two hypotheses that guide the analysis in Chapter 5 are derived and further discussed. In addition, the third part of this chapter develops a definition of social rights. Finally, the research design and methodology are presented.

1.1 Welfare state transformation in healthcare

The history of the welfare state is commonly divided into two parts: the post-World War II golden age, during which welfare programmes and benefits were expanded; and beginning in the late 1970s, the era of austerity, in which welfare states were confronted with various social and economic problems. Welfare states tackled these problems and have enacted numerous reforms since the end of the 1970s. The first part of this chapter describes how these reforms have altered the welfare state in general. The particular challenges facing public healthcare systems are presented in the second part, before an overview of healthcare reforms is given in the third part.

The transformation of the welfare state

The welfare state is in trouble[1] – this insight is not new. Since the late 1970s, the welfare state has faced multiple economic, political and societal challenges.

Processes such as the slowdown of economic growth, rising unemployment, changing patterns of employment, increased capital mobility, demographic ageing, and changing family and social structures have undermined the foundations of the Keynesian welfare state and forced social security systems to adapt to these new conditions (e.g. Butterwegge 2001; Esping-Andersen 1999; Taylor-Gooby 2005).[2] The reforms have altered the welfare state effectively, but the general nature of the change is hard to specify. In the beginning, most academic literature assumed far-reaching welfare state retrenchment, but over the years, as more and more studies were published, a more diversified picture emerged.

Contrary to what race-to-the-bottom theorists had predicted, no drastic reductions in public social spending have occurred. During the 1980s and 1990s, there was even increased social expenditure in nearly all OECD countries;[3] at most, a slowdown in expenditure growth has been witnessed (Castles 2004; Clayton and Pontusson 1998; Starke and Obinger 2009). A massive reallocation of resources between social programmes has also not occurred (Castles 2004). Aggregated spending data, however, gives only a small insight into the mode of welfare state transformation because it is influenced by diverse factors such as economic growth and the number of recipients, which might obscure ongoing transformations (e.g. Kangas and Palme 2007; Korpi 2003; Scruggs 2006).

Analyses of social rights show a different picture. Korpi and Palme (2003) studied income net replacement rates[4] for three social programmes (sick pay, work accident and unemployment insurance) in 18 OECD countries.[5] After reaching a peak between 1975 and 1985, they observe a decrease of net replacement rates in all three programmes in nearly all countries, yet with major differences between countries and programmes. Using a similar research design, but his own data, Scruggs (2006) analysed changes in income replacement rates of public sickness, unemployment and pension programmes from 1971 to 2002. He, too, finds that after peaking in the 1980s, clear signs of retrenchment were evident in nearly all 18 OECD countries studied, but again with major differences between countries.

Expenditure studies, as well as social rights studies, have their limits because welfare state 'recalibration' (Pierson 2001) is a complex, multidimensional process that is hardly captured by quantitative analyses alone (Bonoli and Natali 2012). Moreover, welfare state transformation takes different shapes in different countries and different policy areas since it is heavily influenced by the institutional framework of the particular welfare state or policy area. Despite these differences, some major trends of welfare state reform can be identified.

Many reforms may be described as adaptations to new social needs. The transition to post-industrial society involves various socio-economic changes that create new social risks not addressed by the 'old' welfare state (Rothgang et al. 2010; Taylor-Gooby 2005). One of these changes is the increased labour market participation of women. This has raised the demand for social provisions that allow for the reconciliation of family and work. To address this need, governments all over the OECD realm introduced parental leave schemes and transfer payments, as well as expanded child care provision. The increased labour market participation of women causes a second problem: traditionally, women also cared for the elderly, but with changing employment patterns and family structures, alternative care arrangements are needed. Welfare states responded by adopting long-term care insurance schemes, expanding private or public care services and by introducing diverse other measures. Further new risks arise from structural changes in production. Rationalisation caused by technological progress, together with relocation of companies abroad, decreased the demand for low-skilled workers and heightened their risk of unemployment. At the same time, traditional unemployment insurance and assistance were perceived as inappropriate solutions to long-term unemployment because of their weak incentives for labour market re-integration. In attempting to bring people back into the labour market, activating policies were introduced in nearly all welfare states. While some form of activation such as training schemes or work creation programmes have always been part of most labour market policies (Clasen and Daniel 2006), activation became the leading paradigm of reform. Activation instruments aim at making benefits more conditional by linking them through incentives and sanctions to behavioural requirements (e.g. active job-seeking, participating in job-creation programmes) (Gilbert 2002). Additionally, activation reforms are often accompanied by restrictive measures like the tightening of qualifying conditions or the shortening of the duration of benefits receipt. The expansion of activation policies is impressive: spending for activation measures quadrupled in the EU between 1980 and 1999 (Taylor-Gooby 2005, p. 19).

However, activating policies are far more than just a reaction to changed risks. They express the paradigm shift in social policy which Gilbert (2002) has characterised as 'the enabling state'. The dominant principle of this paradigm – the primacy of the market – has guided various reforms. Capital has been unburdened from taxes and contributions by privatising welfare costs through the introduction of optional or occupational supplementary private insurance schemes (e.g. in pension, health and long-term care). Likewise, following the assumption that private markets work more efficiently than public administrations, public services have been contracted out to private providers and market structures have been introduced into public administration (Gilbert 2002, p. 44). Within this market-oriented approach, benefit recipients are more and more perceived as consumers, and thus many welfare reforms have aimed at strengthening consumer rights in order to enable market participation (Clarke et al. 2007; Gilbert 2002; Needham 2007). The rhetoric of consumer choice and consumer rights has been complemented by the theme of personal responsibility, the support of which has become a main target of the enabling state (Gilbert 2002, p. 43). These transformations indicate a changed understanding of the role of the state and of the relationship between the state and its citizens.

A further reform strategy to be observed in many OECD countries is the restriction of access to welfare through the tightening of eligibility criteria. The aim of these reforms is to target resources to the most needy (Ferrera 2008, pp. 93ff.; Gilbert 2002, p. 44). The tightening of qualifying conditions has also been a strategy with many pension reforms. However, the aim has not so much been to target resources for the needy but to reduce the number of pension beneficiaries in order to stabilise or reduce pension expenditures. Other pension reforms aimed at prolonging the contribution period by postponing retirement age, or by restricting early retirement (Ebbinghaus and Schulze 2008, p. 285).

Challenges facing healthcare systems

The problems welfare states face in the area of healthcare are particularly fierce. In addition to demographic ageing and slowing economic growth, public healthcare systems have had to cope with technological change and medicalisation, both of which have increase demand and boosted expenditures. Furthermore, demographic ageing is especially problematic in healthcare as it has not only an impact on the income base of public healthcare systems, but may also lead to rising expenditures.

When Bismarck introduced the first public health insurance in 1883, average life expectancy was 45 years (Gilbert 2002, p. 32). Today, people live almost 80 years on average (OECD 2012b).[6] In addition, fertility rates have declined, meaning that there are two factors contributing to an ageing population. On the income side, this double burden of demographic change implies that fewer workers must finance a growing share of retirees, which in turn may lead to increased taxes and higher social contributions, and may eventually negatively impact economic growth. To what degree the financial basis of social health programmes is in fact endangered by demographic change depends on the particular type of funding, the develop-ment of economic growth and on the actual effect of labour costs and taxes on competitiveness. In general, contribution-based healthcare systems are expected to be hit more heavily by demographic changes as they are primarily financed from wage deductions and thus funding becomes problematic as the number of wage earners decrease. The problem is less intense with a tax financed healthcare system, because these can resort to a broader source of revenues.

With regard to the expenditure side, increased life expectancy is believed by many health policy actors to boost health spending. This expectation is based on the assumption that older people need more healthcare services (World Bank 1994, p. 4). Yet this assumption is questioned by many experts (e.g. Braun 1998; Reiners 2009). Empirical data indeed shows that health expenditure surges with age, but this can be explained by the proximity of death in old age. A great share of healthcare expenses are generally incurred at the end of life, and because the probability of death increases with age, there is a correlation between age and costs (Dormont et al. 2010, p. 18). Apart from this 'natural correlation' between age and death, it depends on the morbidity of the older population whether growing life expectancy is associated with higher healthcare costs. If people live longer, but at the same time become healthier, costs do not necessarily rise. In fact, empirical findings support the thesis that morbidity is deferred to later phases of life (Dor-mont et al. 2010; Fries, Bruce and Chakravarty 2011). Whether this 'compression of morbidity' thesis remains valid, however, hinges on the health behaviour of the population and thus can be influenced by health policy measures. Summing up the findings on demographic change and health expenditures, it seems that ageing is not a major problem for public healthcare systems. However, reforms result from the perceived need for reform, and demographic ageing has played an important role in legitimising the healthcare reforms of the last decades.

The second highly discussed cost driver is technological change. Usually, tech-nological progress facilitates rationalisations and hence brings about cost savings.

In healthcare, however, technological progress is associated with rising costs. Before shedding light on that puzzle, it needs to be noted that the healthcare sector is very labour intensive, so that rising costs can partly be explained by Baumol's cost disease, i.e. low productivity growth in services leads to rising relative prices and thus to rising costs (Dormont et al. 2010, p. 16; Hacker 2004, no. 12). Gelijns and Rosenberg (1994) addressed the puzzle of mounting costs despite high innovation in healthcare and found several explanations. Many new technologies do not aim at saving costs but at improving the quality of treatment. This is the case because innovation in healthcare often does not occur at the drawing board but comes about through practice (p. 36). However, if a new technology is less expensive than its precursor or than alternative therapies, then aggregate expenditure is also likely to increase due to intensified usage and expanded application. The increased intensity of use can be explained by various factors. One reason is that high-technology medicine is greatly valued in our societies. Hence, its application enhances the professional prestige of doctors, and furthermore, its provision gives hospitals a competitive advantage (p. 34). Moreover, it has been shown that the specialisation of doctors boosts technology-intensive treatment. Intensified usage of high technology, however, might be confined by restrictive reimbursement schemes or cost competition between providers (pp. 34f.). Another reason for mounting expenditure with new technologies is the expansion of application (p. 38). Once on the market, a new technology is often found to be applicable for the treatment of further indications. Furthermore, innovations might allow patients to be treated who formerly were left without treatment either because it was too risky or not even possible. Innovations might also increase application because the new treatment has fewer side effects and thus the risk-benefit analysis becomes positive, even for less serious illnesses (pp. 38f.).

Although less prominent in the public debate, the 'medicalisation' of society certainly constitutes a further factor contributing to rising healthcare expenditure. Medicalisation – understood as a 'process by which nonmedical problems become defined and treated as medical problems' (Conrad 2007, p. 19) – is not a new phenomenon, but in recent decades has assumed vast dimensions.[7] More and more life problems such as menopause, childbirth or sexual dysfunction, for example, have come to be defined as medical problems (Conrad 2007, p. 3), leading to new demands for treatment. Furthermore, '[a]s expectations of health and functioning have risen, conditions that detract even moderately from a sense of optimal human functioning have become interpreted as diseases' (Carpenter 2012, p. 288). Having investigated several cases of medicalisation, Conrad identifies diverse factors driving medicalisation: the medical profession, individuals or groups supporting or opposing certain medical definitions (e.g. Alcoholics Anonymous) and the availability and profitability of treatments (Conrad 2007, p. 22).

As a result of these processes, healthcare spending in OECD countries has been rising continuously. Since the 1970s, total health expenditure has doubled and average public spending on health has increased from 3.4 per cent of GDP in 1970 to 7.5 per cent in 2010 (see Table 1.1), meaning that societies are spending an ever bigger share of their income for healthcare.

Table 1.1 Average healthcare spending of OECD countries 1970–2010[8]

Year	1970	1975	1980	1985	1990	1995	2000	2005	2010
Total expenditure (% GDP)	4.82	6.16	6.68	6.71	7.20	8.13	8.0	9.14	10.09
Total public expenditure (% GDP)	3.41	4.34	4.93	4.90	5.15	5.86	5.85	6.67	7.53

Sources: OECD (2012a), own calculation.

To summarise, healthcare systems face various processes that increase health service consumption and expenditure. Some of these have their origin in more general social and cultural developments, while others stem from the healthcare system itself. The degree to which each country is affected by the above described processes varies and depends, last but not least, on the institutional setting of the particular healthcare system.

Health policy reforms

In reaction to mounting health expenditure, welfare states began to enact health-care reforms at the end of the 1970s. Individual countries have followed diverse reform paths, but some common trends can be witnessed throughout all welfare states. All countries implemented cost-containment as well as structural reforms. In countries with a social health insurance system, cost containment dominated the early reform years, while from the mid-1990s, the policy focus shifted to governance aspects which was hoped would increase efficiency through 'restructuring' (Gerlinger 2009; Hassenteufel and Palier 2008). In contrast, many countries featuring a state healthcare system began structural reforms earlier and concomitantly employed short-term cost-cutting measures.

Amongst cost-containment measures, the increase of private cost sharing and the introduction of budget restrictions have been most common. Most countries have, at some point during the process of reform, introduced or increased co-payments and user charges (e.g. Freeman and Moran 2000; Gerlinger 2009; Starke and Obinger 2009).[9] As a result, private financing rose between 1970 and 2006 from 1.5 per cent of GDP to 2.5 per cent.[10] During this period, various phases can be observed: during the 1970s, public spending expanded from 70.4 to 76 per cent of total health spending; followed by a retrenchment phase during the 1980s and 1990s when the public share decreased to 73 per cent and private contribution rates grew; since the year 2000 public spending has again been on the rise (Schmid, Cacace and Rothgang 2010, pp. 36f.). In addition to co-payments and user charges, many social health insurance systems further privatised costs by freezing the employer's share of contributions.

Another common cost-containment instrument was the introduction and tightening of budget ceilings. Since the ministry (or decentralised state levels) usually controls the health budget and health employment in state healthcare systems, it has been relatively easy to keep the budget in line by fixing it. Most social health insurance countries, in contrast, had to introduce expenditure budgets first. Most

OECD countries established some form of expenditure ceiling, but their organisation (global or sectoral) and level (national, regional or local), as well as the success of these policies, differed between countries.

Cost-containment measures have been accompanied by structural reforms aimed at altering incentive structures for providers and health administrations (Abel-Smith and Mossialos 1994; Freeman and Moran 2000; Gerlinger 2009). Fee-for-service systems, for example, have widely been replaced by prospective capitation payments or other fixed sum payments, because these transfer the cost risk to the provider and deter excessive supply. Yet the key structural reform strategy was the introduction and augmentation of competition and other market instruments (Freeman and Moran 2000, p. 41). Originally, in state as well as in social health insurance systems, market coordination played only a marginal role. Traditionally, state healthcare systems had been characterised by hierarchic state control, while social insurance systems had generally been governed through corporatist self-administration. The introduction of market elements was intended to increase efficiency, improve quality and enhance responsiveness to consumer needs. Which measures were adopted, as well as the degree of marketisation, varied between countries and was influenced by the institutional framework of the given healthcare system and the particular welfare state regime (Giaimo and Manow 1999). Germany and the Netherlands, for example, introduced and fostered competition between health funds as well as between providers (Hassenteufel and Palier 2008, p. 55). Many NHS countries established quasi-markets by splitting state health administrations into providers and payers. Furthermore, they set up managerial control instruments with the intention of enhancing the efficiency of state administrations. The introduction of markets into healthcare was not tantamount to the retreat of the state from healthcare regulation. Quite to the contrary, state governance was strengthened parallel to market expansion in order to organise market regulation (Freeman and Moran 2000; Gerlinger 2009; Giaimo and Manow 1999; Hacker 2004; Rothgang 2009).

This differs with regard to healthcare provision, where private providers now play a more important role. Each country possesses a unique mix of private (for-profit and non-profit) and public healthcare providers. In social health insurance countries, outpatient healthcare is usually provided by private providers (mainly single doctors), and the hospital sector is characterised by a country-specific private-public mix. Contrastingly, in state healthcare systems, inpatient provision is generally public, while outpatient healthcare is provided by private and/or publicly employed general practitioners. It is difficult to establish the exact extent of privatisation in provision because of its various forms. Material privatisation – the sale of publicly owned hospitals and other institutions to private providers – has been limited to sporadic attempts in most countries, with the exception of Germany (Hermann 2007, p. 15). Here, public ownership of all hospitals fell from 46.0 per cent to 32.4 per cent between 1990 and 2007, while private, for-profit ownership rose from 14.8 to 29.7 per cent (Schulten and Böhlke 2009, p. 98).[11] In order to measure privatisation in healthcare, Schmid and Wendt (2010) constructed a service provision index (Public

Service Provision Index, PPI) which calculates the share of public provision throughout all healthcare sectors. They found a general decline in public health service providers between 1990 and 2005, which was more 'substantial' in state than in social insurance systems. However, the comparability of the data used is problematic. The steeper decline of PPI in state healthcare systems can be explained by implicit privatisation, i.e. a shift of resources away from the mainly publicly owned inpatient to the private outpatient sector, which could often be witnessed in state healthcare systems (Schmid and Wendt 2010, p. 69). Another form of privatisation is the contracting out of services only indirectly involved in healthcare treatment such as laundry, catering, cleaning or admin-istration (Maarse 2006, p. 1000). Privatisation of provision is not always the intended goal of policy decisions. In many cases, cost-containment policies and the restructuring of the reimbursement systems triggered privatisation (Maarse 2006; Schulten and Böhlke 2009).

1.2   Research gaps and research questions

In this section, the research gaps in welfare state research, as well as in healthcare system research, are identified. Subsequently, the general research questions of this study are formulated to address these gaps.

Research gaps

As the above presentation has shown, research on welfare state reform is extensive and provides a nearly comprehensive picture of welfare state transformation over the last 35 years. In addition, there exists countless research on healthcare reforms. Nonetheless, the knowledge about welfare state transformation in healthcare is fragmented because most healthcare reform studies have rarely applied welfare state theory, and until now, comparative welfare state research (WSR) has widely neglected public healthcare programmes (Hacker 2004; Moran 2000; Rothgang 2010).[12] What we know about health reform during the past decades has been mainly ascertained by health system research (HSR) specialists. They have pro-duced countless numbers of reports and analyses (e.g. Altenstetter 1997; Busse, Schreyögg and Gericke 2007; Freeman and Moran 2000; Saltman and Figueras 1997). HSR, however, has different goals than WSR, thus posing dissimilar ques-tions and applying distinct analytical categories. HSR primarily seeks to improve health services and health outcomes (WHO 2009). Hence, it is mostly focused on the outcome of reforms with studies targeting the impact that changes in financing, provision and organisation of healthcare have on the performance of the system (Mills et al. 2008; similarly, Velasco-Garrido and Busse 2010). In contrast, WSR strives to explain the formation of, changes to, and differences between welfare state arrangements (Clasen and Siegel 2007, pp. 3f.). Therefore, factors such as institutional characteristics, power relations or normative values typically form the independent variables, while aspects of healthcare systems and healthcare reforms are the dependent variables.

As a result, we know a great deal about reforms of healthcare financing, provision and organisation, but only a little about changes in generosity of healthcare entitlement. The generosity of public healthcare programmes has been the subject of some expenditure studies (e.g. Jensen 2011b), and many healthcare financing studies broached the issue (e.g. Schmid, Cacace and Rothgang 2010). Yet expenditure data cannot reveal qualitative changes, and it furthermore cannot account for shifts in need and demand, thus providing only a fragmented picture. In addition to expenditure studies, social rights studies frequently examine the generosity of welfare programmes. However, no one has so far attempted to systematically examine healthcare entitlement.

Even less is known about the driving forces behind healthcare reform. There is a broad and lively academic debate in WSR about the driving forces of welfare state retrenchment and the resilience of welfare state arrangements (see Chapter 1.5). However, with its focus on outcomes, HSR rarely intended to explain reforms, and thus, it is widely unknown to what degree WSR theories apply to the area of healthcare.

As it is one of the most constitutive elements of the welfare state today (Jensen 2011a; Moran 2000), the nearly complete neglect of healthcare by WSR is distressing. Healthcare is by far the biggest social service, and the second largest spending item of the public purse in OECD countries. In 2009, average public social spending on healthcare amounted to 6.6 per cent of gross domestic product (OECD 2012c). Not only with regard to expenditure is healthcare an important buttress of the welfare state; it is also a crucial factor for its legitimacy. Almost everyone needs medical treatment at least once in her/his life, and thus benefits from these services.

Research questions

This study follows two research aims: first, it adds to the knowledge of welfare state transformation in healthcare by investigating *how healthcare reforms conducted under the conditions of constrained budgets, demographic ageing and rapid medical progress have altered the social right to healthcare over the last 35 years*. Second, the study seeks to explain reforms by examining the driving forces that facilitated or impeded reforms. Hence, the second research question of this study is '*What are the driving forces behind the transformation of the social right to healthcare?*'. The investigation of social healthcare rights reforms is a necessary first step because social rights, which are a classical subject of WSR and usually form the dependent variable of inquiries into the causes of welfare state change, so far have not been systematically researched for the area of healthcare.

As common in traditional WSR social rights studies, this study defines social rights narrowly as the legal entitlement to healthcare.[13] Given this definition, the subject of the study is legal healthcare entitlement regulations, the amendments of which are traced over the last three and a half decades. The first research question is broadly formulated in order to be able to detect any trend in healthcare entitlement regulations. However, given the theoretical background of welfare state transformation, the focus is on retrenchment reforms.

To answer the second research question regarding the driving forces of reforms, the study resorts to classical WSR theories and assesses their explanatory power for the case of healthcare. In doing so, it addresses the WSR debate about the 'new politics of the welfare state'.[14] The 'new politics' approach claims that politics in times of austerity fundamentally differ from politics during welfare state expansion. However, this argument is highly contested within WSR and has so far only rarely been tested for healthcare.

Social rights offer one particular way to conceptualise the welfare state.[15] In my view, they are the most adequate conception for studying welfare state transformation in healthcare because, first, social rights are the dominant form of welfare in modern welfare states and ever more social relationships are structured by legally enforceable rights. Second, social rights are especially suitable for explaining welfare state change because they represent 'the output, or policy, side of the welfare state' (Kvist 2007, p. 201). In contrast to social expenditures or other outcome measures (e.g. income equality, mortality) that are influenced by various other factors, legal entitlements are the direct result of political conflict and struggle (Blank 2007, p. 7), and thus better allow for a causal analysis of the driving forces of reforms. Third, social rights are a broadly used concept in WSR. Thus, results are comparable with research of other welfare areas and contribute to the accumulation of knowledge about welfare state transformation. Last, because social rights embody the normative conceptions of society, an inquiry into social rights reforms allows drawing conclusions about changing normative values and attitudes within society.

The social rights approach, however, has one major shortcoming: it does not reveal anything about the realisation of social rights (Blank 2007, p. 12), i.e. it informs us about formal entitlement, but does not provide evidence as to whether claims have been met in reality. This is especially problematic in the area of social services where, due to the complex organisation of service provision, a gap between legal entitlement and actual access to services often exists. In the long run, however, the real world of a democratic society cannot massively depart from legally guaranteed entitlements, because people would try to enforce their rights by taking legal action, and at the next elections, would hold politicians liable for not fulfilling their expectations.

1.3 Social rights – a definition

The most influential approach to social rights is T. H. Marshall's concept of social citizenship. In his seminal lecture 'Citizenship and Social Class', delivered in 1949, Marshall describes the genesis of social rights in the twentieth century as an inevitable development complementing freedom and political rights as the third constituent of modern citizenship. According to Marshall, it was the establishment of civic rights in the eighteenth century and the expansion of political rights to the general population in the nineteenth century that provided the ground for the emergence of social rights. The basis of civic and political rights is the formal equality of citizens. Once formal equality had been established, an 'urge towards a fuller measure of equality' (Marshall 1950, p. 29) emerged, making equality the guiding principle of social justice (p. 40). Political and collective freedom rights also gave people the necessary means to realise their demands for social equality. However, according to Marshall, social equality is incompatible with the inequalities produced by the market, thus making market restrictions necessary to the fulfilment of social rights. At the same time, Marshall recognises inequality to be a precondition to the functioning of markets because it is a necessary incentive for market participation. Thus, perfect equality is not possible in a capitalist society. The modern welfare state attempts to solve this dilemma by promoting capitalist production, while at the same time regulating and correcting the market. Marshall concludes that, due to its inherent contradiction, this historic compromise is extremely fragile and will not last forever (p. 84).

T. H. Marshall's theory is based on a particular concept of social rights. For him, social rights are a constituent element of citizenship and are thus granted to every recognised member of the state community, irrespective of her/his individual attributes. Marshall leaves open the concrete content of social rights. According to him, social rights cannot be defined ahistorically because in an evolutionary society expectations are rising, and hence, the content of social rights must be constantly adapted to changing prospects, but also to varying resources (p. 59). Marshall was aware of finite resources and competing claims. Thus, he stressed that individual claims cannot be met in every case but must be subordinated, if necessary, to social provisions that aim at improving the general societal wellbeing (p. 59). In other words, Marshall regarded social rights as collective rights that primarily serve society and not the individual. This also becomes apparent in his remarks about the objectives of social rights: these fundamentally redesign the structure of inequality within society and not merely aim at alleviating the worst forms of poverty (p. 46f.). For Marshall, social rights always involved social duties such as paying taxes and school attendance, and he emphasised that if social rights are to exist on a sustained basis, citizens must fulfil their duty to work (p. 77f.). A further characteristic of Marshall's conception is that the main responsibility for the realisation of social rights lies with the state, which he sees as being in charge of redistribution and provision of social services.

Marshall's work has not been spared criticism since its first publication in 1950. One of the bones of contention is the demographic and historic limitation of his depiction of the evolution of citizenship rights. This remains limited to the history of England and does not take into account the chronologies of rights development and the specifications of social rights in other welfare states (e.g. Mann 1987; Turner 1990). Marshall's concept of social citizenship has also drawn feminist criticism for its gender blindness and the ostensibly gender neutral construction of citizenship (e.g. Lister 2003; Orloff 1993). Liberals objected to Marshall's trinity of civic, political and social rights, arguing that social rights cannot be equated with civic and political rights; the latter are negative liberties implying only a duty of non-interference and thus are always enforceable; the former are positive rights involving costs and thus are not always enforceable given the scarcity of resources (Evers and Guillemard 2013; Plant 1998). It is also questionable as to how far Marshall's conception of social rights is still descriptively accurate today. As written above, welfare states are undergoing major transformations, and in particular, the strong role Marshall assigns to the state no longer mirrors reality. Furthermore, several studies have shown that the collective character of social rights described by Marshall is increasingly challenged by individualisation processes (e.g. Bhatia 2010; Redden 2002; Trägårdh and Svedberg 2013). Despite these critiques, Marshall's 'proposition that social citizenship constitutes the core idea of a welfare state' (Esping-Andersen 1990, p. 21) has found many followers, and his theory of social citizenship has become a widely used concept in welfare state research and beyond.

One of the most prominent applications of Marshall's social citizenship theory is Esping-Andersen's welfare regime typology. In comparing types of welfare states, Esping-Andersen (1990) further elaborated the concept of social rights, placing the focus on the de-commodification and stratification effects of social rights. By de-commodification, Esping-Andersen means the degree to which social rights allow an individual to subsist without the need to sell her or his labour on the market (pp. 22, 37). Esping-Andersen's concept of social stratification explains the degree to which social rights modify social structures. In light of these two dimensions and also taking into account the roles of the state, the market and the family in social provision, Esping-Andersen classified, on the basis of empirical data, welfare states into the three well-known welfare state regimes: the social-democratic, the conservative and the liberal. The social-democratic regime type closely corresponds to Marshall's social citizenship ideal, i.e. universal and generous social rights, provided and realised by the state, allowing for a high degree of de-commodification and relatively high levels of equality. Social rights in conservative and liberal regimes, on the contrary, deviate from this model. Social insurances within conservative regimes allow for strong entitlements, but the de-commodification effect is less evident because entitlements depend on contributions from earned income. Furthermore, social rights in conservative welfare regimes are related to class and status and thus replicate the existing social order instead of modifying it. Social rights in liberal welfare states are granted only to the most needy. They are characterised by a low level of generosity and often require prior income or means tests. All other citizens have to rely on the market for social security, which leads to a stigmatisation of beneficiaries and divides society into welfare recipients and non-recipients. With this classification of welfare states, Esping-Andersen reveals Marshall's concept of social citizenship rights to be only one variation of social rights.

A similar conceptualisation of social rights is used by many researchers from the Swedish Institute for Social Research (e.g. Carroll 1999; Kangas and Palme 2007; Korpi 1989; Wennemo 1994).[16] With a theoretical basis in power resource theory,[17] the Swedish researchers see the welfare state as the result of workers' efforts to 'modify outcomes of, and conditions for, distributive processes on markets' (Korpi 2003, p. 427). Hence, social rights do not only aim to redistribute market income, but also to increase the power of workers vis-à-vis capital by allowing them to subsist independently from the market. This explains why their theoretical concept and operationalization of social rights places a high degree of emphasis on de-commodification and wage replacement. With this focus, however, the power resource approach completely disregards social services and hence draws only a fragmentary picture of the modern welfare state (Blank 2007, p. 4).

Social rights research has not been restricted to the power resource approach. There exist several alternative conceptions of social rights, some of which have explicitly been formulated as a critique of the traditional approach, and some refer to earlier works, but depart from them in their definition of social rights. Scruggs (2006), for example, building on the empirical works of the Swedish scholars but leaving aside the theoretical background of power resource theory, understands social rights as welfare commitments affecting people's expectations and incentive structure (p. 351). He acknowledges that social rights follow many different goals, and emphasises that alterations in the design of social rights have an impact on the achievement of these objectives (p. 350).

Clasen and Clegg (2007) criticise the lack of 'salient dimensions' of the social citizenship relationship in the traditional social rights approach (p. 171). They note that the growing importance of responsibilities towards rights is not captured, that social risk categories are taken as a given, and that the individualisation of social rights is not considered. To illuminate these blind spots, the authors propose a complementary approach centred on the conditionality of social rights. Contrary to the view that the conditionality of social rights is a new phenomenon of contemporary welfare state change, they contend that social benefits have always and everywhere been the subject of conditions. In order to capture the conditionality of social rights, Clasen and Clegg developed a framework that differentiates between three different levels of conditionality which are presented in Chapter 1.4.

Blank (2007; 2011) focuses on another blind spot of traditional social rights research: the role of the state in contrast to the private and societal (private non-profit) sector. Referring to the theory of welfare production (e.g. Evers and Olk 1996), he argues that while social benefits can be provided by each of the three sectors, it's a unique feature of the state to grant social rights and thus to guarantee access to welfare goods and services (Blank 2007, p. 6, 2011, pp. 37f.). Blank is right to perceive the state as the single legitimate actor for granting social rights in modern democracies. Yet the task of defining and specifying social rights has been, at least in healthcare, increasingly delegated to non-state actors such as expert bodies or public agencies (Landwehr and Böhm 2011b). The duty of defining the general scope and conditions of social rights remains in the hands of democratic state actors, but the specifics are left to other more or less legitimate actors. This 'fine-tuning' of entitlement can have a major impact on the generosity of and access to social rights and is the reason why non-state actors must also be considered in this study so that no important changes of entitlement are overlooked.

So far, I have referred to positive theories of social rights only, but there exists a lively normative debate about social rights, too.[18] I do not engage in these discussions because the aim of this study is to analyse existing entitlements to benefits. Yet an analysis of substantive rights cannot completely neglect the 'moral' aspect of rights as they 'exist in a fluid or "dialectical" relationship to each other' (Dean 2002, p. 8). This point is best exemplified by the case of human rights. Human rights declarations (e.g. the International Covenant on Economic, Social and Cultural Rights) are 'programmatic' in character (Kaufmann 2003b, p. 40), and reflect the normative objectives of the subscribing nations. Whether or not they become positive rights depends on their national implementation.[19] These 'moral rights' (Dean 2002, p. 11) constitute the basis for claims to concrete entitlements.[20] Conversely, already existing rights influence what a society perceives as morally desirable. Human rights, for example, were postulated after citizenship rights had been more or less fully developed in Western nations. Whether moral claims become substantial rights is decided in 'processes of negotiation and concession' (Dean 2002, p. 11). Hence, legal social rights incorporate those moral convictions that have won recognition in the political process. Due to this interdependence of moral and substantial rights, it is possible to draw conclusions about normative ideas and convictions of the involved actors by analysing positive rights (Blank 2011, p. 30).

T. H. Marshall's conception of social rights as constituent of citizenship and collective right does not depict the variety of forms of social rights in modern welfare states. Therefore, a broader definition of social rights, which is open to different types of social rights, is necessary for this study. Collective social citizenship rights are but one specific kind of social right. They are tightly but not absolutely linked to the social democratic welfare state and constitute a normative goal of many (mainly left-wing) actors. In the tradition of empirical social rights research, social rights are broadly conceived in this study as the legal entitlement to social benefits. Benefits encompass material, immaterial, as well as financial support, and can be provided by both public (which does not necessarily mean state) and private actors. Social rights might be framed as legal rights of individuals, but may also be constituted as collective rights, i.e. general rights of society to be provided with particular benefits, or as legal duties of public or private actors to provide services. I agree with Blank about the state being exclusively responsible for defining the scope and conditions of social rights, because the state is the only legitimate actor to enact law. This does not, however, preclude that the state partly delegates this task to non-state actors. Seen this way, social rights are social constructions (Dean 2002, p. 18) which embody the normative values and attitudes of society. Thus, the decision about which claims are to be met by the welfare state depends on what the society perceives as social need (Esping-Andersen 1999; Jensen 2011b) and accepts as legitimate claim.

This study also does not assume any particular goal of social rights. With the implementation of social rights, various and changing goals are pursued which cannot be assumed *ex ante*, but must be derived from empirical analysis. The content of social rights also cannot be defined ahistorically, as noted by T. H. Marshall and demonstrated by empirical social rights research. The specific content of social rights is repeatedly negotiated, and these negotiations are never free from struggle because social rights redistribute resources and affect the power structures of society. Negotiations thus determine not only who is entitled to what, but also, as Clasen and Clegg (2007) highlighted, the conditions of entitlement. By asking '*who* is entitled to *what*, on *what conditions*?'[21] this study thus takes into account all three aspects of entitlement.

1.4   Assessing retrenchment in healthcare

In order to answer the first research question – how healthcare reforms of the last three and a half decades have altered the social right to healthcare – this study follows traditional social rights research (e.g. Esping-Andersen 1990; Korpi 2003; Scruggs 2006) in applying access and generosity as central categories of investigation. However, to be applicable to healthcare benefits, the analytical categories must be adapted, which is done in this section. In a second step, results from health system research providing some information about changes of healthcare entitlement are presented for each of the analytical categories. From this foundation, more specific research questions are formulated and assumptions about the directions of reforms are made, where possible.

Categories for comparison: access and generosity

In comparative social rights research, generosity of welfare programmes is usually measured by replacement rates.[22] Yet it is not possible to calculate replacement rates for healthcare benefits because they are services and benefits in kind which differ by case. Alternatively, some studies rely on expenditure data (e.g. Jensen 2011a; Jordan 2011). Expenditure data, however, are limited in their depiction of differences and changes in healthcare generosity and 'should not be used as a proxy for the generosity of social rights' (Siegel 2007, p. 51) for two reasons. First, expenditures are usually measured as a share of GDP and are hence influenced by economic up- and downturns. Second, the amount of spending is not only determined by generosity, but also by the degree of need and efficiency of the public healthcare system. Therefore, expenditure data cannot precisely reveal the impact of reforms and thus do not allow for the tracking of driving forces behind single reforms. A third approach to measuring and comparing generosity in healthcare is to evaluate and compare the content of health benefits packages. With the Health-BASKET project,[23] the European Health Management Association attempted to compare the health benefits packages and single healthcare service costs of nine EU countries. The results are disappointing: many countries have only implicitly or vaguely defined benefit catalogues, and all catalogues vary in design and explicitness, rendering conclusive comparison impossible.

But how then should public healthcare retrenchment be studied? Busse, Schreyögg and Gericke (2007) developed a three-dimensional framework for comparing benefits coverage between countries also suitable for the analysis of healthcare entitlement changes within one country. According to the framework, public healthcare entitlement can be described by three coverage dimensions: *population coverage*, *service coverage* and *cost coverage*. Busse and colleagues do not distinguish between access and generosity, but their coverage dimensions can easily be assigned to these two categories. Population coverage defines population groups covered by a public healthcare system, and hence serves to regulate access to the system. Service coverage, together with cost coverage, constitute generosity: the former defines which services and benefits in kind are covered, and the latter determines the share of healthcare costs to be borne by the public healthcare system. This two-dimensional construction of generosity is necessary because the coverage of a particular treatment or service does not always imply the full coverage of costs. Almost all public healthcare systems charge fees or only partly reimburse costs, which may amount to an appreciable financial burden for the patient.

The three analytical categories map the generosity and accessibility of healthcare entitlement, but do not yet capture the conditionality of social rights. Criticising traditional social rights studies for not taking the conditionality of social rights into account, Clasen and Clegg (2007) developed an alternative, three-level framework centred on conditions of benefit receipt. The first level encompasses the mandatory conditions that determine the risk group covered by a particular social programme (e.g. having reached retirement age to be eligible for pension, or, in the case of healthcare, being ill). They call these the 'conditions of category'. The second level addresses 'conditions of circumstance' by assessing eligibility and entitlement criteria. The third level is concerned with 'conditions of conduct', and comprises behavioural requirements and constraints imposed on benefit recipients, for example the new instruments of regulation introduced by activation and personal responsibility policies. Blank (2007) criticises Clasen and Clegg's conditionality framework for not 'distinguishing between a base of entitlement (citizenship, e.g.) and case definition (coming of a certain age)' (p. 9). I take up this critique and exclusively use criteria defining population coverage, i.e. determinants of membership qualification, which I term *population coverage criteria*. Basically, there are three different concepts guiding population coverage in healthcare: citizenship or residence, insurance membership and need (Schmidt 2005b). While citizenship and residency are sufficiently specified coverage criteria, insurance membership, as well as need, must be further defined to be practicable. Common criteria for defining social insurance membership are, for example, membership in a particular occupational group or a certain income threshold.

Population coverage criteria are only one means of defining conditions for healthcare entitlement. Membership in a particular healthcare scheme does not automatically entitle the individual patient to all covered services or to the full reimbursement of costs. In most healthcare systems, entitlement is additionally regulated by *eligibility criteria*, or 'conditions of circumstance' as Clasen and Clegg termed them. Unlike the universal eligibility criteria for cash benefits, eligibility criteria for healthcare are typically defined for single services or single service areas separately. Eligibility criteria may specify characteristics of the person (e.g. age, sex, income) or the disease (e.g. severity) that must be met to qualify as eligible for the receipt of particular benefits. Eligibility criteria may also refer to the behaviour of the patient prior to or during benefit receipt.

Table 1.2 Analytical categories for the assessment of social rights to healthcare

	Access	*Generosity*
Specific analytical categories	*Population coverage*	*Service coverage*
		Cost coverage
Categories of conditionality	*Population coverage criteria*	*Eligibility criteria*

Borrowing from Clasen and Clegg (2007), I term eligibility criteria that define conditions for the patient's behaviour 'conditions of conduct'.[24] Eligibility criteria for service coverage usually differ from those for cost coverage: while the former target services to special groups (e.g. children, the elderly) or diseases, the latter define exemptions from co-payments or entitlement to higher reimbursement percentages. Table 1.2 illustrates the analytical framework for the analysis of healthcare entitlement.

As noted above, the definition and specification of healthcare entitlement is often delegated to specialised bodies. Accepting the assumption that the actor deciding on entitlement makes a difference in decision outcome (Landwehr and Böhm 2011a), this study also takes into account changes in the governance of healthcare entitlement decision-making, as well as changes in the actors granted the decision-making power.

Detailed research questions and assumptions

Since the introduction of national healthcare systems in southern European countries during the 1970s and early 1980s, *population coverage* of public healthcare systems in Europe has been more or less stable at a very high rate of over 95 per cent (Montanari and Nelson 2013, p. 108). Most non-EU welfare states have national healthcare systems and provide universal coverage.[25] Population coverage in Europe further increased towards almost 100 per cent when several European countries with social insurance healthcare systems reached universal coverage in recent years (Busse, Schreyögg and Gericke 2007; Montanari and Nelson 2013).[26] This development is astonishing given the general welfare state crisis, and hence deserves closer attention.

England and Germany, the cases of this study, portray two extremes in the development of population coverage. While the English National Health Service (NHS) granted coverage for all residents from its inception, Germany reached universality only recently, in 2009. Germany is thus a perfect case for tracking the expansion of coverage, and for shedding light on the underlying motivations of expansion. My analysis focuses on regulative reforms that have altered population coverage criteria in Germany. These inform us about who has been granted access to the public healthcare system, and hence might reveal normative criteria guiding expansion. Universal coverage is a core element of the English NHS from which it derives much of its legitimacy. Hence, amendments to the principle of universality are not to be expected.

Concerning the *generosity* of public healthcare systems, much is known about changes in healthcare financing because the OECD maintains a comprehensive long-term database on health expenditures. As described above, research on these data revealed that while overall health expenditure continued to rise, the public share of financing decreased during the 1980s and 1990s. The data, however, do not reveal which charges were increased and which benefits were excluded from public coverage. Charge increases were a very common instrument used regularly by many countries (see above). In addition, some countries have attempted to exclude services and pharmaceuticals from the public health benefits package in order to reduce public spending, but it is not clear to what extent. Most countries have established or expanded positive or negative lists to specify and better control entitlement (Abel-Smith and Mossialos 1994), though that does not necessarily imply a limitation of generosity. Despite a widespread policy discourse about reducing public healthcare to a minimal 'core' package, no country has taken this path so far (Gibis, Koch-Wulkan and Bultman 2004, p. 200). Where services or other benefits have been excluded, cuts seem to have been restricted to certain non-core service areas like dental treatment, plastic surgery or over-the-counter drugs.[27]

Most countries have somehow reduced generosity. I want to find out to what degree generosity of healthcare entitlement has been restrained in the two countries studied. With regard to service coverage, this study investigates which service areas or single treatments have been ex- or included from/into the health benefits package, and which criteria guided exclusions. With regard to cost coverage, the study explores what co-payments (or other cost-sharing arrangements) have been increased or newly introduced.

In contrast to cash programmes, the conditionality of healthcare entitlement has not yet been the subject of research. Hence, we do not know whether conditionality of benefit receipt has been tightened, as was the case with many cash programmes. This book seeks to shed light on the issue, and investigates how eligibility criteria have been modified by recent reforms, or more precisely, it scrutinises whether the generosity of healthcare entitlement has been restricted through the tightening of eligibility. For the purpose of this study, reforms of eligibility criteria are classified as tightening if they reduce the group of patients eligible for a particular treatment, or if they establish conditions for new treatments that exceed the former level of conditionality. With regard to cost coverage, eligibility criteria are characterised as tightening if they result in a more restrictive exemption from charges, i.e. fewer patients are exempted from paying charges.

Given the knowledge from HSR, I expect some retrenchment in service coverage and even greater retrenchment efforts regarding cost coverage. However, overall I expect retrenchment not to be too extensive because healthcare possesses several characteristics making broad retrenchment highly unlikely. First is the universal coverage of most public healthcare systems. Universal coverage implies that in the case of retrenchment reforms, everyone would be affected by cuts and thus opposition to reforms would be broad. Second, due to universal coverage and the fact that public healthcare is financed from contributions or taxes that are paid by (almost) everyone, public healthcare systems enjoy massive public support (Giaimo 2001). Third, because of the vital importance of healthcare, the negativity bias[28] can be expected to be extremely strong in healthcare. Cutting health services might cause at the worst premature death or suffering pain and discomfort, which are high risks that I expect few voters are likely to take. Finally, Western welfare societies in general value health highly (see above) and place a high priority on all provisions that reduce the risk of illness or restore health. In sum, these traits of public healthcare render benefit cuts a highly unpopular reform strategy, and vote-seeking politicians can thus be expected to refrain from deep retrenchment.

There is evidence that the institutional design of decision-making processes has an impact on decision-outcomes for coverage decisions (Böhm, Landwehr and Steiner 2014). Hence, instead of directly curtailing generosity or impeding access to healthcare benefits, reformers might be tempted to alter the institutional design of those bodies charged with the definition of entitlement in an attempt to increase the likelihood of restrictive decisions. In order to detect such 'institutional retrenchment' (Elmelund-Praestkaer and Baggesen 2012), reforms altering the regulation of delegated decision-making in healthcare entitlement are analysed, too.

Table 1.3 gives an overview of the specific research questions and assigns them to the particular analytical categories. Questions about the regulation of entitlement

Table 1.3 Analytical framework and detailed research questions

	Analytical category	*Research questions*
Access	Population coverage	Has access to public healthcare been restricted?
	Population coverage criteria	To whom has access to the public healthcare system been granted and who has been excluded?
Generosity	To what degree has the generosity of healthcare entitlement been restricted?	
	Service coverage	Which service areas or single services have been in- or excluded? What have been the criteria for in- and exclusions?
	Eligibility criteria	Has entitlement to healthcare been restricted through the tightening of eligibility?
	Cost coverage	Which co-payments (or other cost-sharing arrangements) have been increased or newly introduced?
	Eligibility criteria	Have eligibility criteria for the exemption from co-payments been tightened?

Governance-level:
How has the regulation of decision-making for healthcare entitlement been reformed?
Has the authority that defines healthcare entitlement been changed?

decision-making are not part of the analytical framework, but refer to a meta-level concerned with governance issues. For this reason, they have been attached at the end of the table without any reference to the analytical framework.

1.5   Explaining healthcare entitlement reforms

Explaining welfare state transformation has been one of the main tasks of welfare state scholars during the past decades. Amongst the varied attempts, Pierson's 'new politics' approach stands out. He argues that politics in times of austerity completely differ from politics of welfare state expansion and, following from that, new theories for explaining reforms are needed. Pierson's theory has become the reference point for almost all further research on welfare state transformation, but so far, has rarely been tested for the area of healthcare. Selecting some of his central hypotheses, this chapter develops a theoretical framework for the empirical investigation of the driving forces of healthcare entitlement reforms. First, however, Pierson's 'new politics' approach is presented and discussed in detail.

Pierson's 'New Politics' approach and its critique

During the last two decades, much scholarly work has been dedicated to explaining welfare state transformation, or more precisely, much scholarly work has attempted to explain the resilience of welfare states. In the 1990s, scholars were confronted with the conundrum that the radical cutbacks in welfare programmes predicted by the crisis literature did not occur. Instead, welfare states seemed to resist most retrenchment efforts. Pierson addressed this puzzle in his seminal work (Pierson 1994; 1996; 2001) where he made the case that the politics of retrenchment fundamentally differ from the politics of expansion, and thus cannot be explained by the same theories which had helped to explain welfare state growth.[29] According to Pierson, *power resource theory*, which had been very useful in accounting for the differences in welfare state formation, became irrelevant because the power of organised labour declined heavily in most welfare states without bringing about any major retrenchments (1996, p. 150). *Institutionalism* also cannot contribute much to the discussion about welfare state retrenchment. The theory of veto points assumes that fragmented policy systems should decrease the likelihood of retrenchment, while systems with centralised power structures should increase it. According to Pierson, this argument could also be used in reverse: low veto potential not only concentrates authority, but also accountability, thus reducing the possibility of blame avoidance and retrenchment (1996, p. 154). Pierson agrees that previous policies determine the distribution of political resources and thus influence today's policies, but argues that this policy feedback thesis does not allow for any general statement about retrenchment at the welfare state level (1996, p. 154). Yet if adapted to the specific conditions and problems of retrenchment politics, institutionalist theories can be useful for explaining welfare state retrenchment at the programme level (1996, pp. 154f.).

Pierson filled the theoretical gap of common theories to explain welfare state resilience with his theory of the 'new politics of the welfare state'. Referring to Weaver (1986), Pierson claimed that retrenchment politics are predominantly politics of blame avoidance. Because voters show a 'negativity bias', meaning they usually sanction losses more heavily than they reward gains, politicians primarily aim at avoiding policies that are likely to be negatively sanctioned by the voter as opposed to pursuing popular policies. Furthermore, retrenchment policies negatively affect specific groups of voters who are aware of their losses, while reform gains are uncertain and scattered across the population (1996, p. 145). Pierson also argued that the maturity of the welfare state impedes retrenchment because over time, social programmes breed strong interest groups, which then seek to defend existing structures (1996, p. 146). According to Pierson, the design of welfare institutions is also relevant because it determines the ease with which modifications can be made and the visibility of retrenchment reforms (1996, p. 147).

Pierson does not claim that there is no transformation of the welfare state (1996, p. 147). He simply asserts that we should not expect radical retrenchment, and that the new politics are different from the politics of expansion. He expects the new politics to be characterised by the pitting of beneficiary groups against each other and fewer benefit cuts for decisive voter groups. Furthermore, politicians are likely to attempt to keep the visibility of retrenchment low by choosing policies that conceal negative effects, or by diffusing responsibility. Moreover, politicians spread blame by seeking broad coalitions to support reforms. Generally, retrenchment is more likely to occur under the condition of an electoral slack or budgetary crisis (1996, pp. 176f.). In addition, the invisibility of reform and the possibility of 'restructure[ing] the ways in which trade-offs between taxes, spending, and deficits are presented, evaluated, and decided' (1996, pp. 176f.) determine if retrenchment is possible.

Pierson's 'new politics' approach has become the reference point of almost all work on welfare state reform which followed. Besides its wide acceptance, it also had been criticised for its general assumption that the old theories no longer matter. Moreover, alternative measures of retrenchment and updated data have cast doubt on Pierson's thesis of no radical retrenchment. The central thesis of the 'new politics' approach concerning blame avoidance of governments has been proven to be a very good predictor of retrenchment politics. However, there exist some 'anomalies' contradicting its basic assumptions (Bonoli 2012, pp. 95ff.). First, in some cases, politicians have explicitly claimed credit for entitlement cuts. Second, severe retrenchments have been witnessed in sectors usually receiving broad support (e.g. pensions). Third, despite tight social budgets, governments have spent money on the expansion of particular benefits (e.g. active labour policies, childcare), when, according to the logic of blame avoidance theory, they would have fared better maintaining existing benefits insofar as possible. Bonoli explains the first type of anomaly as the congruence of the policy goal of retrenchment with the vote-seeking objective. This might occur in exceptional situations such as a severe budgetary crisis or the existence of a superior policy goal. In these cases, public opinion favours retrenchment and hence, retrenchment can be used for credit claiming (pp. 100f.). In some cases, governments may choose retrenchment reform as the expected 'path of least resistance' (p. 102). Bonoli assumes that politicians not only consider voters' reactions, but are also concerned with the feasibility of a reform. Hence, they choose those reforms which disadvantage groups with weak veto potential or low interest in vetoing reforms (pp. 102f.). The third anomaly – the expansion of benefits despite austerity – usually concerns reforms that promise a win-win situation for both, beneficiaries as well as taxpayers (e.g. 'social investments' such as childcare or activation policies which are supposed to pay out in the long run), and thus most likely receive broad support from various actors. Furthermore, these expansions are very likely to occur in social policy fields with high visibility but low public financial involvement relative to traditional social programmes (pp. 103ff.).

Pierson's assertion about the irrelevance of left-wing actors in times of austerity has been fiercely challenged by power resource scholars. While expenditure studies support Pierson's theory (e.g. Castles 2001; Huber and Stephens 2001), empirical findings of social rights studies not only show significant retrenchment of main replacement rates (see above), but also prove that party politics still matter. The social rights data confirm retrenchment to be more common among centre-right parties than among left parties, while confessional parties fall somewhere between the two (Korpi 2003; Korpi and Palme 2003). Other authors agree on the continuing importance of party politics, but argue that the causal direction has become less clear than it was during the era of welfare state expansion. Ross (2000), for example, points to several cases where left parties had followed the 'Nixon-goes-to-China logic' and introduced major retrenchment and restructuring. The contradictory results of the role of party politics in times of austerity may indicate that politics still matter, but differently than they did during the time of welfare state expansion. There is no simple causal link between party and policies in the sense that the right fosters and the left prevents retrenchment. Instead, which policies the particular party in power chooses to pursue depends on various contextual factors.

Hypotheses

In order to explain healthcare entitlement reforms, I test Pierson's hypotheses for the area of health policy. I am primarily interested in whether his proposition about the irrelevance of power resource theory in times of austerity holds for health policy reforms over the last 35 years. But because Pierson provides strong arguments against retrenchment in general, it is first necessary to explain the occurrence of retrenchment reforms at all. According to Pierson (1996, pp. 176f.), major retrenchment reforms are more likely under the conditions of a severe budgetary crisis, a considerable electoral slack, and where political actors are either able to hide reforms or alter institutional rules to improve justification or shift blame. All four arguments are investigated in Chapter 5 for main healthcare entitlement retrenchment reforms identified in the case studies in Chapters 2 and 3.

In a second step, I examine the role of partisan politics regarding retrenchment reforms in health policy, i.e. I investigate if retrenchment is more likely under a right-wing than under a left-wing party in government. This relationship between partisanship and retrenchment has already been addressed by two recent papers (Jensen 2011a; Jordan 2011). The results of both quantitative analyses confirm the 'new politics' thesis: they do not find any significant effect of partisanship on retrenchment policies.[30] In the absence of alternative data, however, both papers use expenditure data as the dependent variable. We know from similar research on cash programmes that expenditure studies usually confirm a declining role of partisan politics (e.g. Castles 2001; Huber and Stephens 2001). However, spending data is not the best means of tracing the causal link between partisanship and policy output. The actual share of public expenditure is influenced by various factors (see above), and hence is a poor proxy for policy output. Legal entitlement, on the contrary, is usually directly defined in the policy process, and thus better informs us about the influence of partisan politics on policy decisions. Entitlement studies of cash benefits came to different results than did the expenditure studies: left parties are still an important factor for the defence of the welfare state (e.g. Korpi and Palme 2003). So far, however, no one has tested Pierson's hypothesis on healthcare entitlement. Taking the results of the first part as the dependent variable, I attempt to fill this research gap by investigating if retrenchment is enacted likewise by left- and right-wing parties. Table 1.4 clearly represents all hypotheses tested in Chapter 5.

Explaining healthcare reform is a demanding task and in most cases not based on a single variable, but on a combination of many causal factors. Thus, next to partisanship, other factors must be considered as intervening variables. Referring to Ellen Immergut's theory of veto points, I take into account the institutional characteristics of the particular political system. The theory of veto points originates from Immergut's studies on the emergence of public healthcare systems in France, Sweden and Switzerland (Immergut 1992). In this seminal work, she showed that it was not the power of interest groups, but constitutional rules that were decisive for the introduction and various configurations of public healthcare systems. According to Immergut, standard political institutions are very important because they define the 'rules of the game', thereby determining the potential of interest groups to influence the outcome of decisions. She found that although doctors strongly

Table 1.4 Hypotheses

Hypothesis 1
Major retrenchment reforms are more likely to occur . . .
    a) under conditions of severe budgetary crisis.
    b) under conditions of considerable electoral slack.
    c) when reforms can be hidden.
    d) when political actors are able to alter institutional rules to facilitate retrenchment.
Hypothesis 2
Power resource theory does not explain retrenchment: retrenchment is realised regardless of the party in government.

---

opposed a larger role of the state in healthcare in all three countries, they were not able to prevent the introduction of public healthcare in Sweden and France because there were no (Sweden) or only temporary (France) opportunities to veto reforms. In Switzerland, the possibility to call for referenda enabled opponents to successfully veto the introduction of compulsory health insurance. If these findings from the early days of public healthcare systems are still valid, we should expect the existence of many veto points to decrease the likelihood of any type of reform, not just retrenchment reform.

Hacker (2004) studied retrenchment reforms in healthcare and suggested considering, in addition to veto points, the structure of healthcare financing because first, centralised funding schemes face other challenges and demands than decentralised schemes, and second, policy tools for coping with austerity differ between centralised and decentralised funding systems (p. 697). In centralised funding systems such as the English NHS, public health expenses can be directly controlled by political actors. The health budget is part of the general national budget which is every year subject to bargaining in the political arena. In social insurance systems, the overall budget is the result of many decentralised decisions and cannot be directly controlled by political actors. Hence, politicians have to rely on indirect measures to control costs. This may decrease the visibility of cuts, but success of cost containment is uncertain. To what degree the type of healthcare financing affects healthcare entitlement reforms is not clear. Theoretically, there exists a contingency between the health budget and healthcare entitlement: assuming constant need, the budget cannot be reduced without limiting healthcare entitlement. This would mean that in a centralised funding system, budget cuts must always be accompanied by healthcare entitlement cuts. In practice, however, this is not necessarily the case because entitlement is usually not pinpointed but only generally defined and thus must not be adjusted with every budget cut. In a decentralised system where political actors cannot directly control the budget, healthcare entitlement restrictions are a good instrument for reducing expenditures and thus keeping the budget within limits.

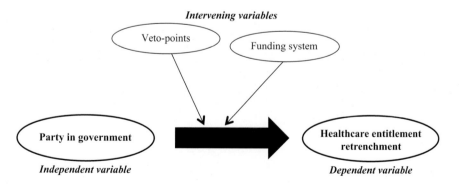

Figure 1.1 Independent and dependent variables – hypothesis 2

1.6   Research design and methodology

The complexity of healthcare entitlement regulation and the fact that little is known about the direction and content of change requires a thorough examination of the transformation process. This limits the analysis to few cases and suggests a case-study design. Case studies are the best means to explore sparsely researched fields (Gerring 2007, p. 40). Such a design is also particularly suitable for this research because case studies allow for the assessment of causal mechanisms (Gerring 2007, pp. 43ff.), especially where causal relations are complex (George and Bennett 2005, pp. 21f.).[31] In this section, I discuss case selection, define the period of investigation, and explain the research methodologies applied.

Case selection

The subject of the study, i.e. welfare state transformation in the area of healthcare, requires cases from the group of advanced welfare states. This reduces possible cases to twenty-some countries.[32] The difficulty with further selection is that the dependent variable is almost unknown, thus case selection according to methodological factors (e.g. typical, deviant or crucial cases) is impossible. This means that irrespective of which countries are chosen, validity of the results is limited.

From the range of possible cases, I have chosen England and Germany for two reasons. First, their healthcare systems are amongst the most studied in HSR because each is a prime example of a particular healthcare system type: the English NHS[33] exemplifies a state healthcare system, while the German statutory health insurance (SHI) represents an archetypal social insurance system (Moran 2000).[34] Thus, there is a broad base of literature on healthcare reform in both countries. Second, because legal entitlement is a constitutional element of healthcare systems, there is a chance that these two countries are also paradigmatic with regard to healthcare entitlement, although entitlement is not part of the ideal type classification.

As is common in welfare state research, one country is treated as one case. Within one case, however, many observations are made.[35] In both countries, government parties changed several times during the period of investigation which allows for studying the impact of partisanship on retrenchment for each case separately. This has the advantage that intervening variables remain more or less constant. Cross-case analysis is of less relevance for the second research question. The primary purpose of the cross-case analysis is to detect similarities and differences of healthcare entitlement reforms in order to gain a more comprehensive picture of healthcare entitlement changes during times of austerity.

Period of investigation

The welfare state crisis is generally recognised to have begun in the mid to late 1970s. Yet the course of reforms differs between welfare areas and welfare states. This is also true for the two countries studied in this book, which is why the starting point of the analysis is slightly different for both countries. In Germany, the first 'cost-containment' health reform was launched in 1977. In England, the first reforms are usually associated with the Conservative rise to power two years later in 1979. The analysis takes into account all reforms adopted up to and including 2013 for both countries.

Methodology

For the first part of the study – the description and analysis of healthcare entitlement reforms – all legislative reforms addressing healthcare entitlement had to be identified as the first step. Although healthcare entitlement is often only vaguely defined, the structure of entitlement regulation can be very complex. Usually, various institutions at different levels and in different areas of the healthcare system are involved in entitlement definition and specification, creating a multilevel structure of regulation. In order to obtain a complete picture of the relevant entitlement regulations, all primary healthcare legislation, as well as potentially relevant secondary legislation and regulations issued by the German joint self-administration for the period under investigation were reviewed. In this process, all regulations defining the goods and services provided by the public healthcare system, as well as regulations specifying beneficiaries of public healthcare, were selected and organised within regulation maps, one for each country for four points in time (depicted in Chapters 2 and 3). In a second step, the most relevant regulations were selected from the regulation maps and their amendments were traced over time.[36] In detail, each amendment of the chosen regulations was looked at in order to determine if the particular reform addressed healthcare entitlement. If it did, the amending regulation was selected for a comprehensive content analysis.[37]

For the content analysis, reform measures were assigned to one of the three analytical categories developed in Chapter 1.4 (population coverage, service coverage and cost coverage). Furthermore, it was evaluated whether generosity was increased or decreased, as well as whether access was expanded or restricted by the particular reform measure. I also noted and categorised which coverage and eligibility criteria were applied. In the course of the analysis, it became evident that service and cost coverage are often determined by characteristics that medical goods and services must fulfil in order to be covered by the public healthcare system (e.g. effectiveness, appropriateness). These 'service criteria' were also noted and categorised, because changes here may strongly impact service or cost coverage. In order to detect variations between service areas and to structure the analysis, the service area(s) affected by the particular reform was recorded. Furthermore, reforms changing the structure or actors of healthcare entitlement decisions were documented. The analysis was conducted with the help of ATLAS.ti, a qualitative data analysis software. Figure 1.2 provides an overview of the main codes used to classify and evaluate healthcare entitlement legislation and reforms. A full set of codes and code description is included in the appendix (Table A.1).

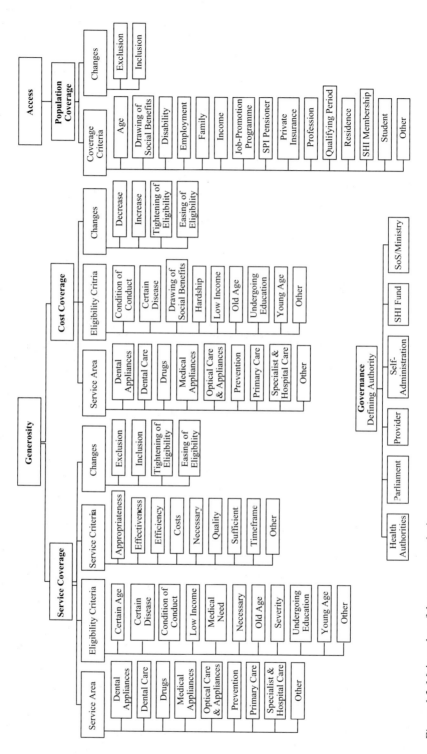

Figure 1.2 Main codes of the content analysis

For the second part – the analysis of the driving forces of reforms – the study relies on different sources. Within the country chapters, background information about the economic and political situations, as well as about important developments in health policy, is given. This information is mainly taken from secondary literature, and the economic data was drawn from national and international (OECD) sources. The causal analysis in Chapter 5 also references secondary literature on healthcare reform. In addition, primary data such as national data on healthcare budgets, polling data or explanatory memorandums of reforms were consulted in order to gain insight into the facilitating and restricting conditions of reforms.

Notes

1   This expression has often been used in literature on the welfare state, e.g. Moran (2000), Rhodes (1996).
2   For an overview, see Ferrera (2008).
3   With the exception of Ireland and the Netherlands.
4   Net replacement rates measure what percentage of work income is replaced by income received from social security programmes after taxes and social security contributions have been paid.
5   See also Korpi (2003).
6   On OECD average in 2010.
7   For a discussion of various aspects of today's medicalisation, see the issue of the British Medical Journal dedicated to that theme from 13 April 2002 (Volume 343).
8   Average health expenditure of countries already members of OECD in 1970.
9   There exists an infinite number of publications on healthcare financing (e.g. Busse, Schreyögg and Gericke 2007; Hermann 2007; Maarse 2006). For an overview, see Schmid, Cacace and Rothgang (2010). The description here is based on Schmid, Cacace and Rothgang (2010) because they have the newest data and most diversified analysis.
10 Private financing also includes private health insurance contributions and other out-of-pocket payments. The increase we see in the share of private financing, however, goes back to an increase in out-of-pocket payments (Montanari and Nelson 2013, p. 107) and hence is at least partly caused by a rise in co-payments and user charges.
11 Additionally, formal privatisation loomed large in Germany: the state region or municipality maintained ownership, but the legal form of the hospital was changed from public to private.
12 Among the few exceptions are: Giaimo and Manow (1999), Hacker (2004), Jensen (2011a), Jordan (2011) and Moran (2000).
13 A more detailed definition of social rights is provided in Chapter 1.3.
14 See Chapter 1.5 for further information on the 'new politics' approach.
15 Social citizenship can be understood as a 'systematized concept' of the broader 'background concept' of the welfare state: While the welfare state is a conglomerate of myriad meanings and understandings, social citizenship is a concrete formulation which grasps the welfare state at a lower level of abstraction (Kvist 2007, p. 201).
16 The Swedish Institute for Social Research at Stockholm University hosts the Swedish Social Citizenship Indicator Programme (SCIP), a database which contains information about replacement rates, the degree of population coverage, and qualifying conditions like waiting days or income ceilings for pension, unemployment, sickness, work accident and family allowance programmes for 18 countries. This builds the basis for Esping-Andersen's de-commodification index and the above mentioned publications. More information about SCIP is available at https://dspace.it.su.se/dspace/handle/10102/7 (16.08.2014).

17 Based on the assumption that capital possesses a structural advantage in distributional conflicts settled in the market arena, and that workers thus primarily rely on the political arena to enforce their interests, power resource theory argues that the outcome of welfare policies can best be explained by the power of parties and organisations representing the interests of the labour force.

18 Leading topics of this debate are, for example, the normative justification of social rights (e.g. Hayek 1976; Nussbaum 2011), the universality of social rights (e.g. Ganß-mann 1993; Lister 2007) and the challenges resulting from globalisation and migration (e.g. Faist 2007; Mau 2007).

19 According to international law, human rights are binding, but the possibility of sanctions, especially in the case of social rights, is limited. They become effectively enforceable only if they are incorporated into national law (Kaufmann 2003a, p. 40).

20 Ronald Dworkin (1977) explicitly uses the term 'background rights' when referring to moral rights.

21 This is a slight modification of Goodin and Rein's definition of regime pillars, which asks 'who gets what on what conditions' (Goodin and Rein 2001, p. 776). For a detailed discussion of my analytical framework, see the following section on access and generosity.

22 Net replacement rates indicate what percentage of income is replaced by social security benefits after taxes and social security contributions, thereby revealing changes in the generosity of benefits.

23 Further information about the HealthBASKET project (2004–2007) are provided on the webpage of the European Health Management Association, http://www.ehma.org/index.php?q=node/81 (21.08.2014).

24 However, unlike Clasen and Clegg, I not only take into account behaviour during benefit receipt, but also that which occurs prior to treatment in order to identify regulations that sanction 'bad' health behaviour of patients.

25 South Korea as well as Japan have SHI systems, and both grant universal coverage. The US remains the only welfare state providing no universal access to public healthcare for its population.

26 Universal coverage has been achieved in the following countries: Belgium in 1998, France in 2000, the Netherlands in 2006 and Germany in 2009. For an overview of coverage development of SHI countries up to the year 2005, see Busse, Schreyögg and Gericke (2007).

27 Freeman and Moran (2000), Gerlinger (2009) and Hacker (2004) find no or only few de-listings of services in the countries they studied.

28 See Chapter 1.5 for a detailed discussion of the negativity bias.

29 I concentrate here on Pierson's arguments that concern power resource theory and institutionalist approaches because these are still relevant to contemporary debates on welfare state transformation. I do not refer to his arguments against economic determinism because this approach is basically no longer relevant.

30 In his quantitative analysis, Jensen (2011a) finds no influence of right-wing governments, but he is aware of the limitation of quantitative studies, and for this reason, conducted two additional case studies. These qualitative studies reveal that right-wing governments in Australia and Denmark have followed a strategy which Jensen calls 'marketization via compensation', i.e. the expansion of private health insurance combined with an expansion of the public scheme. He concludes that 'partisan politics matters – it just does not matter in the way we previously thought' (Jensen 2011a, p. 925).

31 Gerring (2007) argues that causal complexity does not necessarily imply a case study design (pp. 61ff.).

32 In principle, all mature welfare states that provided a social right to healthcare at the end of the 1970s could be chosen, with the exception of Spain and Italy. These two countries completely redesigned their healthcare systems in the 1970s and are hence special cases with regard to healthcare entitlement.

33   When the NHS was founded in 1948, it covered the population of England and Wales. Scotland established its own NHS one year later, and Northern Ireland two years later. For many years, health policy in Wales and Scotland more or less mirrored the English example, with some differences in the administrative arrangements (Hunter 1982). In the course of devolution starting in 1999, the Welsh Government was given full responsibility for the Welsh NHS, and also Scotland and Northern Ireland became completely autonomous in regulating their healthcare systems. Today, the UK has four independent healthcare systems: the NHS England, the NHS Wales, the NHS Scotland and the Health and Social Care in Northern Ireland.

34   Besides the NHS and SHI systems, there is a third ideal type, the private healthcare system. A purely private healthcare system, however, does not provide a social right to healthcare because healthcare allocation is completely left to the market and thus depends on the ability to pay. No such system actually exists among welfare states. The US healthcare system comes close, but it provides public healthcare to a variety of population groups (e.g. the elderly, the poor, the armed forces) (Böhm et al. 2012; 2013). Due to this variety of systems and the fact that concrete entitlement is decided at the state level, healthcare entitlement regulation in the US is extremely complex. For these reasons, I have chosen not to investigate this special case.

35   In principle, each healthcare entitlement retrenchment reform constitutes an observation. Since nearly countless single and often small reforms were made, I have decided to summarise retrenchment reforms per year. Thus, one year is treated as one observation, which amounts to 35 observations for England and 37 observations for Germany. For further details, see Chapter 5.1.

36   Regulations selected for further analysis are marked with an X on the regulation maps.

37   A list of analysed regulations is not provided because, per country, it would fill several dozen pages, but the spreadsheet is available upon request.

2 Healthcare entitlement in England

This chapter presents the social right to healthcare in England and its reforms between 1979 and 2013. After a short introduction to the English healthcare system, the regulation of healthcare entitlement is set out in detail and, structured along government periods, all relevant reforms are described and analysed. For each period, some information about the political and economic background is given, but a detailed analysis of the driving forces behind reforms is reserved for Chapter 5. In England, the courts play a specific role in defining healthcare entitlement, which is highlighted in Chapter 2.6. Delineated in Chapter 2.7 is the influence of EU law on national healthcare entitlement, which is also of particular relevance for the English case. At the end of the chapter, the main findings are summarised and discussed.

2.1 The English healthcare system in brief

The National Health Service (NHS) was launched on the 5th of July 1948. Prior to this date, healthcare in Britain was fragmented and did not meet the health needs of the population (Klein 2010). The national health insurance exclusively covered manual workers and provided general practitioner (GP) services only. Family members of workers and other non-insured individuals had to pay for GP services out of pocket. Hospital care could be received from public and voluntary hospitals, but the latter, suffering from huge financial problems, also charged patients who could afford to pay. Shortly after the war, the newly elected Labour government passed the National Health Service Act 1946, which established a universal and comprehensive national healthcare system in England and Wales that was funded out of general taxes and granted services free at the point of delivery. Despite various subsequent reforms, these core features still characterise the NHS today (Klein 2010).

Moran (2000) has classified the British healthcare system as an 'entrenched command and control state'. A general principle of command and control healthcare states is that decision-making responsibility lies with elected officials while everyday business is delegated to the public health administration (Moran 2000, p. 147). In the NHS, the Secretary of State for Health (SoS)[1] is responsible for the general organisation and provision of healthcare. S/he is in charge of the

Department of Health (DH) and accountable to Parliament. Moreover, the treasury has a say in setting the national health budget. The public health administration is tasked with executing the day-to-day business of the NHS and, in the past, was organised hierarchically at different geographical levels. Since shortly after its inception, the NHS began undergoing numerous reorganisations. These reforms, step by step, transformed the organisational structure of the NHS from a centralised hierarchical command and control system into a 'mimic-market model' (Klein 2007) with decentralised power and contractual relationships amongst manifold actors.

Healthcare in England is financed mainly from public sources. Private funding plays only a minor role and takes the form of private medical insurance (PMI) premiums, NHS user charges and direct payments for private treatment (Boyle 2011, p. 83). Spending on PMI, however, has not yet exceeded four per cent of total health expenditure. Most PMI is supplementary and predominantly covers private acute care. Currently, about 12 per cent of the UK population holds a PMI contract (Boyle 2011, pp. 88ff.). Public funds for the NHS are generated through general taxation and national insurance contributions (NIC) and, to a very small degree, originate from other sources (e.g. capital interests). NIC are compulsory contributions jointly paid by employers and employees, or by self-employed individuals on earned income (Boyle 2011, p. 86). NIC made up approximately 18 per cent of total public spending in 2010/11 (Department of Health 2011b). As Table 2.1 shows, UK health expenditure heavily increased during the period under review. The UK had long been a low spender amongst OECD countries, but caught up to OECD and EU averages during the last decade. Public spending shows a clear downward trend while, at the same time, the portion of out-of-pocket payments has been rising, albeit with some fluctuation over time.

Healthcare provision in England is dominated by public providers (Böhm et al. 2013). Most hospitals are publicly owned. Compared to Germany, hospitals play a more important role in healthcare provision as they provide not only inpatient, but also outpatient specialised services. More than half of the NHS budget is allocated to hospitals (Talbot-Smith and Pollock 2006, p. 48). The provider structure for primary care is more versatile. General practitioners usually work either

Table 2.1 UK healthcare spending 1979–2013

Year	1979	1985	1990	1995	2000	2005	2013
Total health spending (% of GDP)	5.2	5.8	5.8	6.8	7.0	8.3	9.3
Public spending (% of total health spending)	89.6	85.8	83.6	83.9	79.1	80.9	84.0
Out-of-pocket payments (% of total health spending)	8.6[a]	n.a.	10.6	10.9	11.1	9.8	9.0

Source: OECD (2014c).

a Data is provided for 1980, because data for 1979 is not available.

independently or in partnership with other GPs; only 19 per cent are salaried (British Medical Association 2010). GPs provide the so-called 'general medical services' (GMS), which range from preventive services to acute treatment and include almost all ambulatory treatment not requiring specialist attention. Patients have to register with a GP in their area, who then works as a gatekeeper in referring patients to specialised care providers. The work of GPs is supplemented by nurse-led walk-in centres, which offer easy access to treatment for minor diseases and information about healthcare providers (Talbot-Smith and Pollock 2006, p. 52). Dental care and ophthalmic care are provided by private practitioners contracting with the NHS. Similarly, NHS pharmaceutical services can be received from all pharmacies that have contracts with the NHS. Primary care also encompasses community health services provided in community hospitals, hospices, health centres or patients' homes. Examples of covered services include physiotherapy, rehabilitation, continuing care or residential care for the elderly, and are supplied by many different NHS bodies (Talbot-Smith and Pollock 2006, p. 59).

2.2   The English social right to healthcare

Healthcare rights in England closely correspond to an ideal type of social citizenship rights as described by T.H. Marshall: they are universal, i.e. they are granted every English resident. They aim primarily at the wellbeing of society rather than at the wellbeing of the individual, which is best exemplified by the fact that English healthcare law does not grant rights for individual patients, but instead tasks state actors with the provision of a public healthcare system for the English population. Furthermore, the content of healthcare rights is rarely specified in order to allow for continuous adaptation to changing needs and resources. In this section, a general overview of NHS healthcare entitlement is given, and particulars of entitlement as of 1979 are presented according to the analytical categories developed in Chapter 1. The chapter starts with an overview of the laws and regulations relevant to healthcare entitlement in England.

English healthcare entitlement regulations

English healthcare law does not recognise the rights or entitlement of patients. It rarely references patients directly. Instead, the law establishes the duties and responsibilities of the Secretary of State, the NHS administrative bodies and providers. Only recently have the rights of patients been acknowledged and codified, not within traditional healthcare law, but by the NHS's own statutes (e.g. the NHS Constitution). Therefore, an empirical analysis of healthcare entitlement cannot be derived directly from healthcare law, but must be deduced from the duties of the relevant bodies.

The regulation map (see Table 2.2) gives an overview of the regulation of healthcare entitlement in England at four points in time. The primary regulatory legislation of the English healthcare system is the National Health Service Act (NHS Act). It outlines the duties and powers of the SoS, establishes health administration bodies and committees, and defines their responsibilities. Furthermore, it regulates the provision of medical, dental, ophthalmic and pharmaceutical services, including charges.[2]

Table 2.2 Regulation map England – healthcare entitlement regulations 1979, 1990, 2000 and 2013

1979	1990	2000	2013
General Public Acts			
X	X	X	X
The NHS Act 1977	*The NHS Act 1977*	*The NHS Act 1977*	*The NHS Act 2006*
Statutory Instruments			
X	X	X	X
The NHS (General Medical and Pharma. Services) Reg. 1974	The NHS (General Medical and Pharma. Services) Reg. 1974	The NHS (General Medical Services) Reg. 1992	The NHS (General Medical Services Contracts) Reg. 2004
			The NHS (General Medical Services Contracts) (Prescription of Drugs etc.) Reg. 2004
			X — The NHS (Personal Medical Services Agreements) Reg. 2004
X	X	X	X
The NHS (General Dental Services) Reg. 1973	The NHS (General Dental Services) Reg. 1973	The NHS (General Dental Services) Reg. 1992	The NHS (General Dental Services Contracts) Reg. 2005
			X — The NHS (Personal Dental Services Agreements) Reg. 2005
X	X	X	X
The NHS (Dental and Optical Charges) Reg. 1978	The NHS (Dental Charges) Reg. 1989	The NHS (Dental Charges) Reg. 1989	The NHS (Dental Charges) Reg. 2005
		X	X
		The NHS (Pharmaceutical Services) Reg. 1992	The NHS (Pharma. and Local Pharma. Services) Reg. 2013
X	X	X	X
The NHS (Charges for Drugs and Appliances) Reg. 1974	The NHS (Charges for Drugs and Appliances) Reg. 1989	The NHS (Charges for Drugs and Appliances) Reg. 2000	The NHS (Charges for Drugs and Appliances) Reg. 2000

(*Continued*)

Table 2.2 (Continued)

1979	1990	2000	2013
X The NHS (Charges for Appliances) Reg. 1974	The NHS (Charges for Appliances) Reg. 1974	The NHS (Charges for Appliances) Reg. 1974	The NHS (Charges for Appliances) Reg. 1974
X The NHS (General Ophthalmic Services) Reg. 1974	X The NHS (General Ophthalmic Services) Reg. 1986	X The NHS (General Ophthalmic Services) Reg. 1986	X The General Ophthalmic Services Contracts Reg. 2008
			X The Primary Ophthalmic Services Reg. 2008
	X The NHS (Optical Charges and Payments) Reg. 1989	X The NHS (Optical Charges and Payments) Reg. 1997	The NHS (Optical Charges and Payments) Reg. 2003
X The NHS (Remission of Charges) Reg. 1974	X The NHS (Travelling Expenses and Remission of Charges) Reg. 1988	X The NHS (Travelling Expenses and Remission of Charges) Reg. 1988	X The NHS (Travelling Expenses and Remission of Charges) Reg. 2003
			X The NHS (Reimb. of the Cost of EEA Treatment) Reg. 2010
			X The NHS (Direct Payments) Reg. 2013

X: analysed

At a lower level of abstraction are the statutory instruments (SI).[3] These specify access to and generosity of healthcare services. SIs regulate the provision of primary care, dental care, pharmaceuticals and ophthalmic care. Other SIs determine charges for dental care, drugs, medical appliances and ophthalmic care, as well as eligibility for exemption from and the remission of charges.

In addition to primary law and SIs, there is a large body of 'quasi-law'. Quasi-law 'describes rules which may be made without explicit legal authority and which are most important for the guidance they offer rather than the sanctions which follow if they are disregarded' (Montgomery 2002, p. 5). Within the NHS, quasi-law is published by NHS executives with the aim of informing the NHS administration and providers, and to give instructions in the form of directions, circulars or executive letters (Montgomery 2002, p. 15). Quasi-law is binding if primary legislation has granted power to the SoS or other executives to issue legally binding orders. Also relevant to healthcare entitlement are the positive recommendations given by the National Institute for Health and Care Excellence (NICE) within its technology appraisals. Quasi-law, except for the (non-binding) Patient's Charter and the NHS Constitution, is not considered in this study due to its voluminous and detailed nature.

The generally low codification of rights in England is a product of its legal tradition. The British legal system is primarily based on common law, i.e. resting on judicial decisions rather than statutes. Once judges have decided on a case, this judgement sets a precedent and must be followed by succeeding juridical decisions on same or similar matters (Montgomery 2002). For my analysis, this implies that in addition to statutory law, relevant judgements on healthcare entitlement must also be considered, which is done in Chapter 2.6.

Governance – who decides about healthcare entitlement?

Parliament determines the general framework of the NHS while the task of concrete organisation is conferred upon the SoS. S/he is assigned the duty of providing or securing services. For that purpose, the SoS is granted extensive powers by the NHS Act, leaving her/him to determine which services are to be provided by the NHS as well as to decide the particulars of charges:

Secretary of State's general power

(1) The Secretary of State may –
  (a) provide such services as he considers appropriate for the purpose of discharging any duty imposed on him by this Act, and
  (b) do anything else which is calculated to facilitate, or is conducive or incidental to, the discharge of such a duty.
(s. 2 NHS Act 2006)[4]

Historically, there is a difference between general medical, dental, ophthalmic and pharmaceutical services (called part II services due to their regulation in part II of the NHS Act 1977) and other, mainly secondary care services. While the SoS was directly responsible for the secondary care services, responsibility for the organisation and provision of the former was assigned to local health authorities, although without relieving the SoS from her/his general responsibility for these services.

In the course of devolution, more and more responsibilities have been devolved to local health authorities. After the abolishment of primary care trusts (PCTs), the clinical commissioning groups (CCGs) and the NHS Commissioning Board (operating name NHS England) were charged with arranging health service provision, and hence deciding about the scope of services. How they do so differs immensely between local authorities and is not the subject of this study.[5] Since the Health and Social Care Act 2012 has been in force, responsibility of the SoS is limited to the responsibility 'to *secure* that services are provided in accordance with' the NHS Act (s. 1 (1) NHS Act 2006 as amended by 2012 c. 7 sch. 4 s. 1 (1), emphasis added), but s/he remains responsible to Parliament for the provision of health services in England (s. 1 (3)).

As described above, decision-making regarding healthcare provision differs between local health authorities. Furthermore, funds are unequally distributed amongst local areas, additionally increasing geographical differences in provision. As a result, healthcare entitlement varies between regions and hence depends on the domicile of the individual. This local variation in entitlement is possible because no absolute entitlement to healthcare exists in England.

In order to tackle the geographic variation in entitlement, commonly known as 'postcode rationing', the government established NICE[6] in 1999 and tasked it (amongst other things) with specifying healthcare entitlement at the national level. Within its technology appraisal process, NICE assesses single or multiple drugs, medical devices, diagnostic techniques, surgical procedures and health promotion measures, and, based on these assessments, provides recommendations on their funding.[7] Since 2002, positive recommendations resulting from technology appraisals are legally binding, i.e. technologies having been recommended must be made available by all PCTs/CCGs within three months. PCTs/CCGs are free to provide technologies that have been assessed but not recommended for funding.

Access – population coverage

The NHS is a universal system based on the criteria of residence, which means that everyone living in England is covered. This principle was inscribed into the NHS at its beginning and has not been changed. The only difference between 1946 and today is that the English NHS now covers only English residents, while the Welsh have their own NHS which also is based on residency.

The definition of residency is not very clear. As explained above, the content of UK public health law covers the organisation of the NHS and the addressed subjects are NHS bodies and providers. Accordingly, the NHS Act does not explicitly define who is generally entitled to NHS services. Instead, it specifies for whose health the SoS is responsible. Section 1, paragraph 1 of the NHS Act states, '[t]he Secretary of State must continue the promotion in England of a comprehensive health service designed to secure improvement – (a) in the physical and mental health *of the people of England*' (emphasis added). The section on charges furthermore states that 'such persons not ordinarily resident in Great Britain' may be charged for services (s. 175 (2) (b) NHS Act 2006). Who is 'ordinarily resident', however, is not defined by the Act or other regulations. A DH guidance advises NHS bodies to consider a House of Lords judgement on that issue (Department of Health 2011a). According to the judges, 'ordinarily resident refers to a man's abode in a particular place or country which he had adopted voluntarily and for settled purposes as part of the regular order of his life for the time being, whether of short or long duration'.[8] The guidance also makes clear that a British nationality or passport, or the payment of national insurance contributions and taxes, do not constitute a status of ordinarily resident (p. 21).

Persons not ordinarily resident in the UK are termed 'overseas visitors' and are not entitled to free hospital care. However, the National Health Service (Charges to Overseas Visitors) Regulations 2011 lists several exemptions for the healthcare entitlement of overseas visitors. Generally, all persons having lawfully resided in the UK for 12 months or more are entitled (s. 7 (1)). Furthermore, several groups of overseas visitors who are similar to normal UK residents, for example persons employed or self-employed in the UK or full-time students, are exempted from paying for treatment. In addition, the regulation lists numerous further groups that are excluded for humanitarian (e.g. refugees, victims of human trafficking) or other reasons (e.g. UK state pensioners visiting the UK), and numerous diseases for which treatment is generally free (mainly infectious and sexually transmitted diseases). Because the UK is a member of the EU, EU regulations apply and all visitors resident in one of the countries of the European Economic Area (EEA) are entitled to receive free treatment. Moreover, the UK has reciprocal healthcare agreements with several other countries (see schedule 2 of SI 2001/1556) that approve free treatment of visitors from these countries.

Being an ordinary resident is not a pre-condition for receiving primary care. It is at the discretion of any GP to decide whether s/he accepts someone as a registered patient (or temporary resident) or not (Department of Health 2011a, p. 60). Yet there is no legal entitlement to GP treatment for non-residents. Only in emergency cases and when immediate treatment is necessary do GPs and hospitals have a duty to provide treatment free of charge (Department of Health 2011a, p. 60).

In summary, residency is the sole population coverage criterion applied by the English NHS, but it is vaguely defined and not in all cases the pre-condition for healthcare entitlement. Because the coverage criteria have not been changed in the past, and only minor amendments to the exemption criteria have been made, population coverage is not further analysed in the following sections.

Generosity – service coverage

The NHS Act merely sets out very generally which services are to be covered by the NHS. In section 1 paragraph 1, it states that the Secretary of State 'must continue the promotion of a *comprehensive* health service' (emphasis added) without, however, specifying what is meant by 'comprehensive'. Section 3 is more concrete and lists services the SoS is obligated to provide:

   (a) hospital accommodation,
   (b) other accommodation for the purpose of any service provided under this Act,
   (c) medical, dental, ophthalmic, nursing and ambulance services,

(d) such other services or facilities for the care of pregnant women, women who are breastfeeding and young children as he considers are appropriate as part of the health service,

(e) such other services or facilities for the prevention of illness, the care of persons suffering from illness and the after-care of persons who have suffered from illness as he considers are appropriate as part of the health service,

(f) such other services or facilities as are required for the diagnosis and treatment of illness.

(s. 3 (1) NHS Act 2006)[9]

These are quite broad service areas that range from prevention to hospital treatment, and the last subparagraph renders nearly infinite service coverage possible. Yet it makes clear that the listed services must be an integral part of the NHS benefits package. However, the extent of coverage of those service areas is not defined: in the past it was left to the discretion of the SoS and now lies in the hands of the clinical commissioning groups.

Section 3 paragraph 1 does not constitute an individual right to treatment, as case law has confirmed. A group of patients who had been on a waiting list for several years took action against the SoS and their local health authorities, claiming that those bodies had not fulfilled their duty to provide services. The claim was dismissed by the judges, who argued that the particular paragraph does not impose an absolute duty on the SoS because health service provision always depends on the availability of resources, and because resources are limited, all demands cannot be met.[10]

In addition to the services listed in section 3 paragraph 1, the SoS also has the duty to provide high-security psychiatric services (s. 4 NHS Act 2006) as well as medical (and formerly dental) inspection and treatment for pupils, and s/he must arrange the provision of contraceptive services. Furthermore, the NHS Act permits him or her to provide several other services, such as invalid carriages (sch. 1 NHS Act 2006).

The duty to provide general medical care, general dental care, general ophthalmic care and pharmaceutical services is traditionally assigned to local health authorities (part II NHS Act 1977 and part IV to VII NHS Act 2006, respectively). Their duties are – in addition to being generally described by the NHS Act – further concretised by regulations. The content of these regulations in 1979 is presented in detail below, as is the entitlement to other services regulated by the NHS Act in 1979. The following sections then trace reforms of each service area over the last 35 years.

In 1979, healthcare law did not set any eligibility criteria for service coverage. The NHS Act 1977 and its related regulations, however, consistently provided two service criteria for NHS health services: they had to be *appropriate* and *necessary*. Unnecessary treatments or those whose quality was above the necessary level were not allowed to be provided, or the patient had to bear the additional costs by her/himself. Yet the meaning of 'appropriate' and 'necessary' was not further specified, leaving it to the individual health administration and provider to decide if a particular service was appropriate and necessary.

Primary care: According to the NHS Act 1977, it was the Area Health Authorities' (AHAs) duty to arrange with medical practitioners the provision of personal medical services for their area (s. 29 (1)). The Act provided that the conditions of those arrangements, as well as the definition of general medical services, could be further qualified by the Secretary of State within regulations (s. 29 (2)). The definition given by the NHS General Medical and Pharmaceutical Services Regulations 1974, though, was rather general. It stated that the scope of GMS encompasses 'all necessary and appropriate personal medical services of the type usually provided by general medical practitioners' (s. 3 SI 1974/160 as amended by SI 1975/719) and that it included contraceptive services as well as the referral of patients to other NHS services (sch. 1, s. 13).

Pharmaceuticals: In addition to GMS, AHAs were also assigned the responsibility of a 'proper and sufficient' pharmaceutical provision (s. 41 NHS Act 1977). Until 1992, the terms and conditions of pharmaceutical service provision were regulated by the same statutory instrument as GMS (SI 1974/160). This regulation, however, in no way restricted prescription. GPs were allowed to prescribe any drug they deemed appropriate for the patient's treatment (Hartley 1981, p. 713).

Medical appliances: In contrast to pharmaceuticals, NHS provision of appliances was restricted to those items listed in the drug tariff (s. 28 (1) SI 1974/160).

Dental care and appliances: General dental care is the service area where service coverage is most explicitly defined. The duty of dental provision was assigned to AHAs (s. 35 NHS Act 1977), which then contracted with dental practitioners. In 1979, the conditions for those arrangements were specified by the NHS General Dental Services Regulations (SI 1973/1468). Additionally, the SoS issued a 'Statement of Dental Remuneration' that contained a scale of fees, a list of services needing prior approval, and standards and restrictions for material used for treatment.

The regulations generally required NHS dental treatment to be 'clinically necessary for dental fitness' where 'dental fitness means such a reasonable standard of dental efficiency and oral health as is necessary to safeguard general health' (s. 20 and s. 2 SI 1973/1468). At that time, the NHS provided three different types of general dental services (GDS): occasional treatment, prior approval treatment and normal general treatment. The terms of service provided by schedule 1 (SI 1973/1468) listed 12 single services that could be provided occasionally. All those treatments were urgent actions, such as the extraction of teeth or the incision of an abscess, and were allowed to be provided to any patient. Determination II of the Statement of Dental Remuneration contained services that needed prior approval from the Dental Estimates Board – an expert body appointed by the SoS. All other treatment also needed formal approval from the Dental Estimates Board in order to be remunerated, but treatment could be carried out first, before the fee estimate was sent in (sch.1 s. 9). All GDS together with their fees and patient charges were quoted by the scale of fees. This scale can be seen as an implicit positive list because only listed services were remunerated and thus, only those services were provided by dental practitioners. However, the scale did not constitute any individual right to treatment, it merely defined services that could be provided by the NHS.

Ophthalmic care and optical appliances: The provision of sight testing and general ophthalmic services also fell within the duty of the AHAs. In 1979, anyone could receive an NHS sight test free of charge (s. 13 SI 1974/287 as amended 1979). The person providing the sight test, however, had to ensure that the testing was necessary. The ophthalmic statement, issued by the SoS, determined the types and quality of optical appliances to be supplied as part of the general ophthalmic services (s. 10 SI 1974/287). Generally, patients could also receive appliances of a more expensive type than that prescribed, or lenses fitted to a frame not supplied by the NHS, but s/he had to pay the additional costs (s. 14 SI 1974/287). Provision of contact lenses was restricted to clinically necessary cases.

Generosity – cost coverage

In principle, healthcare services within the NHS are to be provided free of charge. Exemptions are allowed only when 'the making and recovery of charges is expressly provided for by or under any enactment' (s. 1 (2) NHS Act 1977 and s. 1 (3) NHS Act 2006 respectively). Concretely, the NHS Act authorises charges for drugs, dental treatment, as well as medical, dental and optical appliances.[11] The specific amounts, as well as eligibility criteria for exemption, are specified by statutory instruments. The content of these regulations in 1979 is presented below.

In addition, a statutory instrument regulates the remission of charges for people with low income or limited resources. In 1979, this regulation exempted members of a family receiving family income supplement or welfare food, people with an exemption certificate issued by the SoS,[12] and people with a weekly income of less than the sum of their weekly requirements (s. 4 SI 1974/1377 as amended 1979) from paying charges for the repair or replacement of appliances (other than dental appliances) necessitated by lack of care of its wearer, and remitted them charges for dentures, drugs, medical appliances and dental treatment (s. 3 SI 1974/1377).

Pharmaceuticals and medical appliances: The National Health Service (Charges for Drugs and Appliances) Regulations specify the concrete conditions for the setting and recovery of charges for these medical goods. In 1979, the regulations determined that for each appliance and drug unit the patient was charged 20p (s. 3 SI 1974/285). Only for elastic hosieries, fabric support and wigs did patients have to pay higher fees. If not explicitly listed by the regulation, children under the age of 16, men older than 65 and women older than 60 years, expectant mothers and women having given birth within the last year, people suffering from certain diseases, as well as people with exemption certificates due to low income, were exempted from paying those charges (s. 6 SI 1974/285). Furthermore, patients requiring a large number of drugs and appliances could buy a pre-payment certificate at a cost of £2 (valid for six months) or £3.50 (valid for 12 months) that exempted them from paying any further charges for drugs and medical appliances.

Dental care and dental appliances: The setting and recovery of charges for GDS is regulated by the National Health Service (Dental Charges) Regulations.

In 1979, charges for general dental treatment amounted to £5. In cases where the fee was less than £5, the charge equalled the fee (s. 4 SI 1978/950). Charges for special dental treatment such as crowns, inlays, pin lays or gold fillings were £10 for each tooth. Charges for dentures ranged between £12 and £36. The maximum charge was £5 per course for general dental treatment and £30 for special dental treatment and dental appliances (s. 5 SI 1978/950). Persons younger than 16, and in some cases 21 years, or persons receiving full-time education, pregnant women and women having recently delivered were not required to pay charges (sch. 12 s. 2 and s. 3 NHS Act 1977; s. 5 SI 1978/950). If patients wanted more expensive dentures, bridges or fillings, inlays or crowns than the clinically necessary ones, they had to bear the additional costs (s. 81 NHS Act 1977, s. 20 SI 1973/1468).

Ophthalmic care and optical appliances: In 1979, sight tests and contact lenses were generally free of charge. For glasses, patients had to pay £2.90 in the case of a single vision lens, £5.50 for a fused glass bifocal lens and £6.15 for a lens of any other description. Children under the age of 16 and older children undergoing qualifying education were exempted from paying charges. If patients wanted a more expensive appliance than the one provided by the NHS they had to pay extra charges, the amounts of which were given by the ophthalmic statement. This statement was issued by the SoS and also defined the charges payable for the repair and replacement of optical appliances.

2.3 Conservative healthcare entitlement reforms 1979–1997

The 1979 general elections marked the beginning of a new era in British politics. Not only was it the start of a Conservative majority lasting four legislative periods, but the election of Margret Thatcher to prime minister also indicated the inception of a new policy paradigm that pursued the ideal of minimal government and free market. Health policy in general, and healthcare entitlement in particular, were not spared by these reforms. In the following section, the general political and economic landscape and relevant events are sketched in order to provide a picture of the changing political powers and potential economic developments that might later help to explain healthcare entitlement reforms. In a second step, the general course of Conservative health policy is outlined, and finally, healthcare entitlement reforms between 1979 and 1997 are covered in detail.

Political and economic background

During her first term in office, Prime Minister Thatcher was forced to cope with major economic problems: double-digit inflation rates accompanied by low or negative economic growth, and steadily increasing unemployment squeezed state budgets. Her remedy against the high inflation was a strict monetarist policy, i.e. reducing the supply of money and government spending (Evans 2004, p. 21). Despite these problems, Thatcher was reelected in 1983. In fact, the Conservatives lost votes but gained more seats because Labour opposition had split off.[13]

With the next elections in 1987, the Conservative majority shrank by 41 seats, but still remained large enough for the party to consolidate power. Invigorated by election victories, Thatcher further limited the power of trade unions and pushed privatisation. Privatisation corresponded with the ideal of a lean state and promised a win-win situation: the state budget would be relieved of the deficits of unproductive public firms, and sales would generate huge income for the public purse (Evans 2004, pp. 34f.). Privatisation was not limited to the denationalisation of state companies, but also included the contracting-out of formerly publicly provided services (e.g. waste disposal) and the retreat of the state from regulation (e.g. transport) (Evans 2004, pp. 34f.). Inflation was tempered, but despite economic recovery at first and an economic boom in the later years, unemployment remained a severe problem.

Thatcher generally received low approval ratings in the opinion polls (Klein 2010), but during the end of the 1980s, support within her own party waned, too. After the resignation of several ministers, a chastening party leadership vote led her to hand power over to John Major in 1990. The new Conservative leader had no problems in winning the next elections in 1992, and gathered more votes than Thatcher had ever managed to win. Major favoured a more consensual leadership style than Thatcher (Evans 2004, p. 124). One of his top priorities was to improve the quality of public services by means of strengthening the citizen's role as consumer (Evans 1999, pp. 156, 174f.). For this purpose, citizen rights to public services were laid down in a Citizen's Charter (HMSO 1991), which was later followed by several specific charters for single public service areas (e.g. the Patient's Charter, the Parent's Charter, the Taxpayer's Charter). During Major's government, unemployment declined slightly, and apart from a small recession early on, he was faced with good economic conditions. Yet the Conservatives struggled with several severe problems (e.g. the Maastricht Treaty and European Monetary Union, the poll tax, as well as significant dissension within the party) and suffered a landslide loss in the 1997 elections (Evans 1999).

Conservative health policy

In order to understand Conservative healthcare reforms, some remarks on the financial situation of the NHS, as well as on the Conservative standing within this policy field are helpful. The competence of Conservatives concerning the NHS has always been perceived by the electorate as low (Klein 2010, p. 113), making health reforms a weak point of every Conservative government. Trust of voters dropped even further when a confidential reform proposal from a government think tank to substitute a private insurance system for the NHS leaked out (Klein 2010, pp. 112f.). For this reason, Conservatives tirelessly repeated that the 'NHS is safe with us' and highlighted the expansion of financial and personal resources under their government. In fact, NHS spending was steadily raised by the Conservative government. During the period 1978/79 to 1991/92, NHS expenditures increased by 50.2 per cent in real terms (Bloor and Maynard 1993, p. 2). Yet there was a permanent perception of 'financial stringency' (Klein 2010, p. 79) for several reasons:

first, due to medical progress and an ageing society, demand was steadily growing. Second, inflation of health service costs was greater than the increase in general retail prices (Rivett 1998, p. 358), which meant that increased financial input did not guarantee growth of real resources. Third, complaints about scarcity seemed to have been one way for NHS staff to demonstrate opposition against Conservative policy, thus providing Labour with a good opportunity to play off the weak point of the Conservatives (Klein 2010).

Following Klein's description of the political history of the NHS, the 18 years of Conservative rule spanned three different periods of health policy-making: the very deedless first Thatcher years, the cautious modifications of the mid-1980s and the big-bang reforms of the early 1990s. With its meek start, the first Thatcher government did not overcome the stagnation that had characterised the increasingly diversified health policy arena present since the major reorganisation of 1974 (Klein 2010, pp. 76ff.). The only appreciable reforms were the restoration of private provision, which had been abolished by the previous Labour government, and the decentralisation of power through the replacement of Area Health Authorities with District Health Authorities.

It was not until 1983 that the Conservatives took more active, albeit very cautious, health reform steps. Thatcher had commissioned Roy Griffiths, managing director of a large UK retail chain, to conduct an NHS management inquiry. In his 1983 report, Griffiths recommended increasing responsibility within the NHS through the introduction of a general management structure, which was almost immediately put into place (Klein 2010, pp. 117f.). These management reforms were only one of several attempts by the second and third Thatcher governments to increase the output of the NHS without spending too many extra resources. Further reforms included the outsourcing of non-clinical services (e.g. cleaning, catering) and the introduction of extensive performance review measures for NHS bodies (Klein 2010, pp. 105ff.). Similar aims were pursued by the new GP contract of 1987, which increased the share of capitation payments, rewarded preventive treatments and attempted to heighten competition between providers through increased information requirements and allowing advertising (Hughes 1993).

The success of these 'politics of value for money' (Klein 2010) of the 1980s remained limited. A severe health financial crisis in 1987, accompanied by NHS staff complaints about the bad condition of the NHS, resulted in intense media coverage (Rivett 1998, pp. 358, 361). This led to a general perception of an NHS crisis and Thatcher, who had so far avoided addressing NHS problems with radical reforms, had no choice but to tackle the problem head on (Klein 2010, pp. 142ff.; Whitney 1988, pp. 9f.). With a radical reform proposal, the 1989 White Paper 'Working for Patients' ushered in a new era in UK health policy. Not only did it propose the adoption of an internal market, but its implementation also helped weaken the broad resistance of doctors and the opposition (Klein 2010, p. 153). The subsequent National Health Service and Community Care Act 1990 implemented the internal market. Health authorities were morphed into 'purchasers' and hospitals and other service providers into semi-independent trusts that had to 'sell' their services to health authorities (Talbot-Smith and Pollock 2006,

p. 6). GP practices were given the opportunity to become GP fundholders with the task of providing and 'purchasing' services for their patients, given a fixed budget (Boyle 2011, p. 27; Klein 2010, p. 146). The adoption of this big-bang reform was Thatcher's last coup. She was followed by John Major as prime minister, whose footprint on health policy was less profound, although not entirely without traces, as is shown below.

Conservative healthcare entitlement reforms

Amongst the various health reforms put into effect by the Conservatives, five addressed healthcare entitlement: the Health Services Act 1980, the Health and Social Security Act 1984, the Health and Medicines Act 1988, the Access to Health Records Act 1990, and last, the NHS Primary Care Act 1997, which was passed shortly before the Conservatives were voted out of office. Most of the relevant changes concerning the generosity of healthcare entitlement, however, were made by the SoS via statutory instruments.

In 1991, an important step in the development of healthcare entitlement in the UK was taken with the publication of the first Patient's Charter. Although the Patient's Charter was not legally binding, it represented a milestone because for the first time, the rights of patients were explicitly spelt out. The Charter embodied a list of 10 patients' rights, of which seven had already been established and three were new. In addition to the list of patients' rights, the Charter defined nine service standards on the national level and committed local health authorities to establish local service standards. These so-called 'Charter Standards' did not constitute any entitlement, but formed 'major and specific standards which the Government looks to the NHS to achieve, as circumstances and resources allow' (p. 6).

Among the seven established rights, only four represented healthcare entitlement as defined in this study:[14] the right to receive healthcare on the basis of clinical need, the right to be registered with a GP, the right to receive emergency medical care at any time and the right to be referred to a consultant or for a second opinion if the GP found it necessary. The Charter newly constituted a guarantee of admission to treatment within two years after being put on a waiting list. Although two years is rather long, this guarantee was revolutionary as it established, for the first time, the right to treatment within a specified period. Additionally, the Patient's Charter established rights to access to facilities, but did not, however, constitute any right to particular services (Klein, Day and Redmayne 1996, p. 39).

In 1992, the Patient's Charter was supplemented by a charter for GP services (Department of Health 1992), and in 1995, an updated version that unified both charters was launched. Although more detailed, the updated version of the Patient's Charter merely listed already existing rights (e.g. pharmaceutical services, dental care, exemptions from paying charges). Its second edition reduced the guaranteed waiting time for all hospital admissions from 24 to 18 months and introduced some new standards. During the 1990s, several Patient's Charters for particular patient groups were published (e.g. maternity care, mental health services).

Governance – who decides about healthcare entitlement?

In 1985, the SoS issued a list of drugs no longer allowed to be prescribed within the NHS (see below). This exclusion of drugs brought about an outcry from doctors and the pharmaceutical industry. Therefore, an expert advisory committee called the 'Advisory Committee on NHS Drugs' was subsequently set up to propose changes to the lists (Collier 1985; Dobbs-Smith 1999, p. 81; Klein 2010, p. 132). Yet the final decision remained with the ministry.

Generosity – service coverage

Various Conservative reforms addressed generosity of healthcare entitlement, but, contrary to what one might have expected, these did not always aim to cut entitlement as the following description of service coverage reforms shows.

Prevention and primary care: Entitlement to primary care was not changed until 1989. But then major amendments were made to general medical services by SI 1989/1897. This statutory instrument introduced child health surveillance services and minor surgery procedures as part of GP services. Additionally, giving advice on healthy lifestyle, preventive examination and consultation and vaccinations against a specified list of diseases were included in the list of services a doctor was required to provide (s. 13 (2) (c) SI 1974/160 as amended 1989). Furthermore, GPs became obligated to provide a comprehensive consultation for all new patients, to offer all patients over the age of 75 a detailed examination and to invite all patients without medical contact over the past three years for consultation. By 1993, this last obligation had already been abolished. Patients remained entitled to such a consultation every three years, but they were required to request it instead of automatically being invited (sch. 2 s. 15 SI 1992/635 as amended by SI 1993/540).

Prevention also became a greater issue in dental care. In the 1980s, NHS GDS were expanded to cover dental prevention with fluoride (SI 1986/1499) and fissure sealants (SI 1987/1512) for children.

Pharmaceuticals: In 1985, NHS entitlement to pharmaceuticals was restrained for the first time in NHS history. The Secretary of State introduced two limited lists for drugs, a black and a grey list. The black list (schedule 3A SI 1985/290) contained about 1800 items for seven different therapeutic groups[15] that doctors were no longer allowed to prescribe. Most of the listed items were drugs for non-severe diseases like cough syrups, pain killers or vitamins and minerals, but the list also forbade the prescription of chocolate biscuits, wine and sun blockers. In 1992, the limited list was extended to cover 10 additional categories of drugs (Dobbs-Smith 1999, p. 82).[16] Including this expansion, more than 1660 new substances were added to the black list between 1985 and 1997, while approximately 190 were delisted. The grey list covers drugs that are allowed to be prescribed only for certain patients given particular conditions specified in schedule 3B (SI 1985/290). In contrast to the hundreds of items on schedule 3A, schedule 3B listed only Clobazam for the treatment of epileptic patients in the beginning and was expanded further by seven substances through 1997.

It is neither stated by the statutory instrument nor by the NHS Act which criteria were used to base the decisions about inclusion of a drug on one of the limited lists. According to the Secretary of State, Kenneth Clarke, clinical need and efficiency guided decisions (Dobbs-Smith 1999, p. 81). These criteria were also given in the terms of reference of the Advisory Committee on NHS Drugs. When evaluating clinical need, the Committee considered the therapeutic action of the product, but also its acceptability and palatability, as well as the range of alternatives available, so as to allow for choice amongst products (Dobbs-Smith 1999, p. 81).

Medical appliances: With the exemption of the introduction of oxygen concentrators for ambulant patients (SI 1985/955), no further appliance has been explicitly in- or excluded by means of statutory instruments during the 18 years of Conservative rule.

Dental care: In the course of the remuneration reform that replaced most fee-for-service payments with capitation payment in 1990, the GDS regulation was completely reorganised (SI 1990/1638). Following the reform, patients had to enrol with a dentist for one year under a continuing care arrangement (adults) or for two years under a capitation arrangement (children). Patients not enrolled could receive occasional treatment only, which was expanded to cover several additional services by the same reform. Later, occasional treatment was further amplified with the inclusion of immediate necessary palliative treatment (SI 1990/2501) and treatment immediately necessary as a result of trauma (SI 1991/1348). The 1990 reform allowed dentists to provide GDS privately as long as they honestly informed their patients about the availability of the treatment as a free NHS service (sch. 1 s. 32 SI 1990/1638).

Ophthalmic care and optical appliances: Ophthalmic care and appliances were subject to far-reaching cuts in entitlement. A first attempt was made in 1980, when the Conservatives tried to exclude free sight tests from the NHS benefits package. However, opposition from their own ranks led them to revoke this passage from the bill (Hockley 2012). The Health and Social Security Act 1984 was more successful; it almost completely withdrew spectacles and lenses from the NHS benefits package and, at the same time, liberalised the market for glasses. In order to provide access to optical appliances to at least children, people with low resources or income and people needing complex appliances, optical appliances vouchers were introduced for this group (SI 1986/976).[17] In the following years, vouchers were slightly expanded to also cover, in special cases, the replacement and repair of optical appliances (SI 1989/396), contact lenses and spectacles with prism-controlled bifocal lenses (SI 1991/583).

Conservatives also cut eligibility to NHS free sight testing. The Health and Medicines Act 1988[18] restricted eligibility to a small population group, which included those eligible for ophthalmic vouchers, people suffering from diabetes or glaucoma, those older than 40 having a near relative diagnosed with glaucoma and people who are blind or partially sighted (s. 13 (1) SI 1986/975 as amended by SI 1989/395). During the 1990s, eligibility for sight testing was slightly extended to cover people receiving a disability working allowance with less than £8,000 of capital resources and to their family members (SI 1995/558). One year later, the income restriction was removed and individuals and families receiving a low income working allowance were once again eligible for sight testing (s. 13 (2) (i) and (j) SI 1986/975 as amended by SI 1996/2320).

Generosity – cost coverage

In 1988, the Remission of Charge Regulation was reformulated (SI 1988/551), but only minor changes were made. The new regulation included the conditions for the refund of traveling expenses, which had so far been regulated by their own statutory instrument. Furthermore, the regulation was simplified, with fewer single regulations for particular groups of charges and persons. Also, the remission of charges became slightly more generous: persons and family members of persons who received income support and family credit were fully exempted from paying charges for drugs, medicines, appliances, pharmaceutical services, and dental appliances and dental treatment. Furthermore, persons and family members of persons whose requirements equalled or exceeded their income and whose capital resources did not surpass a certain capital limit were partly or totally exempt from paying such charges.

Between 1995 and 1997, exception categories for the remission and repayment of charges were broadened in a stepwise fashion. In 1995, people receiving disability working allowance and whose capital did not exceed £8,000 and their family members became eligible for full remission and repayment of charges (SI 1988/551 as amended by SI 1995/642). Also in 1995, following a judgement of the ECJ, the age at which men were relieved from paying charges was reduced from 65 to 60 to equal the age at which women were spared (Hockley 2012, p. 152). In the following year, people receiving an income-based jobseeker's allowance and people entitled to an income-based jobseeker's allowance of less than 10 pence also became exempted (SI 1996/2362). In addition, the capital resource limit was omitted for people receiving disability working allowance (SI 1996/410). In 1997, people living permanently in public nursing care homes and similar public accommodation and who were unable to pay the full costs of their accommodation were fully exempted from paying charges (SI 1997/748). The broadening of exemption categories increased the group of exempted persons to 85 per cent of the population in 1996 (Hockley 2012, p. 152), which meant that only 15 per cent of the population were subject to pay charges.

Pharmaceuticals and medical appliances:[19] Charges for pharmaceuticals and medical appliances were increased sharply by the Thatcher government, especially during their first years in office (see Table 2.3 and Tables A.7 and A.8 of the appendix). At the very beginning of her term, Prime Minister Thatcher more than doubled charges, which had not been raised by the former government since 1972 (Hockley 2012, p. 110), from 20p to 45p. When she left office in 1990, charges had increased from 20p per item to £3.05. Yet charge policies did not change with her successor. The Major governments kept increasing charges above the inflation rate, with the result that the charges patients had to pay for a single pharmaceutical or medical appliance were more than 28 times higher at the end of the Conservative rule than they had been in 1979. Charges for pre-payment certificates were raised accordingly (see Table A.2 of the appendix).

Dental care and dental appliances:[20] Similar to pharmaceuticals, the Thatcher government drastically increased dental charges during their first years in office (see Table 2.4). Charges for general dental treatment, for example, almost tripled between 1978 and 1984 from £5 to £14.50. In 1985, charges for dental treatment,

Table 2.3 Charges for pharmaceuticals and medical appliances 1979–1997

Year	1979	1980	1981	1982	1983	1984	1985	1986	1987	1988	1989	1990	1991	1992	1993	1994	1995	1996	1997
Statutory instr. (No.)	681	264	1503	/	289	306	298	326	432	368	427	419	537	579	365	420	690	643	583 / 559
Charges (per item)	£0.45	£0.70	£1.00	£1.00	£1.30	£1.40	£1.60	£2.00	£2.20	£2.40	£2.60	£2.80	£3.05	£3.40	£3.75	£4.25	£4.75	£5.25	£5.50 £5.65
Charge increase	125%	122%	0%	30%	8%	14%	25%	10%	9%	8%	8%	9%	11%	10%	13%	12%	11%	5%	3%
Annual inflation[a]	13.4%	18%	11.9%	8.6%	4.6%	5.0%	6.1%	3.4%	4.1%	4.0%	5.2%	7.0%	7.5%	4.3%	2.5%	2.0%	2.6%	2.5%	1.8%

a Consumer prices 1979–1984 are estimated values.

Sources: OECD (2014a), own data collection.

Table 2.4 Charges for dental treatment 1978–1997

Year	1978	1979	1980	1981	1982	1983	1984	1985	1986	1987	1988	1989	1990	1991	1992	1993	1994	1995	1996	1997
Statutory instr. (No.)	677	352	307	284	309	299	352	n.a.	n.a.	n.a.	473	394	n.a.	581	369	419	530	444	389	558
Charges																				
General treatment[a]	£5	£7	£8	£9	£13	£13.50	£14.50	£17 + 0.4 × fees	£17 + 0.4 × fees	£17 + 0.75 × fees	£17 + 0.75 × fees	0.75 × fees	0.75 × fees	0.75 × fees	0.75 × fees	0.80 × fees	0.80 × fees	0.80 × fees	0.80 × fees	0.80 × fees
Special treatment[b]	£10	£12	£18	£20	£24	£26	£30	£33	£33	£33	/	/	/	/	/	/	/	/	/	/
Maximum charges																				
General treatment	£5	£7	£8	£9	£13	£13.50	£14.50	£115	£115	£115	£150	£150	£150	£200	£225	£250	£275	£300	£325	£330
Special treatment	£30	£36	£54	£60	£90	£95	£110	£115	£115	£115	/	/	/	/	/	/	/	/	/	/

n.a.: no amendment

a If the authorised fee was smaller than the charge listed here, the patient had to pay charges as high as the fee.

b Special dental treatment (per tooth) included: crowns, inlays, pin lays or gold fillings and fillings, other than root fillings, of any material in a tooth for which crowns, inlays, pin lays or gold fillings is provided as part of the same course of treatment. These treatments were no longer called special dental treatment but became part of GDS with SI 1982/284 but until 1988 (SI 1988/473) different charges for these treatments were applied.

Source: Own data collection.

and then in 1989, charges for dental appliances were completely restructured and thereby increased to 75 per cent of doctors' fees (see Tables A.4 and A.5 of the appendix). The reforms massively simplified charges by substituting a percentage charge for the various fixed amounts. Proportional charges increase with every fee increase, which is good for the health budget because most of the increased costs are borne by the patient, but every fee increase becomes a (hidden) charge increase for patients. Beginning in 1989, patients also had to pay charges for dental examinations (Yule 1993, p. 66). The maximum charge, meant to protect patients from unbearable cost burdens, was raised stepwise from £30 in 1979 to £330 in 1997.

Concerning eligibility for exemption, there has only been a slight restriction of exemptions for young people. Formerly, anyone undergoing qualifying full-time education was exempted from paying charges for dental treatment and appliances. After the reform of 1988, a maximum age of 18 for pupils applied. On the contrary, patients suffering from an oral tumour and having received invasive treatment were exempted from paying charges for dental appliances (s. 2 (4) (b) SI 1988/473; s. 2 SI 1989/394).

Ophthalmic care and optical appliances:[21] In 1982, the three existing charge categories for optical appliances were replaced by approximately 30 new categories, making charges more complex and increasing average charges (SI 1982/284). Furthermore, a maximum charge of £15 was introduced. This sum increased stepwise to £16.50 in 1985, when it was abolished (SI 1985/298). Charges were again slightly increased twice, in 1983 and 1984 (SI 1983/309, SI 1984/299), until they were simplified again by SI 1985/298, which reduced them to five categories.

In 1984, glasses and other optical appliances were excluded from the NHS benefits package and a voucher system was introduced instead (see above). The amount of the voucher depended on the specific optical appliance the patient needed. Altogether, there were eight voucher categories ranging from £14.25 to £66 (in 1986). The value of vouchers was slightly increased every year; however, these increases did not compensate for general price increases. For example, the value of a voucher for glasses with single vision lenses was raised from £14.25 in 1986 to £27.20 in 1997, and vouchers for contact lenses were increased from £25 to £39.80.

Summary

With regard to healthcare entitlement, Conservative reforms can be divided into four phases. Healthcare entitlement reforms of the first Thatcher government remained limited to skyrocketing charges. Hence, the first period of Conservative healthcare entitlement reforms mirrors general Conservative health policy attempts, which Rudolf Klein has described as a 'stalemate' (Klein 2010, p. 76) because all structural reform was missing. During the second period, which lasted the whole of the second and third Thatcher governments (1983–1990), reducing cost coverage remained on the agenda, but charge increases were less intense than during the first Thatcher years. Within this period, Thatcher dared to tackle service coverage, too, and excluded several medical goods and services or tightened eligibility in order to limit access (e.g. the limited list of drugs, exclusion of glasses, reduced access to sight tests). Interestingly, but not surprisingly, the limitation in generosity in the cases of ophthalmic and dental treatment went hand in hand with the privatisation of those services. Contrary to these retrenchment reforms, the Thatcher government expanded service coverage to include ever more preventive measures (e.g. dental prevention in children, prevention by GPs). The third phase of healthcare entitlement reforms spans the first four years of John Major's term in office (1991–1994). During this period, charges were again raised more substantially, increasing at a double-digit rate during each year. At the very beginning of his term in office, Major effected the adoption of the Patient's Charter, a milestone which for the first time defined NHS healthcare entitlement in the language of rights. The last Major years brought about a u-turn in cost coverage policy: charges were increased only moderately and exemption from paying charges was extensively broadened.

Altogether, healthcare entitlement reforms under Conservative rule show a clear retrenchment trend marked by massively increased charges, the exclusion of spectacles, the limitation of adult dentistry and a general lessening in the generosity of NHS entitlement. However, retrenchment was moderate as increased charges applied to only a minority of the population, and cuts were restricted to areas contested since the early days of the NHS; while core areas like GP, inpatient and specialist care remained untouched. In addition to these quantitative shifts, the Conservative reforms also brought about a qualitative change. The introduction of the Patient's Charter, which for the first time in NHS history explicitly set out the rights of patients, marked the beginning of a longer process of individualisation of the English social right to healthcare, as the next chapters will show.

2.4 Labour healthcare entitlement reforms 1997–2010

In 1997, Labour regained power, and with it a new era for the NHS commenced. Labour massively expanded NHS funding, but at the same time fundamentally restructured its organisation. This section assesses the impact of 13 years of New Labour healthcare reforms on NHS healthcare entitlement. It starts with background information on relevant political and economic incidents, proceeds with an outline of main health policy reforms, and then details the content of Labour healthcare entitlement reforms. The section closes with a brief summary of results.

Political and economic background

After 18 years in opposition, Labour succeeded in winning the general elections of 1997. It was a glorious comeback: Labour gained 418 seats and 43.2 per cent of the vote.[22] Conservatives, bitterly divided over Europe and unable to regain the electorate's trust after the economic crisis, won only 30.7 per cent of the vote and 165 seats in Parliament (Thorpe 2008, pp. 250f.). Labour's success, however, was not only a result of the Conservatives' weakness. Tony Blair and his peers had worked hard on a renewal of the Labour party and fundamentally transformed its organisation, as well as its ideology, bringing about New Labour (Chadwick and Heffernan 2003). The world had changed and New Labour attempted to adapt social democratic policies to the new realities of globalisation, post-industrial society and the new political landscape (Blair 1998). Distancing itself from the Old Left, as well as from the New Right, New Labour struck out on a 'Third Way' in which the state's role was to enable the market rather than to command the economy, and civil society was to act as the partner of government (Blair 1998).

During his first term in office, Blair realised several popular reforms pledged during his campaign, such as the introduction of minimum wages and the working families tax credit. Although Labour did not follow up on all its promises, it had no problems winning the elections in 2001 (Thorpe 2008, pp. 262f.). Given a still weak Conservative opposition and faint Liberal Democrats, Labour captured 40.7 per cent of the vote (Conservatives 31.7 per cent) and sustained a majority of 165 seats in Parliament. The results of the following elections in 2005 were less victorious; Labour won only 35.2 per cent of the vote (356 seats). The Conservatives gained slightly with 32.4 per cent of votes, but won only 198 seats. The poor election results, continuing conflicts in Iraq and the Cash for Honours scandal weakened Blair's standing and led him to announce in 2006 that he would step down the following year (Thorpe 2008, pp. 277f.). Gordon Brown, the 'undisputed number two in the government' (Chadwick and Heffernan 2003, p. 3) took over as prime minister.

Labour was blessed with a very good economic climate. For the major part of its three terms, the economy grew steadily, unemployment remained moderate and inflation never exceeded three per cent (OECD 2014a). The tide turned with the global economic crisis in 2008, as GDP growth was negative for the first time under the New Labour government and unemployment rose more than seven per cent during the following year. As a result of the economic downturn, Brown was forced to enact several unpopular policies such as tax increases and spending cuts. However, the bad economic situation was not the only reason for the electoral defeat of Labour in the general elections of 2010. Labour's descent had already begun in 2005: increasing disunity within the party, the lack of a coherent policy programme and a new charismatic Conservative leader contributed to the decline of Labour (Heppell 2013, p. 141).

Labour health policy

When Labour left office in 2010, the NHS only marginally resembled the organisation it was 13 years prior. Labour kept its promise to 'safeguard the basic principles of the NHS' (Labour Party 1997) and to expand NHS spending, but undertook a major revision of its institutions, actors and regulatory processes.

Labour expanded NHS resources from the first year on, starting in 1997 and 1998 with a moderate rise in real prices of two per cent annually, and increasing to four per cent in the following two years (Klein 2010, p. 201). Despite increased resources, the NHS landed in a new crisis with almost daily news coverage of deferred or denied treatment and grievances in NHS hospitals (Ham 2009, p. 58; Klein 2010, pp. 202ff.). In response, Blair announced a huge spending increase in 2000, setting the goal of aligning British health spending with the EU average (Bosanquet 2007; Klein 2010, p. 205). Over the next five years, the NHS budget grew on average 7.6 per cent annually, the highest increase in real terms in the history of the NHS (Harcker 2012).

Labour not only threw money at the NHS, but also undertook major organisational reforms. These reforms completely restructured the NHS hierarchy and devolved most power from the DH to lower levels and arm's length bodies. For example, well-performing NHS trusts were granted the status of NHS Foundation Trusts which allowed them greater autonomy and independence from the DH. They were overseen by Monitor, a newly established independent regulator. The healthcare Commission,[23] another new arm's length public body, was tasked with inspecting and supervising the quality of care and effectiveness of NHS management (Talbot-Smith and Pollock 2006, p. 31).

When Labour regained power, they declared they would eliminate the internal market introduced by the Conservatives. They did so only to replace it with new market elements and institutions, and the purchaser/provider split was maintained (Klein 2010, pp. 193f.). Labour abolished GP fundholding, but introduced a similar concept – 'GP practice-based commissioning' – which assigned practices with an indicative budget for commissioning secondary and community services for their patients (Driver and Martell 2002, pp. 94f.). For the first time in NHS history, these budgets also included prescriptions (Klein 2010, p. 233). The GP practice-based commissioning was overseen by the newly established primary care trusts. PCTs became the 'lead planners for the NHS at the local level' (Talbot-Smith and Pollock 2006, p. 37), tasked with assessing the health needs of the local population, developing annual plans to meet these needs and commissioning services where GP commissioning was not in place. PCTs could contract any provider, private or public, or provide the services themselves. The payment system was reformed accordingly. A national tariff was introduced, which paid all public and private providers the same price for identical procedures. Expanding 'consumer' choice at the same time, this new system was intended to reward good providers, as their income increased with the number of patients treated, and to sanction bad providers, as their income declined if they were unable to attract patients (Klein 2010, p. 233).

Another topic high on Labour's political agenda was the diminution of geographic variations in service provision. Service quality, as well as the bundle of services available, often differed widely between areas, which was, in the eyes of Labour, not acceptable for a national health service (Klein 2010, p. 197). National equality was targeted to be achieved by instituting National Service Frameworks, which set national standards of clinical practice, and with the foundation of NICE, a new arm's length body tasked with fostering evidence-based practice and later, with determining services required to be made available by all PCTs (see below).

Labour healthcare entitlement reforms

Under New Labour, four healthcare reforms addressed healthcare entitlement: the Health Act 1999, the Health and Social Care (Community Health and Standards)

Act 2003, the NHS Act 2006 (which replaced the NHS Act 1977) and the Health Act 2009. Again, many relevant changes were made by means of statutory instruments. The adoption of the European Convention of Human Rights via the Human Rights Act in 1998 had raised many expectations, but was of lower relevance in retrospect (Haggett 2001, p. 6; McHale 2012, p. 552). Nevertheless, it exemplifies New Labour's emphasis on individual rights, which was manifested in the area of healthcare with the adoption of the NHS Constitution in 2009.

The NHS Constitution basically summarises rights already granted by law. Nonetheless, it is a milestone in the development of healthcare rights, because, similar to the Patient's Charter of 1991, it frames matters – previously formulated exclusively as duties of NHS bodies – as the rights of individuals. It therefore partially serves as a counterbalance to NHS administrative law (e.g. the NHS Act) that defines rights and responsibilities of NHS providers and bodies, rarely referencing the patient as subject. However, in contrast to NHS legal regulation, the Constitution has no legal status. Nevertheless, it is not a powerless instrument because each health authority and healthcare provider offering services for the NHS is bound by law to have regard for the Constitution (s. 2 Health Act 2009).

The rights listed in the Constitution are a mixture of general human and anti-discrimination rights (e.g. the right to be treated with dignity and respect), personal freedom rights (e.g. consent to treatment), rights to information and choice (e.g. the right to choose a GP), rights to quality services (e.g. the right to a monitoring of quality) and those that help to enforce patients' rights (e.g. the right to lodge a complaint). As for the definition of healthcare entitlement guiding this study, the Constitution mentions a right to receive services free of charge (with exemptions sanctioned by Parliament), a right to treatment in other European countries, and a right to all drugs and treatments recommended by NICE and to vaccinations recommended by the Joint Committee on Vaccination and Immunisation. The Constitution also takes account of the right of patients to rational decision-making as established by English courts (see Chapter 2.6). In 2010, the rights to be treated within defined waiting time limits for consultant-led treatment, as well as for initial treatment by a cancer specialist were added. Furthermore, patients were given the right to be offered treatment by non-NHS providers if the NHS is not able to offer treatment within the specified time limits. In addition to rights, the Constitution makes various non-binding pledges which do not constitute rights. Following one of the core principles of the Third Way – 'no rights without responsibilities' – the Constitution also sets out the responsibilities of patients. It holds patients responsible for maintaining their own health, keeping appointments, and following the course of treatment.

Healthcare entitlement was heavily influenced by decisions made on the European level. During the late 1990s and the early years of the new millennium, the ECJ delivered several seminal judgements concerning the mobility of patients. In 2002, England took the first step in conforming its healthcare legislation to these rulings (SI 2002/2759), and in 2010, the NHS Act was amended to specify conditions for treatment abroad (SI 2010/915 introduced s. 6A and 6B and amended s. 183 NHS Act 2006).[24]

Governance – who decides about healthcare entitlement?

The Health and Social Care (Community Health and Standards) Act implemented major institutional changes within the NHS also involving important shifts of responsibility within the definition of healthcare entitlement. PCTs and Local Health Boards became responsible for GMS and GDS. PCTs were now to commission those services, hence four kinds of contracts were introduced.[25] These contracts specified, amongst other things, which services must be provided, the standards of services and the persons to whom services are to be provided (s. 28O (2) and 28V (2) NHS Act 1977). Formerly, GPs and general dental practitioners held a direct contract with the SoS that had been negotiated nationally. These organisational changes were a first step in transferring responsibilities for healthcare provision and for the definition of healthcare coverage to the PCTs. In a second step, these responsibilities were then devolved to the contractor. Yet the SoS retained the right to define which services must be provided in primary medical and dental care (s. 16CC (5), (6) and 16CA (5), (6) NHS Act 1977). The NHS Act 2006 established the same institutional arrangement for ophthalmic services.

Following the publication of the NHS Constitution which grants patients the right to transparent decision-making, the SoS committed PCTs to 'have in place arrangements for making decisions and adopting policies on whether particular healthcare interventions are to be made available for patients for which the Primary Care Trust is responsible' (Secretary of State for Health 2009). The same directive also obligated PCTs to provide a rationale for their funding decisions. In addition, the DH published guiding principles for those decision-making procedures (Department of Health 2009a). These principles were not binding, but provide PCTs a framework intended to 'improve the consistency and quality of local decision-making on medicines' (Department of Health 2009a, p. 4).

NHS services had differed between local areas even before PCTs became responsible for healthcare provision. The geographic variation in provision springs from disparate distribution of funds on the one hand, and from differences in local decision making regarding the distribution of funds on the other hand. For Labour, this 'postcode rationing' was no longer acceptable (Klein 2010, p. 197). In order to conform funding decisions, the SoS established NICE in 1999 (SI 1999/220), which he tasked with appraising 'the clinical benefits and the costs' (Secretary of State for Health 1999) of treatments. The treatments are selected by the ministry and then referred to NICE for a technology appraisal. The appraisals were intended to guide funding decisions of PCTs, but in the first years were not binding. It was not until 2002 that NICE technology appraisals became compulsory and PCTs were required to fund drugs and healthcare technologies positively recommended by NICE within three months (Secretary of State for Health 2001). PCTs remained free to fund treatments which were not recommended for provision by NICE. In the past, NICE recommendations had been the subject of several judicial reviews which made clear that directions are binding, but clinicians are expected 'to deviate from or modify its guidance where the circumstances of the individual patient require this.'[26]

Within NICE, it is the technology appraisal committees (TACs) that are in charge of conducting the technology assessments. The TACs are composed of many experts from various academic fields (e.g. health economists, medical doctors, pharmacists and NHS executive staff) and few lay members. In assessing the clinical and cost effectiveness of a technology, NICE must take into account 'the broad *balance of clinical benefits and costs*', 'the *degree of clinical need of patients*', 'the potential for long term benefits to the NHS of innovation', and any guidance of the SoS on that issue (reg. 2 (4) of the Directions 2005, Secretary of State for Health 2005, emphasis in original). Apart from these requirements, NICE is free to decide on the coverage of services. NICE applies a cost-effectiveness ratio of £20,000 per Quality Adjusted Life Year (QALY).[27] If NICE does not recommend funding for a treatment below that ratio, or recommends a treatment that ranges between £20,000 and £30,000 per QALY, it needs good reasons (NICE 2008). In 2009, the maximum threshold for end-of-life treatments was lowered. These may now exceed £30,000 per QALY if particular conditions are fulfilled (NICE 2009).

Generosity – service coverage

The most important Labour reforms concerning service coverage have already been described above – the transferal of coverage decision-making to PCTs and the assignment to NICE of defining the treatments and medicines required for availability throughout the English NHS. Of further note is the implementation of ECJ rulings concerning treatment abroad into English law which is discussed in Chapter 2.7, and the permission of 'top-up payments' for private drugs without losing NHS entitlement. In the past, patients who wanted to receive a medicine not provided by the NHS could purchase it privately, but in doing so, lost entitlement to NHS care. In 2008, the case of a cancer patient who was withdrawn from free NHS treatment after having privately bought a drug not covered by the NHS attracted immense media attention (Klein 2010, pp. 267f.). In response, the SoS commissioned a report, which recommended that 'no patient should lose their entitlement to NHS care . . ., simply because they opt to purchase additional treatment for their condition' (Richards 2008, p. 57), with the caveat that private drugs 'are delivered separately from the NHS elements of . . . care' (Richards 2008, p. 59). The SoS adopted these suggestions and adapted the relevant guidance accordingly, henceforth allowing patients to receive private medicines without losing the right to NHS treatment (Department of Health 2009b).

Prevention and primary care: In the area of prevention, the Labour government followed the Conservatives' policies and further extended preventive measures. For example, pharmacists became obligated to promote healthy lifestyles to their customers in general and to customers with increased health risks such as obesity, diabetes or smoking in particular (SI 2005/641). A minor measure countering this trend was the addition of 12 nicotine substitutes (e.g. nicotine patches and gums) to the black list in 2001.

Pharmaceuticals: Between 1998 and 2004, only 19 items were added to the black list (of which 12 were nicotine substitutes) and 11 substances were removed.

On the grey list, seven drugs for the treatment of erectile dysfunction were added, and two other items were taken from the list. In 2004, the NHS General Medical Services Regulation (SI 1992/635), which so far included the black and grey lists, was replaced by the National Health Service (General Medical Services Contracts) (Prescription of Drugs etc.) Regulations 2004 (SI 2004/629). The new black list (schedule 1) contained 3111 items, or roughly 150 items fewer than the old list (own calculation). The grey list was not amended (schedule 2); it contained the same 12 drugs as the old list. In the years since, no changes have been made to the black list. The grey list was extended to cover Tamiflu and Relenza for the prevention and treatment of influenza in 2004 (SI 2004/3215).

Medical appliances: In 2002, a grey list for medical appliances was introduced that restricted the prescription of specific appliances to particular patient groups (SI 2002/551). These 'restricted availability appliances'[28] and eligibility criteria for prescription were to be specified in the Drug Tariff. However, as of today (2013), the Drug Tariff contains only one group of restricted appliances, namely, vacuum pumps and constrictor rings for erectile dysfunction.

Dental care and dental appliances: In 2001, the General Dental Services Regulation was almost completely rewritten and with it, the range of occasional treatment was extended. Later that year, general anaesthesia was excluded from GDS (SI 2001/3963).

Ophthalmic care and optical appliances: In 1999, Labour partially rescinded the Conservatives' entitlement cuts by extending eligibility for sight testing to cover all people over the age of 60 and those predisposed to glaucoma (SI 1999/693). Similarly as for GDS and GMS, responsibility for ophthalmic care was transferred to PCTs in 2006. The Health Act 2006 established which people had the right to sight tests and constituted the SoS's power to further define eligibility through regulations. Apart from these prerequisites, PCTs were free to provide ophthalmic services as they considered 'necessary to meet all reasonable requirements' (s. 16CD (1) (c) NHS Act 1977).

Generosity – cost coverage

Summing up what follows, it can be concluded that most Labour reforms have expanded generosity in cost coverage, though often in small steps. The income level defining eligibility for a refund of charges and payment of travelling expenses was raised steadily over the years (e.g. by SI 2004/936), adapting it to real prices and thereby avoiding hidden entitlement cuts. Furthermore, in 2009 all patients suffering from cancer were completely exempted from charges (SI 2009/29).

Pharmaceuticals and medical appliances: Labour introduced several exemptions from drug charges. In 2007, patients suffering from tuberculosis were exempted in order 'to encourage [them] to be seen regularly' (explanatory memorandum SI 2007/1975). In the following years, released prisoners continuing to receive medical treatment from the prison health centre, as well as patients under supervised community treatment[29] also were exempted. In the course of the swine flu pandemic of 2009, patients receiving treatment for pandemic diseases were freed from paying charges

(SI 2009/1166), and in addition, the antiviral drugs Zanamivir and Oseltamivir were available free of charge under certain conditions (SI 2009/2230).

Eligibility for the refund of pre-payment certificates (PPCs) was extended by increasing the time period for application, by refunding the remaining value of a certificate in the case of death and by accepting a claim outside the specified time limits in cases where the SoS was satisfied that the delay was for good cause (s. 9 (7) – (15) SI 2000/620 as amended by SI 2001/746). In 2007, PPCs were restructured to cover three and 12 months instead of four and 12 months in order to reduce the initial outlays patients were required to make. For the same reason, instalment payments were introduced for the 12-month PPC (see explanatory memorandum SI 2007/1510). Furthermore, the refund of payments became more generous: formerly, a refund was possible only if the cause for exemption occurred within the first four months of a 12-month PPC, but is now available during the whole period of the PPC.

Charges for drugs and medical appliances in real prices did not increase much during the 13 years of Labour government. In 1998, patients paid £5.80 per item, which increased to £7.20 in 2009 (see Table 2.5). Also, the price increases for PPCs remained moderate (see Table A.3 of the appendix). Only charges for particular medical appliances (e.g. stock modacrylic wigs, particular stockings) were raised above the average (see Table A.8 of the appendix).

Dental care and dental appliances: Charges for dental care and dental appliances remained at 80 per cent of costs until charges were completely restructured in 2005. Between 1997 and 2005, maximum charges increased slightly more than average prices, from £330 to £384 (see Table A.5 of the appendix). With the structural change of dental care reimbursement from an item of services remuneration to an annual payment not related to the dentist's activity, dental charges, which had also been item-based, were completely reformed. The new charge system identifies three categories of charges, called bands, which depend on the complexity of the treatment provided. Because the charge system was completely redesigned, it is difficult to evaluate the cost impact for patients. The explanatory memorandum to SI 2005/3477 states that on average, charges were not increased, yet certain patient groups would have to pay somewhat higher charges (e.g. those seeking a basic assessment), while others would have to pay less (e.g. those with more extensive need for dental treatment). When the old maximum charge for dental appliances of £384 (in 2005) is compared with the new charges that apply to dental appliances (Band 3) of £189 (in 2005), it becomes clear that people in need of extensive treatment were massively unburdened through the reform. Charges for a course of treatment belonging to Band 1 were £15.50, for a Band 2 course of treatment £42.40 and for a Band 3 £189 in 2005, which increased to £16.50, £45.60 and £198 respectively in 2009 (see Table A.6 of the appendix). In the election year 2010, neither dental nor drug charges were raised.

Ophthalmic care and optical appliances: During Labour's terms in office, the coverage of costs for sight tests and optical appliances was increased and eligibility expanded. Vouchers for optical appliances were adapted annually and increased slightly more than average prices. For example, a voucher for single vision lenses amounted to £27.20 in 1997 and increased to £37.10 in 2010. The income level

Table 2.5 Charges for pharmaceuticals and medical appliances 1998–2010

Year	1998	1999	2000	2001	2002	2003	2004	2005	2006	2007	2008	2009	2010
Statutory instrument (No.)	491	767	620	746	548	585	663	578	675	543/ 1510	571	411	/
Charges (per item)	£5.80	£5.90	£6.00	£6.10	£6.20	£6.30	£6.40	£6.50	£6.65	£6.85	£7.10	£7.20	£7.20
Charge increase	2.7%	1.7%	1.7%	1.7%	1.6%	1.6%	1.6%	1.6%	2.3%	3.0%	3.6%	1.4%	0%
Annual inflation	1.6%	1.3%	0.8%	1.2%	1.3%	1.4%	1.3%	2.1%	2.3%	2.3%	3.6%	2.2%	3.3%

Sources: OECD (2014a), own data collection.

at which entitlement to sight testing and to vouchers for optical appliances takes effect was extended from an amount that is equal to (or less than) a person's requirements to that which exceeds requirements by 50 per cent or less of the NHS prescription charge (s. 13 (2) (e) SI 1986/975 and s. 8 (3) (e) SI 1997/818 as amended by SI 2004/936). The decision to abolish vouchers for contact lenses in 2008 stands in contrast to this expansion of generosity (SI 2008/553 omits sch. 1 s. 10 SI 1997/818). Still permissible was the use of eyeglass vouchers towards the purchase of contact lenses, but additional costs are to be borne by the patient.

Summary

During its 13 years in government, Labour steadily expanded the generosity of NHS entitlement and kept entitlement cuts small and rare. The black and grey lists of drugs introduced by the Conservatives degenerated to an unimportant instrument under Labour and charge increases remained very low, rarely exceeding price inflation, with an average of less than two per cent increase per year. Healthcare entitlement reforms thus reflect general, munificent Labour health policy.

   In retrospect, different phases of Labour healthcare entitlement policy can be distinguished. Being bound to the promise to stay within budget, Labour did not conduct any healthcare entitlement reform during its first two years in office. Subsequently, it steadily increased its activity in this field, arriving at a reform peak between 2001 and 2004. Reforms during this period encompassed entitlement enhancements as well as minor retrenchments. Charge increases in these years always remained below 1.7 per cent. The last two years of Blair's term as prime minister, 2005 and 2006, were again characterised by low reform activity. This changed when Brown came into office. Brown almost exclusively focused on charges and, in several steps, massively expanded eligibility for exemption from drug charges. Only one measure slightly reduced generosity: the abolition of vouchers for contact lenses in 2008, which was likely related to the poor economic situation that year. Charges increased more steeply during the Brown years but, compared to the Conservative years, increases were still moderate at 2.3 to 3.7 per cent per year. With the introduction of the NHS Constitution in 2009, Brown influenced healthcare entitlement in the long run. In the election year of 2010, healthcare entitlement reform came to a standstill with the adaption of NHS law to ECJ rulings being the only reform adopted.

   Under Labour, the collective social right to healthcare gradually transformed towards a more individual right. This process was crystallised through three developments: the introduction of NICE technology appraisals, the NHS Constitution and decisions of the ECJ on patient mobility (which are covered in Chapter 2.7). The establishment of the NICE Technology Appraisal Process, for the first time in NHS history, allowed for a specification of entitlement to specific treatments that are to be provided for each patient irrespective of financial resources of PCTs. This specification was a precondition for individuals to claim their rights as they must know about the content of entitlement to be able to claim benefits. In a second step, these and other rights were explicitly framed as rights of patients by the NHS

Constitution. Until its publication, healthcare entitlement could only be derived from NHS administrative law which merely defines rights and responsibilities of NHS bodies concerning the provision of services.

2.5 Conservative–Liberal Democratic healthcare entitlement reforms 2010–2013

The last epoch of healthcare entitlement reforms described in this book is rather short. It covers the first three and a half years of the first British coalition government since 1940.[30] Conservatives and Liberal Democrats had a tough time fighting the economic crisis and pulling through one of the most radical health reforms in NHS history. Following the structure of the previous chapters, the political and economic context is sketched first before the key elements of the structural reform of the NHS are delineated. Again, the focus lies on the analysis of healthcare entitlement reforms in the third part. Finally, reforms are briefly summarised.

Political and economic background

In 2010, after 13 years in government, Labour lost its majority in Parliament. The outcome of the general elections, however, was far from clear cut: Labour lost votes winning only 29.0 per cent, but Conservatives also failed to win a majority, gaining just 36.1 per cent of the vote and 306 out of 650 seats. The Liberal Democrats were voted the third-strongest party with 23.0 per cent and 57 seats (Fisher and Wlezien 2012, p. 1). Despite the huge ideological differences between the two parties (Quinn, Bara and Bartle 2012, p. 178), the Conservatives and Liberal Democrats decided to form a coalition government. Both parties had to make concessions but managed to get most of their priority policies included in the coalition agreement (Quinn, Bara and Bartle 2012, p. 186).

The incoming government faced a miserable economic situation. After two consecutive years of negative growth, GDP had recovered to 1.7 per cent in 2010, but growth remained slow with 1.1 per cent in 2011 and 0.2 per cent in 2012 (OECD 2014a). Unemployment reached a 14-year high of 7.8 per cent in 2010, and grew further to 7.9 per cent in 2012 (OECD 2014b). During the crisis, tax income dropped and public spending increased to 48 per cent of GDP, which led to the annual budget deficit reaching an all-time high of 11 per cent of GDP in the financial year 2009/10 (HM Treasury 2010, p. 8). Overall public net debt amounted to 65.7 per cent of GDP in 2010 (The Guardian 2013).

Given this river of red ink, the Conservatives declared deficit reduction the primary goal of government. With massive spending cuts and tax increases, the new government hoped to find its way out of the budget crisis (HM Treasury 2010). Up to the time of this writing, the Cameron government had already introduced a flood of reforms: welfare benefits and tax credits were fixed at a one per cent increase per year until 2014/15, a welfare benefit cap was introduced, generosity of social housing was lowered and administrative costs of government departments were cut, to name only some of the implemented reforms. The already implemented as well as the envisioned reforms do not only realise substantial cuts in generosity of social programmes, but also contain structural changes that will in the long run lead to a significant modification of the British welfare state into a (neo-)liberal one, as some observers predict (Grimshaw and Rubery 2012, p. 107; Taylor-Gooby 2012).

Coalition health policy

The Coalition had promised in its coalition programme to increase health spending in real terms each year (HM Government 2010, p. 24). However, it did not keep its word and NHS spending declined by 0.2 per cent in real terms during the first Coalition spending period of 2011/12 (Appleby 2013),[31] which is still a rather small decline compared to other welfare areas.

Soon after coming into office, the new government drafted one of the biggest reforms in the history of the NHS (Timmins 2012, p. 14). Their Health and Social Care Bill met broad opposition, not only from the public and health professionals, but also from the Liberal Democrats (Waller and Yong 2012, pp. 181f.). Although the bill was modified and mitigated, the fundamental reforms remained. Due to the comprehensiveness of reforms, a full description cannot be given here. Instead, this section focuses on the main organisational changes and the following section presents in detail the content of healthcare entitlement reforms.

The Health and Social Care Act 2012 completely reshuffled the NHS organisational structure once again: PCTs and Special Health Authorities were abolished and their tasks taken over by clinical commissioning groups (CCGs) and the NHS Commissioning Board. CCGs are GP-led but also involve representatives of the public, nurses and hospital doctors. They are provided with their own budgets with which they commission medical services for their patients from a range of providers. The NHS Commissioning Board (operating name NHS England) commissions specialist services and primary care. It was also assigned several other tasks, including CCG authorisation and quality improvement. The Care Quality Commission and Monitor[32] are responsible for overseeing health service provision. Responsibility for public health was transferred to Public Health England and to local health authorities (The King's Fund 2013). One of the main aims of the reform was to 'to take politics and politicians out of day-to-day management of the NHS' (Lansley, SoS, as cited by Timmins 2012, p. 27;) and to create a service that 'would run more or less on autopilot' (Timmins 2012, p. 124). Therefore, the power of the SoS was curtailed within the NHS Act, which also means that structural reforms in the future cannot easily be reversed by the next SoS but will need to be legislated by Parliament (Timmins 2012, p. 125).

Coalition healthcare entitlement reforms

During the now three and a half years of coalition government, the Health and Social Care Act 2012 has remained the only general health law that affected healthcare entitlement. Due to the fundamental nature of the reforms, almost all secondary health regulation had to be adapted. In addition, the new government revised the NHS Constitution in 2013. They carefully modified the guiding principles (SI 2013/317) and the formulation of patients' responsibilities was softened from 'you should' to 'please, . . .'. Patients' rights were slightly modified too, but with regard to healthcare entitlement as defined by this study, no changes were made.

Governance – who decides about healthcare entitlement?

The 2012 reform made it clear, by changing the particular paragraph in the NHS Act, that it is no longer the duty of the SoS to '*provide* and secure health services' (emphasis added), but to '*secure that services are provided* in accordance with this Act' (s. 1 (2) NHS Act 2006 as amended by the Health and Social Services Act 2012, emphasis added). The SoS, however, 'retains ministerial responsibility to Parliament for the provision of the health service in England' (s. 1 (3) NHS Act 2006). Although in general the CCGs and the Board are free to organise health service provision,[33] the SoS has the power to require them to make available specific services. Moreover, s/he can make provisions to the decision-making processes for coverage and distribution by these health bodies (s. 6E NHS Act 2006).

NICE is responsible for preparing technology appraisals which remain compulsory, although the obligation to fund technologies recommended by NICE was for some time challenged by the new government.[34] The bodies, however, addressed by NICE technology appraisals have changed as a result of NHS restructuring. It is no longer PCTs but CCGs, the Commissioning Board and local authorities that must ensure treatments and drugs recommended by NICE become available for patients within three months (SI 2013/259). In 2013, NICE was additionally tasked with appraising the benefits and costs of highly specialised technologies for the treatment of rare and very rare conditions. Recommended technologies must be provided by the Board, usually within three months (s. 8 SI 2013/259). For this new task, NICE has established a Technologies Evaluation Committee whose composition is quite similar to the TACs.

Generosity – service and cost coverage

With regard to service coverage, the only activities of the Coalition government were smaller modifications of the grey list: eligibility criteria for influenza drugs (SI 2010/2389, SI 2011/680, SI 2010/2389) and for drugs for the treatment of erectile dysfunction (SI 2013/2194) were slightly expanded. Also, amendments regarding cost coverage remained minimal.

Pharmaceuticals and medical appliances: In real terms, charges for pharmaceuticals and medical appliances were not increased during the last four years. They increased between two to three per cent per year, and thus increases equalled or remained slightly below inflation. In detail, the charge per item was £7.20 in 2009, £7.40 in 2011, £7.65 in 2012 and £7.85 in 2013. There was no increase in 2010. Prices of pre-payment certificates were not raised.

Dental care and dental appliances: The policy of the coalition government for dental charges was similar. Charges increased in nominal terms by two to three per cent per year. In detail, charges were raised in three steps from £16.50 in 2010 to £18.00 in 2013 for Band 1, from £45.60 to £49.00 for Band 2 and from £198 to £214 for Band 3 treatments, respectively. In 2013, a new charge that applies where an interim course of dental care treatment is provided to persons receiving primary dental services under the Capitation and Quality Scheme 2 was introduced (SI 2013/364). This Band 1A charge amounted to £17.50 per course of treatment and was later raised to £18.

Ophthalmic care and optical appliances: The old NHS Optical Charges and Payments Regulations (SI 1997/818) were replaced by new regulations in 2013 (SI 2013/641), but with regard to the research question of this study, no major changes occurred. The only noteworthy modification was that the sight test fee is no longer determined within the statutory instrument, but is instead specified by directions of the SoS. The coalition government slightly increased voucher values, but increases were less than the inflation rate.

Summary

Although only in office for three and a half years, the coalition government had an enormous impact on the NHS. The Health and Social Care Act 2012 completely restructured NHS organisation and with it, massively reallocated responsibilities within the system. The Act rarely addressed healthcare entitlement, but as a result of the structural reforms, the actors responsible for defining healthcare entitlement on the micro- and meso-levels changed. Furthermore, the national level retained more power to determine healthcare entitlement with the establishment of the Board and the expansion of NICE competencies. Still to be seen are what effects these changes will have on healthcare entitlement in the long run. Concrete healthcare entitlement reforms remained few with only a very small or no impact on generosity.

2.6   Judicial review of healthcare entitlement decisions

So far, the description of English healthcare entitlement has been concentrated on NHS legislation. Parliamentary acts and secondary legislation, however, form only one part of the English legal system. The other part emanates from the practice of the courts. In common law, legal rules are established through court rulings, which have effect beyond a particular case: in deciding on a case, judges are bound to take into account past judgements of similar cases (Montgomery 2002, pp. 6f.). Over the past decades, the role of the courts has increased as more and more NHS funding decisions have been taken to court. In the following section, the grounds for judicial review of administrative decisions in England are first described before the most important cases of the last two decades are presented.

Decisions about the funding of a particular treatment by the NHS may be challenged through judicial review. An appeal on the merits of a decision is not possible (Syrett 2011, p. 471). During a judicial review, decisions of public authorities are scrutinised by the courts. In doing so, judges cannot provide an alternative decision but only 'quash' the decision of the NHS authority and refer it back for a rehearing (Newdick 2007, p. 60; Sheldrick 2003, p. 152). In general, there are three arguments for judicial review of administrative decisions: illegality, irrationality and procedural impropriety (Newdick 2007, p. 60). *Illegality* is the basis if the authority 'has done something it has no power to do, or failed to do something it is obligated to do' (Newdick 2007, p. 60). The powers and duties of NHS bodies are defined by statutes and secondary legislation (e.g. the NHS Act, statutory instruments), yet often in very general terms.[35] *Irrationality* refers to the 'Wednesbury unreasonableness', which describes a decision that was 'so unreasonable that no reasonable authority could ever have come to it',[36] or as Lord Diplock has phrased it, 'a decision which is so outrageous in its defiance of logic or of accepted moral standards that no sensible person who had applied his mind to the question to be decided could have arrived at it.'[37] Unreasonableness is a very broad concept and might address various aspects of a decision (Montgomery 2002, p. 68). It provides judges with broad discretion and has been employed in a variety of ways, as the cases described below show. The third argument of *procedural impropriety* includes the failure of the decision-making body 'to observe procedural rules that are expressly laid down in the legislative instrument by which its jurisdiction is conferred', a 'failure to observe basic rules of natural justice', and 'a failure to act with procedural fairness' (Newdick 2007, p. 61). Often more than one argument is brought forward when a case is submitted (Newdick 2005, p. 94).

The first relevant judgement on healthcare entitlement was rendered in 1980 when the court of appeal ruled that the duty of the SoS to provide health services (s. 3 NHS Act 1977) is not an absolute duty, but is always contingent upon the resources available.[38] Four patients who had been on a waiting list for orthopaedic surgery for a long time claimed that the SoS did not comply with his duty to provide a comprehensive health service. They accused the SoS of having failed to expand the capacity of the orthopaedic unit of their hospital by not providing sufficient resources. There had been plans approved by the SoS to establish additional orthopaedic services, but they could not be realised because of insufficient financial resources. Lord Denning MR held that '[t]he Secretary of State is not under an obligation to meet all demands for hospital facilities and treatment, but to do what he can within the resources made available to him.'[39] With this judgement, the court made the constraints of healthcare entitlement within the NHS explicit: there is no absolute duty to provide, and hence no absolute right to receive NHS services, but entitlement always depends on the financial resources available.

Having clarified the conditionality of NHS service provision, courts remained rather inactive, and refrained from intervening in resource allocation decisions (Newdick 2005; 2007). During the 1980s, the courts dismissed the applications for judicial review in two similar cases because judges could not find any breach of duties under the law and claimed that they were the wrong body to decide upon the distribution of public resources. In both cases, an operation for a child needing critical heart surgery was postponed several times due to a shortage of intensive care resources, but the judges held 'that this court can no more investigate that on the facts of this case than it could do so in any other case where the balance of available money and its distribution and use are concerned. Those, of course, are questions which are of enormous public interest and concern – but they are questions to be raised, answered and dealt with outside the court.'[40] This view was confirmed by Sir John Donaldson MR: 'It is not for this court, or indeed any court, to substitute its own judgement for the judgement of those who are responsible for the allocation of resources.'[41]

Beginning in the mid-1990s, the attitude of courts towards NHS resource allocation changed and judicial review intensified (Newdick 2007, p. 67). The first case in which this turnaround could be observed is the tragic case of child B, a 10-year-old girl suffering from leukaemia who was, after a relapse, denied further curative treatment by her health authority in 1995. The authority had justified its decision with the arguments that first, the therapy was not in the best interest of the child because of its severe side effects; second, the treatment was experimental; third, the proposed therapy had not been formally evaluated; and last, the substantial costs of treatment given the small prospect of success meant resources could be used more effectively elsewhere. At first instance, the court quashed the decision of the health authority. Referring to the girl's fundamental right to life under Article 2 of the European Convention of Human Rights, the judge deemed that when infringing on that right, 'the responsible authority must . . . do more than toll the bell of tight resources. They must explain the priorities that have led them to decline to fund the treatment.'[42] A second reason for quashing the decisions was that the health authority had not properly accounted for the child's best interest, as it had merely considered medical motives but not the family's view. The court of appeal, however, objected to the decision of the court of first instance.[43] It found that the child's interest had been properly considered and that it was not practical to list exactly how funds are distributed.

The first case of denied funding ever decided in favour of the patient occurred in 1997 (Newdick 2005, p. 100; 2007, p. 67).[44] The patient took legal action because his health authority had refused to fund a new drug (beta-interferon) for the treatment of multiple sclerosis, despite the fact that the SoS had issued a circular requesting the health authorities to make the drug available to their patients. The circular merely provided guidance to the health authorities and, as such, did not need to be followed, but only taken into account. The court judged the decision unlawful because the health authority disregarded the guidance. Furthermore, it ruled that the reasons given by the health authority were 'irrational'. The health authority had argued that it had only £50,000 and that it could not distribute the money fairly, i.e. according to clinical need, but only on a first-come, first-served basis and hence decided it was better not to provide the treatment at all.

In 1998, three patients suffering from gender identity dysphoria also successfully took legal action against their PCT after it had refused to pay for transsexual surgery. The PCT gave this treatment low priority because it was considered to be clinically ineffective. The court of appeal quashed the decision, arguing that the policy adopted by the PCT was a 'blanket policy'.[45] Although ostensibly the health authority acknowledged transsexualism to be an illness, 'it did not in truth treat it as such', and thus there had never been a real chance of the patients receiving this treatment – not even in exceptional circumstances such as overriding clinical need.

The rise of the new millennium saw a flood of legal disputes on healthcare entitlement which cannot all be presented here. The following paragraphs concentrate on two cases in which judicial review overrode decisions of health authorities to not fund treatment, and where judgements extensively defined which criteria for the allocation of funds are valid. In 2006, a woman suffering from breast cancer took legal action against the decision of her PCT to not fund an adjuvant therapy with trastuzumab (trade name Herceptin).[46] Herceptin is a type of monoclonal antibody effective against a certain type of breast cancer, namely HER2-positive cancer cells. The problem with Herceptin at that time was that it had not yet been licensed for adjuvant treatment, but only for secondary or late-stage breast cancer. However, there was significant evidence that women suffering from HER2-positive breast cancer could benefit from early treatment with that drug. As it was not licensed, NICE had not yet given a recommendation, and thus PCTs had to decide individually on funding. Swindon PCT decided to apply the normal policy for off-license drugs to Herceptin, i.e. to individually review each case for which treatment had been recommended by the managing clinician, and to grant funding only in exceptional circumstances. Mrs Rogers appealed the denial of funding, but the PCT sustained its refusal. The court also dismissed her claim, as it could not find that Swindon's policy was arbitrary or irrational and thus unlawful. The judge in the second instance, however, dissented from that view and quashed the decision. He argued that because the PCT treated financial considerations as irrelevant, 'the only concern which the PCT can have must relate to the legitimate clinical needs of the patient . . . . Where the clinical needs are equal, and resources are not an issue, discrimination between patients in the same eligible group cannot be justified on the basis of personal characteristics not based on healthcare.'[47] Furthermore, there was no evidence that supported a distinction between patients within the eligible group on the basis of exceptional clinical circumstances and thus, 'the only reasonable approach was to focus on the patient's clinical needs and fund patients within the eligible group who were properly prescribed Herceptin by their physician.'[48]

A similar case was brought to trial in 2007.[49] A women suffering from metastatic colorectal cancer received a colectomy and was treated with chemotherapy. Her liver tumours were too big to be resected and they did not respond to chemotherapy. Therefore, her doctor decided to treat the patient with an additional cancer drug named Avastin. Avastin was not licensed in England and thus it was not regularly funded by the NHS. The treating clinician requested funding from the patient's PCT which had a Difficult Decisions Panel to handle such decisions for non-standard drugs. The panel applied its normal decision-making framework, and on the basis of the criteria given in their framework (e.g. equity, evidence of effectiveness), refused funding. The judge, however, held the opinion that the decision of the panel was irrational and thus unlawful for several reasons: the panel had not taken into account the fact that there were no other treatments available 'within normal National Health Service standards which were likely to have any benefit for'[50] the patient. Furthermore, the judge accused the panel of not having considered 'the slim but important chance that treatment including Avastin could prolong [the patient's] life by more than a few months.'[51]

One particular case stands out in several respects. First, it was not a claim of patients against their health authority, but of a pharmaceutical company against the SoS. Second, it did not address secondary care, as had all the other cases, but primary care. And third, the claim was based on EU law. In 1998, the SoS issued a circular which advised GPs not to prescribe Viagra (a drug for the treatment of erectile dysfunction) other than in exceptional circumstances until the minister made a final decision regarding reimbursement of the drug. In response, the manufacturer (Pfizer) sued the SoS, arguing that the circular contradicted the statutory obligations of GPs as set out in the terms of service (sch. 2 SI 1992/635) and, furthermore, infringed on EU law. The court agreed with the claimant's opinion and held that the circular was unlawful because 'the advice was given in a manner which meant that GPs would inevitably regard it as overriding their professional judgement.'[52] With regard to European law, the judge deemed that the circular restricted Community trade (Art. 28 of the Treaty) and in addition, also violated the Transparency Directive (89/105/EEC). The Transparency Directive requires Member States, in the case of an exclusion of a medical product from the coverage of the public healthcare system, to publish in an appropriate publication a statement of reasons based upon objective and verifiable criteria (Art. 7 (1) 89/105/EEC). According to the court, the SoS had failed to comply with the requirements set out by the Directive.

Shortly after the judgement, the SoS put Viagra on the grey list of drugs, which are to be prescribed in special circumstances only (see Chapter 2.4). Pfizer challenged this policy too, claiming again that it was in breach of the Transparency Directive. Meanwhile, however, the UK had provided the European Commission with criteria for the exclusion of medicinal products from NHS coverage:

> A medicinal product or a category of them may be so excluded where the forecast aggregate cost to the NHS of allowing the product (or category of products) to be supplied on NHS prescription, or to be supplied more widely than the permitted exceptions, could not be justified having regard to all the relevant circumstances including in particular: the Secretary of State's duties pursuant to the NHS Act 1977 and the priorities for expenditure of NHS resources.[53]

The court held that these criteria were sufficient to fulfil the requirements of the Transparency Directive, and an analysis of competing priorities as demanded by the claimant must not be provided.

The second Viagra case is of particular importance because it is the first that addressed NICE decision-making, albeit only casually. During the process, the SoS clarified the role of NICE and judges upheld his opinion: it is the task of NICE to assess the cost-effectiveness of treatments and drugs, but it is not within its scope to decide on their affordability. This is the responsibility of the ministry, which, in selecting the medical technologies that are referred to NICE for technology appraisal, defines priorities of the NHS. The judges once again made clear that the setting of priorities and decisions about the allocation of NHS resources is a 'political decision to be taken by government.'[54]

In 2007, NICE was challenged directly for the first time (Syrett 2011, pp. 476f.). The year before, NICE had issued a guideline on the treatment of Alzheimer's disease with a particular group of drugs. The guideline recommended that these drugs be provided only for patients with moderately severe Alzheimer's disease. One of the manufacturers sought judicial review on several grounds.[55] First, it accused NICE decision-making of being procedurally unfair because NICE had not provided the fully executable economic model on which its decision was based. This argument was dismissed by the first judge, but the court of appeal acknowledged that fairness required access to the full model because only in that way are the manufacturers able to question the reliability of the model and hence give intelligent responses.[56] Second, it was claimed that the formulation of the guidance was too rigid and, as a result, discriminated against a particular group of patients. The judge held that NICE decision-making was unreasonable and unlawful because NICE did not consider its duties 'to promote equal opportunities and to have due regard to the need to eliminate discrimination.'[57] Grounds three to six were all based on irrationality and referred to different aspects of the decision-making process. All four grounds were dismissed by the judge and not appealed by the claimant.

Invoking almost the same grounds, another manufacturer challenged NICE in 2009.[58] Again, the court held that NICE had failed to provide information on the economic model and forced it to do so. The claim on grounds of irrationality was again dismissed, and this time the judge did not find NICE guidance to be unlawfully discriminatory against particular patient groups. A similar case was taken to court the same year,[59] but this time the manufacturer's demand for a disclosure of the economic model was not successful. In this case, the manufacturer also claimed the NICE guidelines to be in breach of the Transparency Directive. Discussing this argument, the judge held the view that a positive recommendation of a drug by NICE is tantamount to putting the drug on a positive list.[60] Although it agreed that the Transparency Directive applies to NICE guidelines, the court dismissed the claim because it could not find any infringement of the Directive.

Summing up the judicial review of coverage decisions, a clear trend towards a greater willingness of judges to challenge decisions of health authorities can be observed. Prior to 1995, courts altogether refused to scrutinise allocation decisions, but starting with the child B case, they regularly questioned the reasonableness of decisions taken.[61] Courts thereby established several principles decision-makers must take into account when making funding decisions. First, decision-makers must provide a rationale for their decisions. Second, they need always allow for exceptional circumstances: blanket bans are unlawful. Third, decision-makers must take into account all relevant aspects of a case. And fourth, discrimination between patients, other than on medical grounds, is unlawful. The judges, however, made it plain that it is not the role of the courts to decide about the distribution of health resources, and in each of the cases described above referred the issue back to the health authority for reconsideration. Judges dealt with the wave of manufacturer claims against NICE in a similar vein. Here, most claims succeeded on procedural grounds, and neither the TAC decision-making process in principle, nor the applied criteria, were subject to judicial scrutiny.

Over the last several decades, NHS resources were massively expanded, which has resulted in increasing numbers of people receiving ever more NHS services. At the same time, more and more patients are taking legal action against denied funding. What might explain this greater willingness of patients to challenge decisions of NHS bodies? Perhaps one of the main reasons for this is increased patient expectations and a greater sense of entitlement. Today, almost one third of citizens expect the NHS to provide 'all drugs and treatments, no matter what the costs', and 40 per cent demand that the NHS provide at least 'those that are most effective' (Rankin, Allen and Brooks 2007, p. 28). If these expectations are not fulfilled, people feel treated unfairly and will challenge the decision. Another reason is that allocative decisions have become more visible as NHS bodies at various levels of the system have set explicit restrictions on the treatments and services they provide (Syrett 2004, p. 294). In the old system of implicit rationing, patients often did not realise that they were denied treatment, and even if they did, it was almost impossible for them to ascertain the responsible body or person (Syrett 2004, p. 296). Finally, a juridical claim might provide wider benefits than the outcome of the actual trial. For example, cases of denied funding often attract broad media coverage and public attention, which in some instances has prompted health authorities to provide funding despite the case being lost by the patient (Montgomery 2002, p. 68). Or, as in the child B case, private donors cover the costs of treatment. However, there is one problem with solving allocative problems through legal action: 'only the most empowered patients' (Ford 2012, p. 328) are able to enforce their rights this way.

2.7   The impact of EU law on English healthcare entitlement

In principle, the organisation and delivery of public healthcare falls under the sole authority of the Member States (Art. 168 No. 7 TFEU, formerly Art. 152 (5) TEEC). Yet persons, goods, services and capital are free to move between EU countries, and these freedoms have an impact on various aspects of the national organisation of public healthcare systems (e.g. the application of competition law, the approval of qualifications). The following section focuses on the rights of patients to receive treatment within an EU country other than their own, and answers the question of how EU law regarding patient mobility has affected English healthcare entitlement.

If a patient seeks treatment abroad in another Member State, s/he can do so on the basis of two legal grounds: first, the EU regulation concerning social security coordination (883/04/EC, formerly 1408/71/EEC) and second, EU regulations and case law arising from the fundamental principles of free movement of goods and services (Palm and Glinos 2010, pp. 514f.).[62] The former is based on Article 42 EC and primarily aims to secure the social security of migrant workers and their family members (Palm and Glinos 2010, p. 514). Article 19 grants the right to treatment when an illness occurs during a temporary stay or holiday abroad. Of more importance is Article 20 (formerly Art. 22, 1408/71/EEC), which regulates those cases in which patients travel to another Member State specifically to seek treatment there (also known as E112 scheme). Under the E112 scheme, prior approval is required and must be granted if treatment cannot be provided in the home country 'within a time-limit which is medically justifiable, taking into account his current state of health and the probable course of his illness' (Art. 20 (2), 883/04/EC). Furthermore, the treatment must be part of the benefits package of the public healthcare system of the home country. If these conditions are fulfilled, the patient is entitled to receive treatment in another Member State as though s/he were covered by the public healthcare system of that country.

The second legal option allowing for treatment abroad is based on Articles 28 and 49 EC – the free movement of goods and services – and has been developed stepwise by decisions of the ECJ. In 1998, two similar cases of patients from Luxembourg were brought before the ECJ: Mr *Kohll* had sought orthodontic treatment in Germany, and Mr *Decker* had bought spectacles in Belgium without gaining prior permission.[63] The patients held the opinion that the prior authorisation process hinders free movement of goods and services and hence contravenes Articles 28 and 49 EC. Several nation states, including the UK, however, brought forward the argument that healthcare services provided by a public healthcare system were not economic goods and services and thus did not fall under Articles 28 and 49 EC (Mossialos and Palm 2003, p. 9). The ECJ followed the patients' view and held that the right to free movement also applies to medical goods and services for which reimbursement is granted by a public healthcare system. Only in the event of 'overriding reasons in the general interest', such as the securing of the financial balance of the social security system for example, might a restriction of these freedoms be justified. But this was not present in the given cases.

The Kohll and Decker judgements raised more questions concerning patient mobility than they answered, and thus it was not long until the ECJ had to decide the next case. In the *Geraets-Smits and Peerboom* ruling,[64] the ECJ clarified that not only services which are reimbursed by a public healthcare system, but also services provided as benefits in kind by a social-insurance system, are services within the meaning of Article 50 EC, and hence are subject to Article 49. The ECJ furthermore made clear that Article 49 applies to hospital care, too. But this time the court held that a prior approval process is justified because 'overriding reasons in the general interest' were given. The judges argued that if patients were free to choose their hospital, this would undermine hospital planning, which is necessary, otherwise the ability of the system 'to guarantee a rationalised, stable, balanced and accessible supply of hospital services would be jeopardised at a stroke' (para. 81). Outpatient services are another matter. In the *Müller-Fauré and Van Riet* case,[65] the ECJ held the opinion that the abolition of prior authorisation for outpatient services does not give rise to patients travelling to other countries in such large numbers, despite linguistic barriers, geographic distance, the cost of staying abroad and lack of information about the kind of care provided there, that the financial balance of the social security system concerned would be seriously upset and that, as a result, the overall level of public health protection would be jeopardised (para. 95).

The judges of the Geraets-Smits and Peerboom cases accepted prior approval for inpatient care, but laid down criteria that prohibit rejection. With regard to the criteria of 'normal treatment' and medical necessity, which the Netherlands health funds usually applied in deciding on treatment abroad, the court deemed:

> that authorisation cannot be refused on that ground where it appears that the treatment concerned is sufficiently tried and tested by international medical science, and authorisation can be refused on the ground of lack of medical

necessity only if the same or equally effective treatment can be obtained without undue delay at an establishment having a contractual arrangement with the insured person's sickness insurance fund.

(para. 108)

In reaction to the Geraets-Smits and Peerboom rulings, England adapted its national regulations to allow for treatment abroad for English (and Welsh) patients (SI 2002/2759). This did not, however, prevent an English case from ending up at the ECJ in 2004. Mrs *Watts*, an elderly woman who suffered from osteoarthritis in her hips and therefore needed a hip replacement, had been put on the waiting list for hip surgery. As her case was not classified as urgent, she was expected to wait approximately 12 months for the operation. Mrs Watts applied for treatment abroad under the E112 scheme, but her PCT refused permission because her case was not specifically supported by the consultant orthopaedic surgeon and because it was a routine operation for which the expected waiting time did not amount to an 'undue delay' (McHale 2007). Although her case was reassessed after judicial review and her medical need was reclassified as 'soon', thus shortening her expected waiting time to three or four months, she went to France for immediate treatment. Back home, she requested reimbursement for the cost of the operation from her PCT, but her claim was rejected. Again, she took legal action with the argument that her claim was supported by Article 49 EC (free movement of services). Furthermore, she referred to Article 22 of the Council Regulation No. 1408/71 (now Article 20 883/04/EC, see above) and to the European Convention on Human Rights, Articles 3 and 8. In the first instance, Mrs Watts lost the case.[66] Though the high court held that Mrs Watts's case was subject to Article 49 EC, it stated that a waiting time of three months cannot be seen as 'undue delay'. Both Mrs Watts and the SoS appealed this judgement.[67] The SoS did so because he challenged the court's view that the English NHS falls within the scope of Article 49 EC. Due to its wide-ranging policy implications, and because the applicability of former ECJ rulings to the English NHS were not clear, the court of appeal decided to stay the proceedings and to refer open questions in the Watts case to the ECJ. The ECJ held that NHS hospital services do fall under the freedom to provide services as laid down in Article 49 EC. National authorities, however, are allowed to make reimbursement of hospital treatment subject to prior approval. It also made clear that an application for hospital treatment abroad, no matter if made under Article 49 EC or under Article 22 of the Council Regulation No 1408/71, cannot be rejected merely on the grounds that there is a waiting time in the home country. Instead, the health authority

is required to establish that that time does not exceed the period which is acceptable on the basis of an objective medical assessment of the clinical needs of the person concerned in the light of all of the factors characterising his medical condition at the time when the request for authorisation is made or renewed, as the case may be.

(para. 79)

With this judgement, the ECJ constituted an entitlement to hospital treatment in an EU Member State at the cost of the public healthcare system of the home country in cases where the waiting time is not medically acceptable. In other words, the ECJ created a right to hospital treatment within a medically acceptable time in the UK. This right must be granted by the NHS, either at home or abroad.

As a reaction to the Watts case, the DH issued an advice to healthcare commissioners on how to organise and grant authorisation for treatment abroad (Department of Health 2007). It took a further three years before the judgement was fully implemented into English law. The National Health Service (Reimbursement of the Cost of EEA Treatment) Regulations 2010 (SI 2010/915) amended the NHS Act 2006 accordingly and specified conditions for treatment abroad. According to the new regulation, treatment abroad is reimbursed if the service was necessary 'to treat or diagnose a medical condition of the patient', and if the service was the same as or equivalent to a service that is provided by the English NHS (s. 6A (3) and s. 6B (5) NHS Act 2006). For normal services (i.e. outpatient services), no further requirements apply. In the case of special services, such as hospital treatment or specialised treatment that involves anaesthesia or the use of specialised or cost-intensive medical infrastructure or equipment, prior approval is necessary. In addition to the conditions described above, approval is granted only if the Secretary of State or a responsible authority cannot provide the service 'within a period of time that is acceptable on the basis of medical evidence as to the patient's clinical needs, taking into account the patient's state of health' (s. 6B (5) (c) NHS Act 2006). While the SoS must authorise medical treatment and diagnosis if all these conditions are fulfilled, s/he might allow treatment or diagnosis abroad for services that are not generally available in the NHS (s. 6B (4) (b) NHS Act 2006). In general, the reimbursement for services abroad can be limited to the costs that would have been incurred for the same service in the NHS. Furthermore, if patients would have had to pay charges for the service in England, this amount can be deducted from the reimbursed sum.

In 2011, the European Parliament and the Council passed a legal regulation codifying ECJ case law on patient mobility. The Patients' Rights Directive (2011/24/EU)[68] in principle sums up all prior ECJ rulings on that issue. In some aspects, however, it goes beyond the content of ECJ rulings. Of relevance here are further grounds for a justified denial of treatment abroad that requires prior approval. According to the ECJ rulings, authorisation may be refused only if the treatment the patient seeks is available in the home country without 'undue delay' (see above). In addition to this reason, an approval may now be rejected if there is a possible health risk for the patient, if public health is endangered, or if there are 'serious and specific concerns relating to the respect of standards and guidelines on quality of care and patient safety' (Art 8 (6) (a) – (d) 2011/24/EU). Furthermore, the Directive establishes new rights that do not result from case law on free movement, but define the responsibilities of the Member State providing treatment (Sauter 2011, pp. 8f.). In particular, Member States must ensure that patients have access to information on quality and treatment standards, that patients receive all relevant information necessary 'to make an informed choice', that transparent complaint procedures and systems of professional liability insurance or similar arrangements are in place, that privacy of data is protected and that access to medical records is given (Art. 4 (2) (a) – (f) 2011/24/EU). The Directive was incorporated into national law in 2013 by SI 2013/2269.

The UK long refused to acknowledge ECJ jurisprudence, arguing that the rulings did not apply to the NHS because of its differing structure and provisions (Davis 2007, p. 158; McHale 2007, p. 102). In fact, there are several aspects of the ECJ rulings and the Patients' Rights Directive that clash with fundamental principles of the NHS and that might, in the long run, transform the social right to healthcare in England. First, EU law provides patients with an exit option. The ECJ judgements and the Directive constitute a new legal right to access hospital and other special treatment within a medically acceptable time, which theretofore had not been part of NHS entitlement (Veitch 2012, p. 390). There was no explicit right to hospital treatment, but only an obligation of the SoS and health bodies to provide such services. If they failed to do so, the only option patients had was to file for judicial review. Now, patients can go abroad if they cannot get services at home, hence effectively sanction malfunctioning of the NHS. It remains to be seen to what extent patients will in fact use this opportunity, and to what extent the mere existence of an exit option for patients will put pressure on NHS providers and commissioners.

Second, EU law demands an increased specification of healthcare entitlement. Member States indeed remain free to determine service coverage (Art 7 (3) 2011/24/EU), and treatment abroad must only be reimbursed to the extent that it is provided at home. But in order to determine if patients are entitled to a particular treatment abroad, it must be known if they are entitled to this treatment at home. This poses a problem for the NHS, which so far had not, or only rarely, defined healthcare entitlement explicitly. NHS healthcare entitlement usually is concretised on a day-to-day basis and subject to available resources. EU law now leads to an increased necessity for the specification of provided services as Elisabetta Zanon, Director at the NHS European Office, has noted: 'a key issue will be for commissioners to have a clear "list" of the types of healthcare they do and do not provide. This will be crucial for minimising uncertainty for commissioners and patients, and for reducing the possibility of legal challenge from patients who want to access treatments that are not routinely available on the NHS' (Zanon 2011, p. 35).

Third, the EU law follows a clear individual approach to social rights, and thereby triggers further individualisation of the social right to healthcare in the NHS. This is perhaps the most important aspect of the EU patients' rights law, since it carries several profound implications for the NHS. As described above (see Chapter 2.2), NHS law rarely establishes rights of patients, but only obligations of NHS bodies to provide services. The EU law, however, 'speaks with the voice of the patients – it is their rights it clarifies' (Zanon 2011, p. 34). It is not the formulation of healthcare entitlement as individual rights, per se, that clashes with NHS entitlement, but the fact that the rights granted by EU law amount to absolute rights. This becomes most apparent with regard to waiting lists. Waiting lists used to be a common instrument for priority setting in the NHS, and restrictions on waiting times were, if at all, set by national regulations defining general maximum waiting times for particular treatments (e.g. the Patient's Charter, the NHS Constitution). In contrast, the definition of 'undue delay' applied by the ECJ and the Directive, refers to the situation of the individual patient in order to determine if a waiting time is too long and thus, if entitlement to treatment abroad must be granted. With it, access to NHS treatment is no longer determined according to financial resources and societal preferences, but according to the medical need of the individual patient (Newdick 2006, p. 1657). As a result, waiting lists can no longer be used to regulate access and set priorities (Davis 2007, pp. 160f.; Veitch 2012, p. 378). The UK government was well aware of this problem and therefore strongly argued against such a construction of 'undue delay' in the Watts case, but without success.

2.8 Discussion

First of all, some notes about the limitation of this analysis are necessary. English healthcare entitlement is rarely specified by law but is defined in day-to-day activities, where it is subject to actual need and available resources. Hence, generosity results from resources available rather than from legislative rights. For this reason, this analysis of legal entitlement reforms did not mirror the full extent of changes in generosity. Nevertheless, it disclosed several important modifications in the regulation of entitlement and, furthermore, revealed a fundamental transformation of the social right to healthcare.

The heydays of healthcare entitlement retrenchment were in the 1980s and the first half of the 1990s. During that period, the Conservatives sharply increased co-payments and excluded several services (e.g. optical appliances, particular drugs). Exclusions of services, however, were few and remained limited to non-core service areas, and eligibility for exemption from charges was widened. Labour, as well as the new government coalition, adhered to co-payments but increased them only with or slightly above inflation. They also refrained from broad service exclusions and instead relied on health technology appraisals by NICE in order to regulate entitlement.

The most important changes of the last 35 years, however, modify the basic principles of the English social right to healthcare. Rudolf Klein, an acknowledged UK health policy expert, noted in 1996: 'Essentially, then, one of the defining characteristics of the NHS – in contrast to many other healthcare systems – remains its repudiation of any notion of entitlement' (p. 39). Today, almost 20 years later, this assessment requires revision. Beginning in the early 1990s, the social right to healthcare underwent a fundamental transformation. Several processes at different levels have led to an individualisation of the former collective social right, bringing about individual entitlement and absolute rights to treatment.

The first tentative step towards individualisation was taken in 1991 with the publication of the Patient's Charter. For the first time in NHS history, this document explicitly spelt out the rights of patients, albeit to a very limited extent. The rights listed included, for example, the right to receive healthcare on the basis of clinical need, the right to be registered with a GP and the right to access hospital treatment within two years. The latter was revolutionary as it set limits on waiting times for the first time. What the Patient's Charter did not do, however, was grant rights to particular treatments. Moreover, the Patient's Charter itself was not a legal document but merely put legal obligations of health bodies into rights language. Nonetheless, it marks the start of the individualisation process because it was the first document that spoke about rights of individuals with respect to the NHS.

It took another 10 years before entitlement to particular treatments was established. In order to develop a common standard of healthcare provision within the NHS, the government founded NICE and tasked it with making recommendations on the provision of medical technologies (e.g. drugs, medical devices). Since 2002, treatments positively recommended by NICE technology appraisals must be provided by the NHS for all patients. As a consequent next step, the entitlement resulting from the obligation to fund treatments positively recommended by NICE was explicitly framed as a right of patients to receive these treatments through the NHS Constitution of 2009. NICE technology appraisals contribute to the individualisation of the social right to healthcare with regard to two aspects: first, they specify entitlement to concrete treatments, thus rendering healthcare entitlement explicit and transparent; second, and even more importantly, they constitute an absolute entitlement to these treatments as funding of recommended technologies is obligatory.

During the first decade of the new millennium, individualisation of healthcare rights also was advanced by processes emanating from the EU level. In its judgements on patient mobility, the ECJ established an almost unlimited right to treatment abroad for individual patients. There are only two restrictions: first, the services received abroad need not be reimbursed by the NHS if they exceed service provision at home (i.e. treatments that are not provided by the NHS need not be financed by the NHS if they are consumed by an English resident abroad); second, hospital and special treatment is subject to prior approval. Approval must be granted, however, if the service cannot be provided by the NHS within a timeframe that is medically acceptable. EU law thus constitutes an individual and absolute right to treatment for English patients.

Not only courts on the European level, but courts in the UK as well, had a share in promoting individualisation. Over time, judges were ever more willing to intervene in allocative decisions of PCTs and accepted individual claims that challenged decision-making. So far, however, courts have merely overturned funding decisions and referred the decision back to the relevant health authority for reconsideration. The increased willingness of courts to challenge allocative decisions accompanies a greater willingness of patients to take legal action if they are denied funding. Since the early 1990s, patients have been offered an individual rights perspective by the NHS (e.g. by the Patient's Charter), which it seems they have accepted and now call in.

To conclude, the English social right to healthcare underwent major transformations over the last 35 years. As expected, some retrenchment occurred, but explicit entitlement cuts remained within limits. Of more relevance, however, were the qualitative changes that fundamentally altered the basic characteristics of the English collective social right to healthcare and led to an individualisation of rights. This individualisation process is analysed in more detail in Chapter 4, while the driving forces and effects of this transformation are further discussed in Chapter 5.

Notes

1 For the period from 1968 to 1988, the Ministry of Health and the Ministry of Social Services were merged into the Department of Health and Social Services with one Secretary of State being responsible for all social services (Boyle 2011, p. 26). For convenience, this book exclusively uses the terms 'Secretary of State for Health' and 'Department of Health'.

2 Further matters regulated by the NHS Act are the property and finance of NHS bodies, the cooperation with local authorities and, in its amended version of 2006, public involvement and the protection from fraud and other unlawful activities. These aspects of the Act are not relevant to this study.

3 Statutory instruments are secondary legislation compiled by the DH and are approved or rejected by Parliament without debate (Montgomery 2002, pp. 9f.).

4 As of 2012, without amendments made by 2012 c. 7 sch. 4 s. 1 (1).

5 Decision-making within PCTs and CCGs respectively is not a subject of this study. For information regarding these processes, see Robinson et al. (2011).

6 At the time of founding, NICE was named 'National Institute for Clinical Excellence'. Its name was changed to 'National Institute for Health and Clinical Excellence' in 2005, and mirroring its new tasks, it was again renamed in 2013 and is now called 'National Institute for Health and Care Excellence'. Its abbreviation NICE has always remained the same.

7 Further details about the tasks of NICE and its technology appraisal process are provided in Chapter 2.4.

8 *R v Barnet LBC ex p. Shah (Nilish)* [1983] 2AC 309 HL.

9 Section 3 has remained nearly unchanged since 1977. Paragraph (b) formerly listed ophthalmic services and within paragraph (d) and (e) the words 'services or' and in paragraph (f) the words 'facilities or' were inserted. Since the introduction of the Health and Social Care Act 2012, it is the clinical commissioning groups instead of the SoS who are responsible for the provision of services. Section 13 (2) (a) of the Health and Social Care Act 2012 changes the section accordingly, but leaves the list of services unchanged.

10 *R v Secretary of State for Social Services, W. Midlands RHA and Birmingham AHA (Teaching), ex p. Hincks* (1980) 1 BMLR 93.

11 Charging is regulated by Part IX of the NHS Act 2006. The respective sections in the NHS Act 1977 were s. 77 and schedule 12 s. 1 for drugs, appliances and pharmaceutical services, s. 78 and schedule 12 s. 2 for dental and optical appliances, and s. 79 for dental treatment.

12 Under the provisions of regulation 6 (1) (i) of the National Health Service (Charges for Drugs and Appliances) Regulations 1974 (as amended).

13 Conservatives received 42.4 per cent of votes in 1983, compared to 43.9 per cent in 1979. They gained 397 seats (339 in 1979), while Labour received 209 (269 in 1979) mandates (Butler and Kavanagh 1997).

14 The remaining three rights concerned the information of patients (right to an explanation of treatment, right to access to health records) and inscribed the individual freedom right to decisions about treatment (right to choose whether to participate in medical research and medical student training).

15 The therapeutic groups were: antacids, laxatives, analgesics used for mild to moderate pain, cough and cold remedies, bitters and tonics, vitamins, benzodiazepine tranquillisers and sedatives.

16 The pharmaceuticals that became excluded were anti-diarrhoea, drugs for allergic disorders, hypnotics and anxiolytics, appetite suppressants, drugs for vaginal and vulval conditions, contraceptives, drugs used in anaemia, topical anti-rheumatics, drugs acting on the ear and nose, and those acting on the skin. Coincident with the expansion of excluded drugs, the process of switching a drug's status from 'prescription only medicine' to 'freely available at pharmacies' was eased with the aim of enabling patients to buy those items out of pocket at the pharmacies (Hockley 2012, p. 148).

17 s. 39 (2A) NHS Act 1977 as amended by Health and Social Security Act 1984 and SI 1986/976.

18 s. 38 (1) NHS Act 1977 as amended by Health and Medicines Act 1988, further specified by SI 1989/395.

19 Charges for drugs and medical appliances had been regulated by SI 1974/285 until the regulations were replaced by SI 1980/1503 in 1980, which for their part were substituted by SI 1989/419 in 1989.

20 Charges for dental and optical care had been regulated by SI 1978/950 until 1988, when the regulation of dental charges was separated from the regulation of charges for optical appliances (SI 1988/473). Major restructuring of charges made it necessary to widely renew regulations again one year later (SI 1989/394).

21 After the division of regulations for dental and optical charges in 1988, charges for optical appliances were regulated by SI 1989/396 until 1997, when regulations were replaced by SI 1997/818.

22 All general election results in this section are drawn from Thorpe (2008, appendix 1).

23 The healthcare Commission was replaced in 2009 by the Care Quality Commission that had also taken on the tasks of the Commission for Social Care Inspection and the Mental Health Act Commission and is now, besides Monitor, the most important regulatory body.

24 For a detailed description of ECJ rulings and adaptations of English healthcare law, see Chapter 2.6.

25 The four contracts were, in detail: a new GMS/GDS contract between practices and trusts, an alternative provider of medical/dental services contract, a locally negotiated personal medical services or personal dental services contract and fourth, a PCT medical services contract or PCT dental services contract that allowed PCTs to employ GPs and general dental practitioners directly (Pollock et al. 2007, p. 475).

26 *R (on the application of Eisai Ltd.) v NICE* [2007] EWHC 1941 (Admin), 9.

27 QALY is 'a generic measure of health-related quality of life that takes into account both the quantity and the quality of life generated by interventions' (NICE 2005, p. 37).

28 ' "Restricted availability appliance" means an appliance which is approved for particular categories of persons or particular purposes only' (SI 2002/551).

29 Supervised community treatment was a new programme for the care and treatment of certain patients in the community. Patients taking part in that programme had been detained for treatment for a mental disorder, and were required to comply with certain conditions while in the community, amongst which one condition may be the taking of medication.

30 All reforms and amendments made before 31 December 2013 were analysed.

31 Whether there was a breach of promise depends on how you read the figures. Including the part of the budget that was transferred to communities and local governments, NHS spending increased by approximately 0.4 per cent (Appleby 2013).

32 Monitor is a non-departmental public body, which was already established under Labour (see Chapter 2.4).

33 The NHS Act 2006 secures the autonomy of the health authorities and providers (s. 1D NHS Act 2006).

34 See Chapter 5.2 for further information on that issue.

35 See chapters 2.2 to 2.5 for a detailed description of the rights and responsibilities of NHS authorities and providers.

36 *Associated Provincial Picture Houses v Wednesbury Corporation* [1947] 2 ALL ER 680, [1948] 1 KB 223.

37 *Council of Civil Service Unions v Minister for the Civil Service* [1985] 1 AC 374, 410.
38 *R v Secretary of State for Social Services, W. Midlands RHA and Birmingham AHA (Teaching), ex p.* Hincks and others (1980) 1 BMLR 93.
39 Ibid. 93.
40 *R v Central Birmingham HA, ex p. Walker; R v Secretary of State for Social Services and another, ex p.* Walker (1987) 3 BMLR 32.
41 *R v Central Birmingham HA, ex parte* Collier (1988), unreported.
42 *R v Cambridge HA, ex p. B.* (1995) 25 BMLR 5.
43 *R v Cambridge HA, ex p. B.* [1995] 2 FCR 485 CA.
44 *R v North Derbyshire HA, ex p.* Fisher (1997) 38 BMLR 76.
45 *R v NW Lancashire HA, ex p. A, D and G* (1999) 53 BMLR 148 CA.
46 *R (on the application of Rogers) v Swindon NHS PCT* [2006] EWHC 71 (Admin).
47 *R (on the application of Rogers) v Swindon NHS PCT and another* [2006] EWCA Civ 392, (2006) 89 BMLR 211, 236.
48 Ibid. 237.
49 *R (on the application of Otley) v Barking and Dagenham PCT* [2007] EWHC 1927 (Admin), 98 BMLR 182.
50 Ibid. 191.
51 Ibid. 191.
52 *R v Secretary of State for Health, ex p. Pfizer Ltd.* (1999) 51 BMLR 189, 199.
53 As cited in *R (on the application of Pfizer Ltd.) v Secretary of State for Health* [2002] EWCA Civ 1566, 70 BMLR 219, 222.
54 Ibid. 226.
55 *R (on the application of Eisai Ltd.) v NICE* [2007] EWHC 1941 (Admin).
56 *R (on the application of Eisai Ltd.) v NICE* [2008] EWCA Civ 438.
57 *R (on the application of Eisai Ltd.) v NICE* [2007] EWHC 1941 (Admin), para. 96.
58 *R (on the application of Servier Labratorie Ltd.) v NICE* [2009] EWHC 281 (Admin).
59 *R (on the application of Bristol-Myers Squibb Pharmaceuticals Ltd.) v NICE* [2009] EWHC 2722 (Admin).
60 Ibid. 41.
61 Only in *R v North Derbyshire HA, ex p. Fisher* and *R v Secretary of State for Health, ex p. Pfizer Ltd.* judges also declared the decision to be illegal.
62 Cases heard by the European Court of Human Rights are not addressed because these had no impact on healthcare allocation decisions (Ford 2012, p. 321).
63 Case C-120/95 *Decker v Caisse de Maladie des Employés Privés* [1998] ECR I-1831; Case C-158/96 *Kohll v. Union des Caisses de Maladie* [1998] ECR I-1931.
64 Case C-157/99 *Geraets-Smits v Stichting Zieckenfonds; Peerbooms v Stichting CZ Groep Zorgverzekeringen* [2001] ECR I-5473.
65 Case C-385/99 *Müller-Fauré v Onderlinge Waarborgmaatschappij OZ Zorgverzekeringen UA and E.E.M. van Riet v Onderlinge Waarborgmaatschappij ZAO Zorgverzekeringen* [2003] ECR I-4509.
66 *R v Bedford PCT, v the Secretary of State for Health, ex p. Watts* [2003] EWHC 2228 (Admin).
67 *R (on the Application of Watts) v Secretary of State for Health* [2004] EWCA Civ 166.
68 The full name of the Directive is 'Directive of the European Parliament and of the Council on the application of patients' rights in cross-border healthcare'.

3   Healthcare entitlement in Germany

This chapter presents the social right to healthcare in Germany and explores healthcare entitlement reforms conducted between 1977 and 2013. Analogous to the English case study in Chapter 2, a brief introduction to the German healthcare system is given before the characteristics of the German social right to healthcare are described in more detail. In a next step, healthcare entitlement reforms are analysed for each government period, preceded by information about the economic and political background and general health policy. The joint self-administration plays a particular role in the definition of healthcare entitlement in Germany. This role is explained and discussed in a separate section. Finally, a brief conclusion on the main findings is drawn in the last section. The forces driving these reforms are not a subject of this chapter. These are analysed for both case studies in Chapter 5.

3.1   The German healthcare system in brief

In 1883, Germany was the first country to introduce social health insurance. In reaction to the rising socialist movement that threatened the existing social order, the government strived to improve the living conditions of workers by setting up a system of social insurances covering the main work and life risks (Rosenberg 1969). Social insurance membership was compulsory but restricted to particular groups of workers. The new health insurance was built upon already existing institutions such as mutual societies and contributory funds of companies and municipalities. These remained independent, but became subject to national regulation. Funding was stipulated to be shared between workers and employers at a ratio of two to one, and the amount of contributions was determined by the funds. Funds had to offer a minimum benefit catalogue defined by law, but could provide more generous benefits (Busse and Riesberg 2004, p. 14). Over the course of its now 130 years of existence, the German statutory health insurance (SHI) massively expanded population coverage as well as benefits. Starting from initially 10 per cent of the population, SHI today covers about 86 per cent. In the beginning, the main goal of SHI was to secure income maintenance during illness. With the years, however, the focus of SHI switched from cash benefits to the provision of medical care (Busse and Riesberg 2004, p. 16; Rosenbrock and Gerlinger 2014, pp. 42f.).

The 14 per cent of the population not covered by SHI are either insured with special public schemes or private health insurance, or both. Civil servants, for example, receive between 50 and 80 per cent of healthcare costs paid by their public employer (*Beihilfe*) and most of them insure the remaining costs privately. Persons not obligated to insure with SHI and not covered by other public schemes (e.g. self-employed) were free to insure privately or to pay health costs out of pocket until 2009, when a general obligation to insure was implemented. Since then, all persons not obligated to insure with SHI have to take out private insurance. Private health insurance funds now are committed to provide a basic insurance tariff with a legally determined benefits package and premiums, and to accept anybody who cannot insure with SHI. Because SHI covers the majority of the population, this study exclusively deals with SHI.

The German social healthcare system is characterised by its corporatist governance (Moran 2000). One of the core elements of this system is the self-administration of funds, i.e. health funds are governed jointly by elected representatives of the insured and employers.[1] The self-administration wields wide-ranging powers: they decide about benefits exceeding the legally defined minimum, about organisational matters, and in the past, they also determined the contribution rate (Rosenbrock and Gerlinger 2014, p. 134). A second core element is the 'joint self-administration' of SHI funds and providers. In brief, payers and providers jointly organise and regulate the public healthcare system. The most important body of the joint self-administration at the national level is the Federal Joint Committee (FJC, *Gemeinsamer Bundesausschuss*),[2] in which the national associations of providers (the National Association of SHI Physicians, the National Association of SHI Dentists and the German Hospital Federation) together with the National Association of SHI Funds decide about SHI benefits and organisational matters of the public healthcare system. Similar self-administration structures do exist at the federal states level (*Länder*). In general, the state's role (at the national, as well as at the federal states level) is restricted to setting the regulatory framework and supervising self-administration bodies (Rosenbrock and Gerlinger 2014, pp. 16ff.). In the course of the expansion of competition and market governance, however, the joint self-administration, and in particular the health funds, lost some of their autonomy while the regulatory power of the state increased (Gerlinger 2009; Moran 2000; Noweski 2004).

German SHI is predominantly financed from contributions paid on gross earned income. Further sources are a tax grant (since 2003) and co-payments made by patients out of pocket. For many years, contributions had been equally shared between employer and employee.[3] Since 2005, however, employees have been forced to contribute an ever growing share. First, employees' contributions were increased to be 0.9 percentage points higher than the employers' contributions in 2005. Then, a so called 'additional premium' (*Zusatzbeitrag*) was introduced in 2009.[4] This additional premium varies between funds and is to be paid by the employees alone. With the same reform, a general contribution rate applying to all funds equally was implemented. Furthermore, all contributions and the tax grant were pooled together within one financial fund (*Gesundheitsfonds*) and are

Table 3.1 German healthcare spending 1977–2013

Year	1977	1985	1990	1995	2000	2005	2013
Total health spending (% of GDP)	8.3	8.8	8.3	10.1	10.4	10.8	11.3
Public spending (% of total health spending)	78.7	77.4	76.2	81.4	79.5	76.6	77.1
Out-of-pocket payments (% of total health spending)	10.2	11.2	11.1	10.0	11.4	13.5	12.9

Source: OECD (2014c).

distributed amongst SHI funds according to age, gender and health status of the insured. If SHI funds do not make ends meet with this money, they have to levy the additional premium.[5] The fixed general contribution rate together with the additional premium will lead to future health expenditure increases being borne entirely by the employee. As Table 3.1 shows, health spending increased in Germany as it did in every advanced welfare state over time. While Germans spent 8.3 per cent of GDP in 1977 for health, this amount increased to 11.3 per cent in 2013. Out-of-pocket spending rose from 10.2 per cent to 12.9 per cent of total spending.

Healthcare provision in Germany is pluralistic with a clear dominance of private providers (Böhm et al. 2012, p. 44). Ambulatory care is almost exclusively provided by private physicians. In contrast to England, ambulatory specialist treatment is usually carried out by private doctors in their practices and not in hospitals. Hospitals in Germany can be found in public, private non-profit and for-profit ownership, the latter with an increasing market share: while in 1991 15.25 per cent of hospitals were owned by private for-profit providers, this share had more than doubled to 32.7 per cent in 2010 (Bölt and Graf 2012). Access to medical treatment is nearly unrestricted. Patients are free to choose their general and specialist doctors, and only for hospital treatment (with the exemption of emergency treatment) is a referral needed. Traditionally, there is a strong separation of ambulatory and hospital care which recent reforms have attempted to mitigate, but with limited success. Around 98 per cent of ambulatory medical doctors are SHI-accredited (*Vertragsärzte*), and thereby compulsory members of the Association of SHI Physicians, which has a legal monopoly on SHI treatment (Rosenbrock and Gerlinger 2014). Similarly, only SHI-accredited hospitals (*Vertragskrankenhäuser*) are allowed to provide treatment for SHI members. The Associations of SHI Physicians are legally obliged to secure ambulatory provision, and the federal states are responsible for sufficient hospital provision. For this purpose, the federal states compile regional hospital plans and partly cover investment costs of the hospitals listed in the plan.

3.2   The German social right to healthcare

In Germany, there exist different social rights to healthcare for various population groups. In the following analysis, I concentrate on the social right to healthcare as granted by the German SHI which covers the majority of the population.

Healthcare rights of other population groups are broached only in the case of very important reforms. This chapter provides a general overview of SHI healthcare entitlement and presents the particulars of entitlement as of 1977. The presentation is structured along the analytical categories developed in Chapter 1, and an overview of relevant healthcare entitlement regulation for the whole period of investigation is given.

German healthcare entitlement regulations

The right to healthcare is constituted by public social law and specified by directives of the joint self-administration. The regulation map below (Table 3.2) gives an overview of relevant public laws and ministerial orders regulating SHI healthcare entitlement in Germany at four points in time. The main law concerning social security in general, and statutory health insurance in particular, had been the Imperial Insurance Code (*Reichsversicherungsordnung*, RVO) until its regulations were transferred stepwise into single social code books. In 1975, Book I was the first to be established and comprises general principles concerning all social insurances. Book V (*Fünftes Sozialgesetzbuch*, SGB V) was introduced in 1988 and contains all relevant regulations with regard to SHI. Besides the SGB V, further separate regulations for particular population groups (e.g. artists, farmers) exist. Health insurance of the unemployed had been regulated by the Employment Promotion Law (*Arbeitsförderungsgesetz*, AFG) until it became included into the SGB V in 1997.

Ministerial orders play only a minor role in the regulation of healthcare entitlement in Germany because specification of entitlement is in most cases delegated to the joint self-administration. The joint self-administration defines particulars of service provision and entitlements within directives issued and amended by the Federal Joint Committee (formerly the Federal Committee of Physicians and Sickness Funds, *Bundesausschuss der Ärzte und Krankenkassen*, BAÄK). The directives are part of the general contracts between the Federal Association of SHI Physicians and the health funds, and are thus binding for all providers and funds. The directives are too numerous and detailed for an in-depth analysis, but a short overview of them is given in Chapter 3.8. The various reimbursement regulations are also not considered because the primary purpose of these documents is to determine reimbursement and not to define entitlement, albeit services not reimbursed are not likely to be provided.

Healthcare rights are legally enforceable in Germany. Hence, a near infinite number of court decisions on healthcare entitlement exist. Yet, other than in England, these decisions are not binding for future cases since Germany has no case law. For this reason, decisions of the social courts are not studied. The only cases considered are those decided by the Federal Constitutional Court (FCC, *Bundesverfassungsgericht*) because these are binding for all constitutional bodies, the federal states, the courts and public administration.

Table 3.2 Regulation map Germany – healthcare entitlement regulations 1977, 1990, 2000 and 2013

1977	1990	2000	2013
	General Public Laws		
X Imperial Insurance Code *Reichsversicherungsordnung (RVO)*	X Imperial Insurance Code *Reichsversicherungsordnung (RVO)*	X Imperial Insurance Code *Reichsversicherungsordnung (RVO)*	
X Social Code Book I – General Principles *Sozialgesetzbuch I (SGB I)*	X Social Code Book I – General Principles *Sozialgesetzbuch I (SGB I)*	X Social Code Book I – General Principles *Sozialgesetzbuch I (SGB I)*	X Social Code Book I – General Principles *Sozialgesetzbuch I (SGB I)*
	X Social Code Book V *Sozialgesetzbuch V (SGB V)*	X Social Code Book V *Sozialgesetzbuch V (SGB V)*	X Social Code Book V *Sozialgesetzbuch V (SGB V)*
Law on Health Insurance for Farmers *Gesetz über die Krankenversicherung der Landwirte*	2. Law on Health Insurance for Farmers *2. Gesetz über die Krankenversicherung der Landwirte*	2. Law on Health Insurance for Farmers *2. Gesetz über die Krankenversicherung der Landwirte*	2. Law on Health Insurance for Farmers *2. Gesetz über die Krankenversicherung der Landwirte*
Law on Social Insurance for Mineworkers *Reichsknappschaftsgesetz*	Law on Social Insurance for Mineworkers *Reichsknappschaftsgesetz*		
Law on Social Insurance of the Disabled *Gesetz über die Sozialvers. Behinderter*			
	Law on Social Insurance for Artists *Künstlersozialversicherungsgesetz*	Law on Social Insurance for Artists *Künstlersozialversicherungsgesetz*	Law on Social Insurance for Artists *Künstlersozialversicherungsgesetz*
Employment Promotion Law *Arbeitsförderungsgesetz (AFG)*	Employment Promotion Law *Arbeitsförderungsgesetz (AFG)*		

Ministerial Orders

1974 National Order on Hospital Rates *Bundespflegesatzverordnung* (BPflV)	1986 National Order on Hospital Rates *Bundespflege-satzverordnung* (BPflV)	1994 National Order on Hospital Rates *Bundespflege-satzverordnung* (BPflV)	1994 National Order on Hospital Rates *Bundespflege-satzverordnung* (BPflV)
	X 1989 Order on Medical Aids with Little Therapeutic Benefits or Low Price *Verordnung über Hilfsmittel von geringem therapeutischen Nutzen oder geringem Abgabepreis in der GKV*	X 1989 Order on Medical Aids with Little Therapeutic Benefits or Low Price *Verordnung über Hilfsmittel von geringem therapeutischen Nutzen oder geringem Abgabepreis in der GKV*	X 1989 Order on Medical Aids with Little Therapeutic Benefits or Low Price *Verordnung über Hilfsmittel von geringem therapeutischen Nutzen oder geringem Abgabepreis in der GKV*
	X 1990 Order on Inefficient Drugs in SHI *Verordnung über unwirtschaftliche Arzneimittel in der GKV*	X 1990 Order on Inefficient Drugs in SHI *Verordnung über unwirtschaftliche Arzneimittel in der GKV*	
		1993 Order on Co-Payments for Pharmaceuticals and Bandages in SHI *Verordnung über die Zuzahlung bei der Abgabe von Arznei- und Verbandmitteln in der vertragsärztlichen Versorgung*	

X: analysed

Governance – who decides about healthcare entitlement?

Healthcare legislation is part of the concurrent legislation, meaning that the national and the federal states level (*Länder*) share responsibilities. Concerning healthcare entitlement, however, the parliament (*Bundestag*) and the federal government (*Bundesregierung*) are competent to decide without approval of the federal council (*Bundesrat*), the representation of the Länder. In principle, the *Bundestag* is free to specify healthcare entitlement, but it usually defines healthcare entitlement only generally and leaves its specification to the joint self-administration.

The responsible committee of the joint self-administration is composed of representatives of providers' and health funds' associations. The actual composition, the particulars of the decision-making process and the tasks of the committee have been reformed several times over the last decades (see Chapters 3.3 to 3.8). In 1977, the BAÄK was merely responsible for entitlement definition of ambulatory services. Its sister committee, the Federal Committee of Dentists and Sickness Funds (*Bundesausschuss der Zahnärzte und Krankenkassen*, BAZÄK) was responsible for entitlement definition in dental care. Entitlement to hospital care was not further specified by the joint self-administration until the year 2000. The RVO authorised the BAÄK to issue any directive it deemed necessary for the 'sufficient, appropriate and efficient' provision of ambulatory services (§ 368p (1) RVO). In particular, the BAÄK was tasked with deciding about new diagnosis and treatment methods, services in kind prescribed by a doctor, the prescription of drugs and remedies, hospital referrals, occupational stress tests and therapy, and about the assessment of work incapacity (§ 368p RVO). By 1977, the BAÄK had not passed directives on every theme. At that time, the directives were not legally binding (Döhler and Manow-Borgwardt 1992a, p. 582). Providers and SHI funds were merely requested by law to 'pay regard to the directives' (§ 368p (3) RVO).

Access – population coverage

Population coverage of SHI in Germany is quite complex. Historically, population coverage was organised along different employment groups, and this still informs coverage criteria today. With the gradual expansion of SHI and the inclusion of additional population groups, coverage regulation grew ever more complex. A full description of SHI membership eligibility would take several pages to explain. In order to be able to trace changes over time, this study concentrates on the main insurant groups and disregards all exceptions.[6]

The primary coverage criterion for all social insurances in Germany is residence. Only ordinary residents in Germany are eligible for social insurance coverage (§ 30 (1) SGB I). In addition, each social insurance branch has its own conditions of membership. Statutory health insurance differentiates between two member groups: mandatory and voluntary insured. Criteria for defining mandatory and voluntary membership have been changed several times since 1977. Therefore, this section describes the situation in 1977, and membership reforms are then presented in the respective chapters below.

In 1977, SHI was mandatory for all blue-collar workers, white-collar workers with an income threshold below 30.600 DM per year, pensioners receiving benefits from statutory pension insurance, students, certain population groups taking part in job promotion programmes and particular self-employed workers (e.g. artists, midwives, nurses) earning less than the income threshold (§§ 165, 166 RVO). Unemployed workers receiving unemployment benefits were automatically covered by SHI (§ 155 (1) AFG). Becoming a voluntary member of SHI was possible for white-collar workers with an income above the threshold, trades- and craftsmen and persons attending vocational schools whose earnings did not exceed the income ceiling, surviving and divorced spouses of insured members, children of insured members not eligible for family allowance and severely disabled persons (§ 176 RVO). Persons who had been mandatorily insured but were no longer obligated to stay within the SHI system (e.g. students leaving university) could also voluntarily remain SHI members (§ 313 RVO).

One of the core solidarity elements of SHI is the contribution-free insurance of dependent family members. In 1977, dependent family members (spouses and children) of SHI members not fulfilling the conditions of insurance membership themselves, received a family allowance (§ 205 RVO). They were not entitled to benefits themselves; rather the contribution-paying insurant was entitled to obtain benefits for his/her family. Service coverage under family allowance, however, was almost identical to that of SHI members, with the exception of sick pay. Altogether, 91.6 per cent of the German population was secured by SHI in 1975 (Rosenbrock and Gerlinger 2014, p. 43).

Generosity – service coverage

SHI healthcare rights are explicitly framed as rights of the insured, and these are generally defined by the Social Code Book I (SGB I): 'Persons being insured by social insurance . . . do have the right to necessary measures for the protection, the preservation, the improvement and the recovery of their health and capacities' (§ 4 (2) No. 1 SGB I, author's translation). The SGB I also lists all service categories and cash benefits to which SHI members are entitled. In 1977, these included:

1 Examinations for the early detection of diseases;
2 Preventive regimens and other benefits aiming at the prevention of diseases;
3 In the case of illness: healthcare, hospital care, treatment at a health resort or other specialised facility, sick pay;
4 In the case of maternity: medical and midwife attendance, pharmaceuticals, remedies and dressings, maternity care at a maternity centre or hospital, maternity pay;
5 Sick pay in the case of leave of absence from work because of an ill child that needs to be looked after;
6 Home help;
7 Farm assistance for farmers;
8 Burial allowance.

(§ 21 (1) SGB I, as amended 1977, author's translation)

Until 1988, the content and conditions of service coverage were specified by the second book of the RVO (§§ 179–224 RVO), and since 1989, they are defined by the Social Code Book V (§§ 11–68 SGB V). The concrete content of the RVO concerning service coverage in 1977 is described for each service area below. In general, SHI members are entitled to medical treatment, 'if the treatment is necessary to detect or to cure an illness, to prevent aggravation, or to alleviate pain' (§ 27 SGB V, author's translation).

Healthcare services and goods must meet particular criteria to be provided under the SHI system. The 'economic imperative' (*Wirtschaftlichkeitsgebot*) determines that SHI services must be *sufficient, appropriate* and *efficient*, and they are not allowed to exceed the *necessary* level (§ 12 (1) SGB V, formerly § 368e and § 182 (2) RVO). The German law differentiates between economic[7] and efficient: efficiency describes the relation between costs and benefits and is one criteria of the economic imperative. In order to be economic, a medical good or service must be efficient, and in addition, must meet the other three principles stated above. If no treatment alternative exists, and the treatment is necessary, sufficient and appropriate, the treatment is economic irrespective of its costs (Engelhard 2012).

The requirements of the economic imperative are rather general and are not further specified by law. The specification of its principles is delegated to the joint self-administration, which concretises entitlement in its directives. Apart from these directives, the decision as to whether a particular treatment meets the requirements lies within the hands of single doctors.[8] The above named criteria had applied to ambulatory care[9] only, until their scope of application was extended to cover all SHI services in 1989.

Service coverage differs at least slightly between SHI funds. In principle, all funds must provide the SHI benefits package as defined by law. Beyond this, funds can provide additional benefits.[10] These are, however, restricted to benefits explicitly named by law.[11] In order to avoid major differences in coverage of additional services, the RVO stated that services must be 'comparable' (§ 259 RVO) between funds. Furthermore, funds were bound by law to cut the additional benefits so as to obviate contribution increases (§ 391 RVO). As a result, differences in service coverage between funds were marginal (Reiners et al. 1977, p. 54). Thus, the following description of service coverage in 1977 concentrates on general SHI benefits.[12]

Prevention: Given its historical roots as 'sickness' insurance, prevention plays only a minor, albeit increasing, role in German SHI. In 1977, SHI merely covered two secondary preventive measures: preventive medical examinations for children younger than four years that aim at detecting diseases which might endanger the physical or psychological wellbeing of the child; and one preventive medical examination per year for the detection of cancer in women over the age of 30 and men over the age of 45 (§ 181 RVO). The BAÄK was assigned with defining further details of these medical examinations in their Paediatric Directive and their Cancer Screening Directive, respectively. In addition, the Minister for Labour and Social Security was authorised by the RVO to determine additional preventive medical examinations (§ 181a RVO), but the minister never exercised this option (Heinze 1976, no. 103).

Primary and specialised ambulatory care: In 1977, SHI covered all 'treatment by medical doctors and dentists' (§ 182 (1) No. 1a RVO) that fulfilled the above named conditions. This included: medical treatment, diagnosis, the prescription of drugs, remedies, dressings, medical aids, glasses, supportive treatment by other health personnel and hospital care. Services provided by health personnel other than doctors were covered only if they were either supervised by a doctor (e.g. a practice nurse), or authorised by a doctor via prescription (Heinze 1976, no. 114/7).

Maternity care was regulated within a separate part of the RVO because maternity was not seen as an illness, but as a normal state of life and as such, was not among the original services of sickness funds (Heinze 1976, no. 199, 202). Yet maternity care was provided by SHI. The RVO generally defined the range of covered maternity services (§§ 195ff.) and the BAÄK specified entitlement through its Maternity Directive.

Hospital care: One of the principals of SHI service coverage is the primacy of ambulatory over hospital care (§ 39 SGB V). In 1977, this principle was not yet set out by law. The RVO merely required SHI hospital care to be 'necessary' (§ 184 RVO). It did not specify the services to be provided by SHI hospitals.

Pharmaceuticals: In 1977, pharmaceutical coverage was virtually unrestricted (§ 182 (1) No. 1b RVO). Ambulatory pharmaceutical prescription was regulated by the Pharmaceutical Directive 1976, which defined the principles of an 'appropriate, sufficient and efficient' pharmaceutical provision. The Pharmaceutical Directive listed several substances forbidden to be prescribed at the costs of SHI, but this list rarely contained real pharmaceuticals (e.g. wine, cosmetics and dietary products). Coverage of hospital drugs was not regulated at all.

The German system differentiates between drugs and remedies ('Heilmittel'). Remedies are substances or objects that primarily affect the body externally, like for example a mudpack application or a clinical thermometer (Heinze 1976, no. 114/9). According to § 368p RVO, the BAÄK was supposed to establish further regulations concerning the prescription of remedies, but it was not until 1982 that it issued such a directive. Hence, it often remained to the courts to decide which remedies must be reimbursed by SHI (Heinze 1976, no. 114/9).

Medical aids and appliances: In principal, artificial replacements, orthopaedic and other medical appliances are covered by SHI if they are necessary 'to prevent disability, to secure the success of treatment or to compensate a disability' (§ 33 SGB V, formerly § 182b RVO). Entitlement also includes the modification, repair, replacement as well as the instruction in the usage of the appliance.

Dental care and appliances: Dental care and appliances were part of the German benefits package in 1977. Entitlement to dental care was generally regulated by § 182 (1) No. 1a RVO and specifically by the Dental Care Directive 1962. The directive described in detail the diagnosis measures and treatments allowed, and explicitly excluded dental hygienic products, as well as restorative and nutrient substances from coverage.

In contrast to most other SHI benefits, dental appliances were not provided as services in kind. Instead, costs were partially or totally refunded by SHI. The amount of cost coverage was determined by the statutes of each health fund (§ 182c RVO). Coverage of dental appliances was specified by the Dental Prostheses Directive 1977.[13] This directive described the extent of treatment, as well as general and specific eligibility criteria for bridges, crowns, dentures and other prosthodontics. In principal, dental appliances were considered necessary if one tooth or several teeth were missing, and as a result, functional capability was reduced (No. 4). SHI, however, bore only the cost of the 'most efficient' replacement. If the patient wanted a more expensive one, s/he had to pay the additional costs (No. 7).

Ophthalmic care and optical appliances: Ophthalmological services provided by doctors are covered under SHI. Glasses (lenses and frame) belonged to the SHI benefits package in 1977, but only 'necessary' frames were reimbursed. Patients choosing more expensive ones had to bear the additional costs (Heinze 1976, no. 114/21). Contact lenses were covered too, but only if they were medically necessary or if they were required for one's work.

Other benefits: The RVO listed some additional benefits to be provided in the case of illness, for example homecare if hospital care were not possible (§ 185 RVO), home help (§ 185b RVO), regimens (§ 184a RVO) and occupational therapy (§ 182d RVO). Furthermore, SHI covered catering and accommodation expenses incurred as a result of medical treatment for the patient and one assistant (§ 194 (1) RVO). The SHI benefits package also included medical advice on family planning, as well as the examination and prescription of contraceptives. The contraceptives themselves, however, were not reimbursed (§ 200e RVO). Moreover, SHI covered sterilisation and legal abortion (§ 200f RVO). To keep the analysis manageable, these other benefits are not considered further.

Generosity – cost coverage

Similar to the case as is in England, SHI benefits are generally free of charge, but co-payments apply for some goods and services. In contrast to England, the principle of free healthcare is not constituted by law. In 1977, patients had to share at least part of the costs of pharmaceuticals, remedies, dressings and dental appliances. For the first three of these services, patients had to pay 20 per cent of costs but not more than 2.50 DM per receipt (§ 182a RVO). One receipt could contain more than one prescription. Pensioners, individuals at least 50 per cent work disabled, persons receiving sick pay and children were generally exempted from this charge. Cost-sharing for dental prostheses and crowns differed between SHI funds and was defined within the statutes of the funds (§ 182c RVO).

3.3   Social–Liberal healthcare entitlement reforms 1977–1982

Since the foundation of the German social health insurance system, its expenditures have steadily increased. With the economic recession of the mid-1970s, however, this growth was increasingly perceived as problematic, and health policy turned from an era of expansion to an era of 'cost-containment' (Gerlinger 2002; Vincenti 2008). The following investigation of German healthcare entitlement reforms starts in 1977 with the passage of the first major health reform of this new era, and ends in 1982, the year the Social–Liberal coalition was superseded by the Christian Democrats and Liberals coalition. As background information, this section starts with a short overview of the political and economic conditions at that time and very briefly discusses general health policy of the Social–Liberal coalition. The detailed analysis of healthcare entitlement reforms builds the core of this section. It is followed by a short summary.

Political and economic background

Germany had been governed by a coalition of Social Democrats (SPD)[14] and Liberals (FDP)[15] since 1969. After the resignation of the social democratic Chancellor Willy Brandt, Helmut Schmidt, former Minister of Finance, assumed office in 1974. The electorate had broad confidence in Schmidt's ability to solve the economic crisis in the aftermath of the first oil price shock and confirmed the Social–Liberal coalition in the general elections of 1976 (Thränhardt 1996, pp. 207f.). In fact, compared to other OECD countries, Germany mastered the economic crisis of the mid-1970s very well: during this period, GDP shrank only once, unemployment never exceeded five per cent, and inflation peaked at seven per cent, which was quite low compared to the double-digit inflation rates of other countries.

The Social–Liberal coalition was reelected in October 1980. The SPD faired similarly as they had in 1976; the FDP improved their results, drawing in more than 10 per cent of the vote. The Christian Democrats achieved their worst result since 1953.[16] This time, however, the government was less able to tackle the problems of the second oil price crisis. It had already adopted an expansive trade cycle policy in order to boost the world economy, and thus there remained limited room for manoeuvre (Thränhardt 1996, pp. 258f.). The economy suffered from stagflation, and unemployment rates climbed to formerly unknown heights. The coalition partners could not agree about the right approach to crisis management. The FDP favoured supply side economics, tax reductions and social cuts, which contradicted the social democratic credo. Nonetheless, the SPD approved several Liberal retrenchment reforms, thereby increasing voters' dissatisfaction with the party (Thränhardt 1996, pp. 261ff.). In September 1982, the two parties could no longer manage the discord and all FDP ministers resigned. The FDP defected and took up negotiations with the Christian Democrats. One month later, the opposition, for the first time in German history, successfully called a constructive vote of no confidence against the Chancellor, which resulted in Helmut Kohl being elected the new German Chancellor.

Many laws in Germany require the consent of the *Bundesrat* in addition to approval from the *Bundestag*. Often majorities in both bodies are opposed, as was also mostly the case during the Social–Liberal coalition. The Christian Democrats had held the majority in the *Bundesrat* since 1972 and could thus block reforms. Only between January 1977 and July 1978 were there unclear majorities because two *Länder* were governed by a coalition of Christian Democrats and Liberals. Given opposed majorities in both bodies, most reforms required consensus of all parties and hence, radical reforms were hardly possible.

Social–Liberal health policy

Since the mid-1970s, the health policy discourse in Germany centred on the 'cost explosion' in healthcare (Vincenti 2008, p. 521). SHI expenditures had increased between 15 and 20 per cent per capita per year during the first half of the 1970s, and contribution rates had climbed from 8 per cent in 1970 to around 11 per cent in 1976 (Rosewitz and Webber 1990, p. 231; Vincenti 2008, pp. 522f.). It was feared that these 'high' rates were hindering economic development and reducing German competitiveness in the world market. Therefore, stability of contribution rates became the prime goal of health policy (Vincenti 2008, p. 555).

In the late 1970s, the statutory pension insurance (SPI) suffered a huge budget deficit which the government wanted to tackle through a reduction of SHI contributions paid by SPI. In order to avoid subsequent SHI contribution increases, cost-reduction measures had to be implemented in the health sector (Vincenti 2008, pp. 526f.). The Health Insurance Cost Containment Act 1977 (*Krankenversicherungs–Kostendämpfungsgesetz*, KVKG) thus imposed a capped budget for ambulatory medical treatment and for pharmaceuticals, both of which were to be defined in negotiations between the associations of SHI funds and of SHI physicians (and dentists) at the national level (Vincenti 2008, p. 531). Furthermore, the KVKG introduced several measures addressing the service and cost coverage of SHI (see below).

The KVKG, together with the voluntary income restraint of doctors, successfully kept expenditure increases low, and thus contribution rates could be kept stable between 1977 and 1980 (Vincenti 2008, p. 533). But already in the second half of 1980 and in 1981, expenditures rose again and another cost-shifting, this time from the general state budget, made new cost-containment reforms necessary (Vincenti 2008, p. 535). The Health Insurance Cost Containment Amendment Act 1981 (*Kostendämpfungs–Ergänzungsgesetz*, KVEG) expanded the corporatist budget negotiations to include medical aids and appliances. Moreover, the KVEG further increased the cost burden of patients through new as well as higher co-payments and service exclusions (for details see below).

Faced with poor economic development, the government envisaged a next round of cost-shifting between social insurance sectors and set out to increase co-payments of patients once again (Vincenti 2008, pp. 537f.). These plans, however, could not be realised because of the unexpected change of government in 1982.

Social–Liberal healthcare entitlement reforms

During their last six years in government, the Social–Liberal coalition carried out two main health reforms, the Health Insurance Cost Containment Act 1977 (KVKG) and the Health Insurance Cost Containment Amendment Act 1981

(KVEG). Both reforms addressed healthcare entitlement in various dimensions. Although individual competencies were shifted between the joint self-administration and the ministry, the general governance structure of healthcare entitlement remained untouched. Hence, there is nothing to report for this period and this category was omitted.

Access – population coverage

The KVKG severely restricted conditions of SHI membership for pensioners. In the past, all persons receiving a pension from SPI were automatically insured through SHI (Zipperer 1978, p. 12). With the KVKG, former SHI membership became a pre-condition of SHI membership for pensioners: compulsory coverage now required a minimum period of SHI membership equalling half of one's working life (§ 1 No. 1a KVKG),[17] and voluntary membership was restricted to pensioners who had been voluntary members of SHI during their working lives as well as having joined SHI during the first month of retirement (§ 1 No. 3 KVKG).[18] A further reform tied SHI membership for the disabled to a required minimum previously insured period of five years (Art. 1 No. 1 KVEG).

The conditions of family allowance were tightened, excluding family members with earnings above a defined income ceiling (§ 18 KVKG). Formerly, dependency on the insured in conjunction with no own SHI membership had been the single criteria for eligibility (§ 205 RVO). As a countermeasure, voluntary SHI membership was extended to cover spouses of SHI members not eligible for family allowance (§ 1 No. 4 KVKG). Furthermore, children lost entitlement to family allowance if one parent was not an SHI member and earned more than her/his SHI insured spouse (§ 18 KVKG).

Generosity – service coverage

Although cost containment was high on the political agenda, restrictions of SHI service coverage remained few.

Pharmaceuticals and remedies: During the late 1970s and the whole of the 1980s, the ministry, the parliament, the joint self-administration and the pharmaceutical industry struggled with the introduction of a pharmaceutical (and remedies) negative list. In a first attempt, the joint self-administration was tasked with deciding on the exclusion and restriction of pharmaceuticals and remedies being used for the treatment of minor diseases (§ 1 No. 38b KVKG). The BAÄK prepared a list of pharmaceuticals as requested, but it was not approved by the ministry. For the following reform, the power of decision regarding the exclusion of pharmaceuticals and remedies was delegated to the ministry (§ 1 No. 2a and No. 6 KVEG), but it was not until 1990 that the ministry issued the first negative list (see Chapter 3.4).

Medical aids and appliances: Medical aids considered as 'common articles of daily use' were officially excluded from public reimbursement in 1981 (§ 1 No. 4 KVEG). Yet this was merely a codification of common and legal practice. In 1976, the Federal Social Court had already ruled that SHI entitlement does not include articles of daily use (Die Ersatzkasse 1978, p. 430).

Ophthalmic care and optical appliances: In 1981, coverage of optical appliances was tightened by setting a timeframe of three years for new glasses for persons older than 14 years. This timeframe, however, applied only if eyesight remained constant (§ 182f RVO, introduced by § 1 No. 6 KVEG).

Generosity – cost coverage

The first two austerity reforms drastically increased the share of costs borne by the patient:

Pharmaceuticals, medical aids and appliances: Charges for pharmaceuticals, remedies, medical aids and appliances were restructured by the KVKG. Instead of paying 20 per cent of costs and at the most 2.50 DM for all items prescribed at the same time, patients had to pay 1 DM for each item without any limitation. This reform particularly increased the cost burden of the chronically ill, because now co-payments rose with the quantity consumed. Furthermore, eligibility criteria for the exemption of co-payments were tightened by limiting exemption to hardship cases, which were to be defined by each health insurance fund separately. Formerly, all pensioners, all persons with a reduced ability to work of more than 50 per cent and persons receiving other social benefits due to illness had been exempted from paying charges (§ 182a RVO).

With the KVEG, co-payments for pharmaceuticals and dressings were increased to 1.50 DM per item. In addition, the definition of hardship cases was changed to make clear that the requirement of many drugs was not sufficient grounds for exemption. In addition, the income of the patient had to be low enough to make co-payments an 'unacceptable burden' (§ 1 No. 3 KVEG). However, the same reform freed self-insured persons younger than 16 years from paying charges.[19]

Dental care and appliances: While health funds had formerly been totally free to determine cost coverage of dental appliances, the KVKG, in a first step, capped their subsidies at 80 per cent of total costs (§ 1 No. 6 and 7 KVKG). Moreover, exemptions formerly defined individually by health funds were limited to hardship cases. In a second step, the KVEG reduced maximum cost coverage of dental appliances to 60 per cent of total costs. At the same time, treatment by a dentist in the course of the provision of dental prosthesis and crowns became a service in kind, which diminished the effective costs of treatment for the patient (§ 1 No. 2b and 2c KVEG).[20]

The KVKG gave SHI funds the opportunity to levy co-payments of up to 20 per cent of costs for orthodontic treatment with a maximum of 25 per cent of the reference income (462.50 DM in 1977). SHI funds could make the co-payments contingent upon the completion of treatment in order to sanction the discontinuation of orthodontic treatment (§ 182e RVO, introduced by § 1 No. 8 KVKG). Co-payments and their modalities had to be regulated by each fund within its statutes.

Ophthalmic care and optical appliances: The KVKG introduced a general co-payment for spectacles of 4 DM (§ 1 No. 6 and 7 KVKG). Only children and hardship cases were exempted from paying these charges.

Summary

All healthcare entitlement reforms of the Social–Liberal coalition can be clearly characterised as retrenchment. Without any noteworthy exception, the reforms restricted population coverage and cut generosity.[21] Generosity was constrained mainly through measures affecting cost coverage: co-payments and charges were introduced and/or raised and exemptions from paying charges were limited. In contrast, restrictions of service coverage remained few. The exclusion of drugs for the treatment of minor diseases was decided but not carried into effect. In order to present a balanced evaluation of Social–Liberal reforms, it must be noted that entitlement to core services such as ambulatory medical care and hospital care were spared from retrenchment.

3.4   Christian Democratic–Liberal healthcare entitlement reforms 1982–1998

The 16 years between 1982 and 1998 are in Germany generally referred to as the 'Kohl era'. Neither before nor after has one person held the office of the Federal Chancellor for such a long time. Despite this stability in government, the 16 years were anything but constant: they were marked by the German unification, rapid progress in European integration and the implementation of structural reforms in the area of healthcare after long years of mere cost-containment policies. Healthcare entitlement policies during the late 1980s and1990s cannot be fully understood without the political and economic context. For that reason, a more detailed description of the central political events and economic conditions is given in the first part of this section. It is followed by an outline of Christian Democratic–Liberal health policy that focuses in particular on the genesis of reforms in order to show how prone to conflicts health policy was during this period, and to reveal the important role of veto players in the German system. As before, healthcare entitlement reforms are the main subject and hence are described in detail. The section ends with a short summary.

Political and economic background

The new Christian Democratic (CDU/CSU)[22] and Liberal (FDP) government had a rough start. Besides the poor economic performance and therefore precarious budget situation, the legitimacy of the government was contested because of the defection of the FDP. In order to increase its legitimacy, and to retain support for their far-reaching reform plans, the government decided in 1983 to dissolve the *Bundestag* and call early elections (Schmidt 2005a, pp. 12f.). The electorate confirmed the Christian Democratic–Liberal government with 48.8 per cent of votes for the CDU/CSU and 7.0 per cent for the FDP. The SPD share of the vote declined sharply (to 38.2 per cent) and its power was further weakened as it had to share opposition with the Green Party (*Die Grünen*), which entered the *Bundestag* for the first time in 1983.[23] Despite numerous corruption affairs and a huge party financing scandal, the Christian Democrats and Liberals managed a repeat of their success in the general elections of 1987 and again formed the government.[24]

The economic situation was especially poor during the first years of the CDU/CSU/FDP government. Stagflation and high unemployment squeezed state budgets necessitating immediate intervention. In response, the new government implemented a multitude of retrenchment measures through the Accompanying Budget Laws (*Haushaltsbegleitgesetze*, HBeglG) of 1983 and 1984. Measures included, amongst others, an increase of pension and unemployment contribution rates, an increase in the value added tax, cuts in public financial support for students, and cuts of social assistance and unemployment benefits. The German economy recovered during the 1980s, but unemployment remained high and never fell below 7.9 per cent. The government attempted to reduce unemployment rates through early retirement policies and a moderate deregulation of the labour market (Jochem 1999, pp. 11ff.). With economic recovery in the second half of the 1980s, the financial scope of the public budget rose, resulting in some expanded social benefits (e.g. child rearing allowance, housing allowance), but retrenchment reforms were not withdrawn.

The fall of the Berlin Wall on 9 November 1989 marked a fundamental break in German political history. After the opening of the border, events came thick and fast, and exactly 11 months later, the German Democratic Republic (*Deutsche Demokratische Republik*, DDR) acceded to the Federal Republic, and Germany was unified. For several years, the German unification dominated the political agenda and all other themes were put on hold.

The German unification was an enormous organisational task: public administration had to be built up, the economy privatised, infrastructure modernised and the social security system adapted – to name only some of the main remits. Above all, the unification posed a huge financial challenge. Almost immediately after the unification, great parts of the eastern economy broke down, and around four million workers lost their jobs (Ritter 2007, p. 70). The high unemployment meant a huge financial burden not only for the public budget, but also for the social insurance systems, which had been conferred from West Germany to the eastern part.

During the first two years of unification, the economy of western Germany experienced a 'unification boom', and in total grew more than five per cent per year (OECD 2014a). However, it could not escape global recession for long and in 1993, GDP growth became negative. The economy recovered slowly, but growth rates during the last years of the Kohl era never exceeded 2.5 per cent. As a result of the recession, unemployment rose in western Germany, too. Unemployment peaked at 12.7 per cent in 1997, reaching 19.1 per cent in eastern and 10.3 per cent in western Germany (Statistisches Bundesamt 2014).

Policy-making in the aftermath of the unification was difficult and prone to conflicts (Jochem 1999). The CDU/CSU managed to win the 1990 and 1994 elections[25] and again formed a coalition with the Liberals, but the two parties had lost majority in the *Bundesrat* in March 1991.[26] However, there was also no majority within the opposition because several *Länder* had mixed coalition governments, thereby necessitating broadly negotiated agreements between all parties for each reform. A tactic for coping with these difficult majority constellations was the splitting of reforms: one part required approval by the *Bundesrat*, and a second part could be passed without it. Because consent of the Social Democrats was often required, the ruling government parties were forced to make concessions to them, which in turn increased dissent within the CDU/CSU and FDP coalition (Jochem 1999, p. 36). Despite these difficult majorities, the Kohl government realised several retrenchment reforms during its last period in office which were designed to fill the budget holes torn into the finances of the state and the social insurances after unification, and in order to meet the Maastricht criteria. For example, the duration of unemployment benefits was reduced and replacement rates cut in 1993, the average level of SPI pensions was reduced stepwise, and in 1997, the retirement age was raised (Jochem 1999, pp. 31 ff.). However, one reform stands out because it extensively expanded social rights – the introduction of statutory long-term care insurance in 1994. With it, a fifth pillar was added to the German social insurance system providing social security in the area of elderly and social care.

Christian Democratic–Liberal health policy

During the first decade, the Christian Democrats and Liberals followed the path of their predecessors by continuing cost-containment policies. They passed their first cost-containment reform and other social cuts with the Accompanying Budget Laws of 1983 and 1984. Most of the measures addressed service and cost coverage and are described in detail below. In 1988, the new coalition agreed on its first major healthcare reform, the Statutory Health Insurance Reform Act (*Gesundheitsreformgesetz*, GRG). Even though the CDU/CSU and Liberals still held majorities in both parliamentary bodies, they did not succeed in implementing major structural reforms due to the interventions of powerful interest groups (primarily healthcare providers and funds) (Bandelow 1998, p. 194; Wasem and Greß 2005, p. 409). Furthermore, most hospital reform measures had to be abandoned due to pressures imposed by the CSU (Perschke-Hartmann 1994). Nevertheless, the GRG was highly relevant because it re-codified SHI law by establishing the Social Code Book V. Moreover, the GRG introduced a reference pricing system for pharmaceuticals, dressings and medical aids, several instruments to better integrate hospital and ambulatory medical care, and various measures that limited healthcare entitlement (described below). Although the primary goal of the GRG was to stabilise contribution rates (Deppe 2000, pp. 99ff.) – it even inscribed the principle of contribution rate stability into law – and although it had introduced budget limits for various health sectors, the reform had only a minimal impact on SHI finances. In 1989, SHI expenditures fell by 3.7 per cent, but grew again the next year, causing contribution rates to rise above pre-GRG levels to 13.1 per cent of gross income (Wasem and Greß 2005, pp. 413f.; Wasem, Greß and Hessel 2007, p. 670).

Rising contribution rates called for further health reform, particularly because a further increase would have reduced pension growth in the following year,[27] an effect politicians were keen to avoid given upcoming general and *Länder* elections (Wasem, Greß and Hessel 2007, p. 671). However, majorities in the *Bundesrat* had changed, and there was little prospect for comprehensive reform. Only because the SPD opposition decided to cooperate could a far-reaching joint reform, the health-care Structure Act 1992 (*Gesundheitsstrukturgesetz*, GSG), be passed (Wasem, Greß and Hessel 2007, p. 672). In contrast to the GRG, interest groups in this case were not given opportunity to influence decision-making (Bandelow and Schubert 1998, p. 119; Wasem, Greß and Hessel 2007, p. 675). The GSG signified a 'para-digm shift' from cost containment to structural reform (Gerlinger 2002; Noweski 2004; Urban 2001). One of the core elements of the reform was the expansion of competition between health funds brought about by allowing (almost all) insured to freely choose between SHI funds as of 1996. Another core area was the hospital sector, which had previously been spared from most reforms because these had been blocked in the *Bundesrat* (Busse and Riesberg 2004, p. 168). In addition to structural reforms, the GSG also implemented various traditional cost-containment instruments (e.g. fixed budgets, increased co-payments) (Deppe 2000, pp. 112ff.; Wasem, Greß and Hessel 2007, p. 675). Despite these substantial cuts, the GSG had only a mixed impact because, in bowing to pressure from the Liberals, budget limits were widened, and several measures were not implemented or abolished afterwards (e.g. the pharmaceutical positive list, the reference pricing system for drugs with patent protection) (Deppe 2000, p. 131).

The consensus between the government and SPD opposition did not last for long and already the next reform attempt, the so called 'third step' of health reform, was blocked by the *Bundesrat*. For this reason, reforms were again split into reform laws needing approval of the *Bundestag* and those that did not (Ban-delow 1998, pp. 219ff.). In September 1996, prior to the next reform step, the government passed another cost-containment reform as part of a massive austerity package.[28] This reform stipulated that funds had to reduce contribution rates by 0.4 per cent in 1996, and once again called for severe cuts in services and cost cover-age of public healthcare (described below). The third reform step was realised in 1997 by two reform laws which required no approval from the *Bundesrat*. The First SHI Restructuring Act 1997 (*1. GKV–Neuordnungsgesetz*, 1.GKV–NOG) linked co-payment increases to contribution rate increases (for details, see below) with the purpose of further intensifying competition between funds (Deppe 2000, p. 137). The Second SHI Restructuring Act 1997 (*2. GKV–Neuordnungsgesetz*, 2.GKV–NOG) once again implemented co-payments and increased established ones. Elements formerly unique to the private health insurance sector, such as franchise, premium refund, and choice between reimbursement of costs and ben-efits in kind, were introduced into the social health insurance system, and a greater diversification of service coverage between funds was permitted (Deppe 2000, pp. 139f.).

Christian Democratic–Liberal healthcare entitlement reforms

During their 16 years in office, the Christian Democratic–Liberal government passed 13 reforms affecting healthcare entitlement (see Table 3.3). The GRG 1988, the GSG 1992 and the 2.GKV–NOG 1997 were major health reforms, while the

Table 3.3 Reforms affecting healthcare entitlement, Germany 1982–1998

Law German short title	Adoption Commencement	Abbreviation
Accompanying Budget Law 1983 *Haushaltsbegleitgesetz*	20.12.1982 *01.01.1983*	HBegleitG 1983
Statutory Health Insurance Reform Act *Gesundheits-Reformgesetz*	20.12.1988 *01.01.1989*	GRG
KOV–Adjustment Act *KOV–Anpassungsgesetz*	26.06.1990 *01.07.1990*	KOV–AnpG
Second SGB V Amendment Act *Zweites SGB V Änderungsgesetz*	20.12.1991 *01.01.1992*	2.SGBVÄndG
Help for Expectant Mothers and Families Act *Schwangeren- und Familienhilfegesetz*	27.07.1992 *05.08.1992*	SFHG
Healthcare Structure Act *Gesundheitsstrukturgesetz*	21.12.1992 *01.01.1993*	GSG
Fifth SGB V Amendment Act *Fünftes SGB V Änderungsgesetz*	18.12.1995 *01.01.1996*	5.SGBVÄndG
Eighth SGB V Amendment Act *Achtes SGB V Änderungsgesetz*	28.10.1996 *01.11.1996*	8.SGBVÄndG
Health Insurance Contribution Rate Exoneration Act *Beitragsentlastungsgesetz*	01.11.1996 *01.01.1997*	BeitrEntlG
First Statutory Health Insurance Restructuring Act *1. GKV–Neuordnungsgesetz*	23.06.1997 *01.07.1997*	1.GKV–NOG
Second Statutory Health Insurance Restructuring Act *2. GKV–Neuordnungsgesetz*	23.06.1997 *01.07.19977*	2.GKV–NOG
First Social Code Book III Amendment Act *Erstes SGB III Änderungsgesetz*	16.12.1997 *01.01.1998*	1.SGBIIIÄndG
Act on the Professions of Psychological Psychotherapists and Children and Teenager Psychotherapists and SGB V and Other Laws Amendment *Gesetz über die Berufe des Psychologischen Psychotherapeuten und des Kinder- und Jugendlichenpsychotherapeuten, zur Änderung des SGB V und anderer Gesetze*	16.06.1998 *01.01.1999*	PsychThG/ SGB5uaÄndG
Ninth SGB V Amendment Act *Neuntes SGB V Änderungsgesetz*	08.05.1998 *01.01.1999*	9.SGBVÄndG

other laws either addressed only one or few aspects, or had short-term cost containment as their sole aim (HBegleitG 1983, BeitrEntlG). The GRG not only introduced various health reform measures, but also reorganised healthcare entitlement regulation. It replaced the Imperial Insurance Code (*Reichsversicherungsordnung*, RVO) with the Social Code Book V (*Fünftes Sozialgesetzbuch*, SGB V). In the course of the introduction of compulsory long-term care insurance in 1995, long-term care was massively expanded. However, as care services were shifted from SHI to the new insurance branch, they no longer fell under SHI entitlement and thus are not considered in the following sections.

Differences in generosity between health funds were at first decreased and later increased again. In 1989, the GRG initially abolished differences in cost coverage and reduced service coverage variations. In 1997, the 2.GKV–NOG again permitted differences between SHI funds in order to strengthen competition between them. In addition to a differentiation of co-payments, the reform allowed SHI funds to exceed the SHI benefits package within clearly defined limits. These so called 'amplified services' (*erweiterte Leistungen*), however, were financed from additional contributions paid solely by the fund's members (§ 56 SGB V introduced by Art. 1 No. 14 2.GKV–NOG).

Governance – who decides about healthcare entitlement?

Under the Kohl government, the competencies of the joint self-administration were extensively increased (Döhler and Manow-Borgwardt 1992a; Urban 2001). In particular, the BAÄK was assigned several new tasks regarding the definition of service coverage (details below). In order to enable the BAÄK to meet its responsibilities, the binding nature of its directives was strengthened by the GRG in 1988. In the past, BAÄK directives had been tantamount to (non-binding) recommendations to members of the joint self-administration. The GRG made directives binding for all SHI providers and SHI funds (Döhler and Manow-Borgwardt 1992, p. 587). The legal enforceability of directives was confirmed by several judgements of the Federal Social Court (FSC) during the 1990s. The court also made clear that directives are not only legally binding for SHI providers and funds, but also for the insured (Zimmermann 2012, pp. 51ff.). Moreover, the GRG expanded the scope of application of the directives to apply to substitute funds (*Ersatzkassen*), too (§ 91 (1) SGB V).

Access – population coverage

With regard to population' coverage, the GRG enacted one of the most significant reforms of the period under investigation: it expanded SHI membership to family members of SHI members. Formerly, they received only a family allowance, and entitlement was mediated through the insured member. With this reform, family members of SHI members became insured themselves, which meant they became bearers of rights and could thus claim entitlement autonomously and independently from the insurant (see explanatory memorandum BT–Drs. 11/2237, p. 161). However, more coverage criteria applied to this new group of SHI members than had applied to recipients of family allowance.

The GRG implemented a second important change by eliminating the requirement differences between blue-collar and white-collar workers. Formerly, blue-collar workers were compulsorily insured no matter how high their income. After the reform, the same rules as for white-collar workers applied to blue-collar workers: if they earned above the income ceiling,[29] they were freed from compulsory membership (§ 6 (1) No. 1 SGB V). The GSG then further increased equality by allowing all insured to freely choose their health fund, which formerly had been an exclusive privilege of white-collar workers.

Aside from those fundamental alterations, population coverage reforms under Kohl were rather restrictive. First came the limitation of eligibility for voluntary insurance. The GRG now demanded previous minimum SHI membership of 12 months within the five years prior to withdrawal of SHI membership, or six months immediately before withdrawal as pre-conditions for voluntary membership (§ 9 SGB V). These qualifying periods were doubled by the GSG (Art. 1 No. 2). According to its explanatory memorandum, the reason behind the linkage of voluntary membership to previous SHI membership was to protect solidarity by preventing persons from joining when they are in need without having paid beforehand (BT–Drs. 11/2237, p. 160). Moreover, the GRG restricted eligibility to voluntary membership to include fewer population groups, e.g. voluntary membership was no longer possible for pensioners and self-employed (§ 9 SGB V, formerly §§ 176–178 RVO). With this provision, the Christian Democratic–Liberal coalition pursued the strict policy against pensioners begun by the Social–Liberal coalition. It further restricted access for pensioners through the GSG, which allowed only persons formerly compulsorily insured to join SHI as pensioners. Pensioners who had been voluntarily insured during their working life could remain voluntarily insured but had to pay full contributions (Art. 1 No. 1 GSG).[30]

In addition to the voluntarily insured and pensioners, students also became subject to restrictions. Compulsory membership of students was limited to students below the age of 30 having completed 14 or fewer semesters of study (§ 5 SGB V). Students not fulfilling these conditions can either insure privately or voluntarily with SHI, but must pay at least the minimum contribution rate which is more than double the rate of compulsorily insured students.

In one aspect, the Christian Democrats and Liberals expanded SHI membership, at least de jure. The GSG allowed for the inclusion of those receiving social assistance (*Sozialhilfe*) into SHI as of 1.1.1997 (Art. 28 GSG). However, this reform, although laid down by law, has not been realised to this day.[31]

Generosity – service coverage

In the course of the changeover from the RVO to the SGB V, important alterations regarding the constitutive criteria of service coverage definition were implemented. First, the service criteria that had in the past exclusively defined SHI coverage of ambulatory services were applied to all SHI benefits. Hence, since 1989 all services covered by SHI must be *sufficient, appropriate, efficient* and they are not allowed to exceed the *necessary* level (§ 12 SGB V).

Second, a principle of 'personal responsibility for health' (*Eigenverantwortung*) was constituted by SHI law. Unknown to the old RVO, the SGB V centrally highlights:

> The insured are co-responsible for their own health; in following a health-conscious lifestyle, participating in preventive programmes and by actively contributing to healthcare treatment and rehabilitation, they shall contribute

to avoid the occurrence of diseases and impairments or to overcome their consequences.

(§ 1 SGB V, author's translation)

In accordance with the principle of personal responsibility, SHI coverage was restricted to those services not belonging to the 'sphere of individual responsibility of the member' (§ 2 SGB V). Thereby it made clear that not all goods and services benefiting health are covered under SHI, and established the basis for several exclusions (see below). Based on similar arguments of individual responsibility, patients having caused their illness deliberately became obligated to pay part of the treatment costs (§ 52 SGB V).

Under the GRG reform, it was determined that in case necessary treatment were not available in Germany, SHI funds could agree to pay all or part of the costs of treatment abroad (§ 18 SGB V). This measure, however, constituted a voluntary guideline for the funds and did not guarantee any entitlement to treatment in a foreign country.

Prevention: Historically, prevention was not part of SHI. This changed radically with the GRG, which made health promotion and general prevention a primary task of SHI funds (§§ 20–24 SGB V). Providing information and consultation on health hazards and disease prevention was made compulsory for all funds (§ 20 (1) SGB V), while health promotion and primary prevention were discretionary, and each fund could establish its own measures (§ 20 (3) SGB V). The GRG also introduced entitlement to biennial examinations for the early detection of diseases for adults over the age of 35 (§ 25 (1) SGB V). The concrete content of the examinations was to be specified by the BAÄK. Furthermore, the age limit for preventive medical examinations in children was increased from four to six years (§ 26 SGB V).

Prevention played a less dominant role in the succeeding reforms. Only two additional measures were introduced: the GSG allowed SHI funds to sponsor self-help groups with prevention or rehabilitation goals (Art. 1 No. 8b), and the 2.GKV–NOG extended check-ups for children, adding another check-up for 10 year olds (Art. 1 No. 3a). Prevention was even restricted somewhat: the GSG explicitly forbade health funds to finance vaccinations for private journeys (Art. 1 No. 8a); and in 1996, health promotion, which had been introduced by the GRG, was again eliminated from the SHI benefits package (Art. 2 No. 1a BeitrEntlG) because, according to the explanatory memorandum, health funds had often used health promotion measures for marketing purposes and expenses had increased immensely over the years (BT–Drs. 13/4615, p. 9).

Accompanying medical prevention, the GRG also implemented several dental preventive measures: health insurance funds became responsible for general preventive dental care in children under the age of 12, to be provided as group prevention (§ 21 SGB V). Furthermore, young adults between the ages of 12 and 20 became entitled to a preventive dental examination once per year (§ 22 SGB V). In the following years, preventive dental care was further expanded. The GSG lowered the age limit for the annual individual preventive dental treatment of children from 12 to six years. In addition, it extended entitlement to cover fissure seals of the molars for children and teens. Moreover, the GSG expanded group preventive measures to also include the detection of dental diseases (Art. 1 No. 10 GSG). The 2.GKV–NOG then added preventive dental examinations for children younger than six years to the covered preventive measures (Art. 1 No. 3b). Preventive dental care was not only augmented for children, but also for adults, who became entitled to individual preventive dental care (Art. 1 No. 2 2.GKV–NOG), the concrete content of which was to be specified by the BAZÄK.

Primary care and specialised ambulatory care: The GRG implemented a major coverage restriction for new diagnosis and treatment methods in ambulatory care. It determined that new services in the ambulatory sector may be provided only if the BAÄK has positively decided on their effectiveness and issued obligatory quality requirements (§ 135 (1) SGB V). This regulation is equivalent to a positive list: only treatments having been checked and positively recommended by the joint self-administration are admitted under SHI. The 2.GKV–NOG increased the hurdle by demanding that new treatments must also be efficient and medically necessary (Art. 1 No 50). Moreover, it was determined that these criteria applied to all services provided in the ambulatory sector.

Over the years, several single services were added to the SHI benefits package by law. In 1990, artificial insemination became part of the SHI benefits package (§ 27a SGB V introduced by Art. 2 No. 2 KOV–AnpG). In 1991, service coverage was extended to socio-paediatric treatment for children (notably, psychological, therapeutic pedagogical and psycho-social services) not provided by, but overseen by a doctor, if treatment was necessary in order to detect a disease or to draw up a treatment plan (§ 43a SGB V introduced by Art. 1 No. 12 2.SGBVÄndG). In 1998, psychotherapy provided by psychotherapists was added (§ 92 (6a) SGB V introduced by Art. 2 No. 10 PsychThG/ SGBVÄndG),[32] and the BAÄK was assigned with defining further details of service provision within its Psychotherapy Directive.

Hospital care: In order to add authority to the primacy of ambulatory care and to avoid unnecessary costs, the GSG introduced a mandatory check of eligibility before each stationary admission (Art. 1 No. 23).

Stationary and day care hospice services were added to the SHI benefits package (§ 39a SGB V introduced by Art. 1 No. 12 2.GKV–NOG). However, costs were only partly refunded, and only if treatment or care at home was not possible. The exact degree of cost coverage was to be defined by each health fund within its statutes.

Pharmaceuticals and remedies: One of the first laws the new government realised stemmed from its predecessor and excluded pharmaceuticals for the treatment of minor diseases such as colds, constipation or traveling disease (Art. 19 No.4 HBeglG 1983). Only children and young adults below the age of 16 remained eligible for those pharmaceuticals. The GRG furthermore extended the power of the ministry to exclude drugs: it determined that, besides pharmaceuticals for the treatment of minor diseases, the ministry could also exclude pharmaceuticals which were 'not economic' (*unwirtschaftlich*)[33] (§ 34 (3) SGB V). The ministry issued the first negative list via ministerial order in 1990.[34] The order generally excluded drugs with more than three active pharmaceutical ingredients and those containing a combination of particular active pharmaceutical ingredients. It further specified that drugs containing one or more unnecessary active pharmaceutical ingredient (listed in annex 2 of the order) were not to be reimbursed by SHI. Most of the ingredients listed in annex 2 were homeopathic or herbal substances. The GRG furthermore restricted the provision of new remedies in ambulatory care by introducing an approval process similar to that for new diagnosis and treatment methods in ambulatory care (§ 138 SGB V).

As a result of SPD demands, the GSG contained provisions for the introduction of a positive list of pharmaceuticals (Art. 1 No. 21 GSG; Wasem, Greß and Hessel 2007, p. 673). The positive list, though, has never been created. Bowing to pressure from the Liberals, whose demands had largely been overlooked in the big GSG compromise, but who later successfully managed to advance the interests of their voters, the 5.SGBV-ÄndG revoked all provisions for the pharmaceutical positive list (Deppe 2000, p. 131).

Medical aids and appliances: The GRG established a negative list of medical aids. According to the principle of personal responsibility (§ 2 SGB V), the ministry was granted the power to exclude medical aids offering minimal medical benefit as well as inexpensive ones. Furthermore, it could exclude medical aids for which effectiveness was not sufficiently proven (§ 34 (4) SGB V). The ministry issued the first negative list in 1989.[35] [36] It contained nine items that were excluded for reasons of minimal or contested effectiveness (e.g. articles for compression, abdominal fasciae) and 20 low cost items (e.g. rubber gloves, urine bottles). In 1995, the list was changed once when breast pumps were removed from it.[37]

Dental care and appliances: Similar to ambulatory medical care, the GRG introduced coverage restrictions for new diagnosis and treatment methods in ambulatory dental care: the BAZÄK had to attest the effectiveness of the new method and to issue obligatory quality requirements before provision was permitted (§ 135 (1) SGB V).

The GSG draft had intended to split dental appliances, as well as orthodontic treatment, into basic and elective services, but the idea failed due to opposition from the Social Democrats (Wasem, Greß and Hessel 2007, p. 673). Instead, entitlement to dental appliances (with the exception of urgent treatment) was made conditional upon a minimum membership period of one year for SHI members who had previously not resided in Germany, as well as for asylum seekers and displaced receiving social assistance (Art. 1 No. 14b GSG). In the course of the reform, bridges replacing more than four teeth were excluded from coverage (Art. 1 No. 17a GSG).

In a next step, the BeitrEntlG almost entirely eliminated dental appliances from the SHI benefits package for persons born after 1978. Only in cases where accidents or other diseases caused the loss of teeth did dental appliances remain covered (Art. 2 No. 7). According to the explanatory memorandum, the age limit was set because people born after this date had received preventive dental care and were thus less likely to need dental appliances. The legislator assumed that those requiring dental appliances had not taken care of their teeth (BT–Drs. 12/3608, p. 80). Furthermore, artificial dentition based on implants was excluded for all insured. The exclusion was slightly diminished by the 2.GKV–NOG (Art. 1 No. 4) which allowed the provision of these implants, but only in exceptionally severe cases which were to be defined by the BAZÄK.

Coverage of orthodontic treatment was also greatly restricted. Firstly, the GRG limited entitlement to specific cases defined by the BAÄK. Furthermore, it changed entitlement from a benefit in kind to a reimbursement system.[38] Secondly, orthodontic treatment for adults was also almost completely excluded from the public benefits package. Only cases of severe anomalies of the jaw requiring a combination of surgical and orthodontic treatment were still covered (Art. 1 No. 15 GSG).

Ophthalmic care and optical appliances: Following in the footsteps of the Social–Liberal coalition, the GRG further reduced coverage of optical appliances. Persons older than 14 years received new glasses only if their eyesight had changed more than 0.5 dioptres (§ 33 (4) SGB V). Entitlement to lenses was restricted to 'urgent necessary exceptional cases' (§ 33 (3) SGB V). Care products for contact lenses were excluded entirely as were eyeglass frames (Art. 2 No. 9 BeitrEntlG).

Generosity – cost coverage

The Kohl government instituted a massive increase in co-payments. In order to reduce the cost burden for the most vulnerable, exemption policies were completely reformed. Formerly, the definition of 'hardship case' for exemption from co-payments had been left to the discretion of each health fund. With the change-over from RVO to SGB V in 1989, eligibility criteria for the exemption from co-payments were united within one regulation that applied to all SHI funds. The SGB V differentiated between full and partial exemption. Full exemption from all co-payments for pharmaceuticals, remedies, medical aids and appliances (including optical appliances), dental appliances, hospital treatment and all travelling costs was granted if the patient would have suffered an 'unacceptable burden' from co-payments (§ 61 SGB V). An unacceptable burden was determined to exist in cases of low income or the receipt of other social benefits (e.g. unemployment allowance). If the conditions of full exemption were not met, co-payments for pharmaceuticals, remedies and traveling costs had to be borne, up to a certain threshold, by the patient (§ 62 SGB V): low income earners had to make co-payments until the sum of co-payments reached two per cent of their income; for high income earners, a maximum threshold of four per cent of income applied. Children and young adults were generally exempted from paying charges. The 1.GKV–NOG (Art. 1 No. 1) amended the maximum co-payment threshold by switching the eligibility criterion from income to disease: a general threshold was set at two per cent of income for all income groups; only for patients suffering from a chronic disease did a lower threshold of one per cent apply.

The first and second SHI Restructuring Act implemented several reforms addressing cost coverage that never took effect because they were abolished by the new government directly after it came into office. First, the 2.GKV–NOG

(Art. 1 No. 19) provided for an automatic increase of co-payments for preventive and other regimens, pharmaceuticals, stationary rehabilitative services and traveling expenses as of 1.1.1999. The amount of the yearly increase was thereby determined by the increase in aggregated wages. Second, co-payments were pegged to the contribution rate: increases of the contribution rate of 0.1 percentage point caused all absolute co-payments to rise by 1 DM and all relative co-payments by one per cent (Art. 1 No. 4 1.GKV–NOG). Third, SHI funds were allowed to individually increase co-payments for their members (Art. 1 No. 15 2.GKV–NOG).

Primary care and specialised ambulatory care: In the course of the introduction of ambulatory psychotherapy by psychotherapists (see above), a co-payment of 10 DM per session for adults was introduced in 1996. For these co-payments, another maximum threshold of two per cent of the patient's income for the first, and one per cent for the following years was set. Children were exempted from paying charges, as well as pregnant women and young mothers, if their need for psychotherapy was related to their pregnancy or the birth of their child (§ 62 (1a) SGB V introduced by Art. 1 No. 4 9.SGBVÄndG).

Hospital care: Formerly unknown to the German SHI, the HBeglG 1983 introduced co-payments for hospital treatment for the first time.[39] Adult patients had to pay 5 DM per day for a maximum of 14 days per year (Art. 19 No. 5 HBeglG 1983). In 1991, charges were doubled (§ 39 (4) SGB V). They were further increased to 11 DM in 1993, to 12 DM in 1994 (both increases, Art. 1 No. 23c GSG) and to 17 DM in 1997 (Art. 1 No. 11 2.GKV–NOG).

Pharmaceuticals: The HBeglG doubled charges from 1 DM to 2 DM per item (Art. 19 No. 3). The GRG raised charges to 3 DM and arranged for a restructuring of co-payments as of 1 January 1992. There was a plan to introduce a 15 per cent co-payment for up to a ceiling of 15 DM for all drugs with no reference price (see below, § 31 SGB V). This plan was first postponed to 1 July 1993 with the 2.SGBVÄndG and then completely abolished by the GSG. The age ceiling for co-payment exemptions was increased from 16 to 18 years by the GRG (§ 31 SGB V). The 2.SGBVÄndG reduced the maximum co-payment for drugs and dressings from 15 DM to 10 DM (Art. 1 No. 8) in an attempt to keep the burden on the weakest members of society within limits, as the explanatory memorandum argued (BT–Drs. 12/1154, p. 5). The GSG then finally reformed co-payments: during the transition period (1.1.1993 – 31.12.1993), patients had to pay 3 DM per item for drugs and dressings equal to or less than 30 DM, 5 DM for items equal to or less than 50 DM and 7 DM for all items costing more than 50 DM (Art. 1 No. 18b GSG). As of 1 January 1994, patients were charged 3 DM for small packages, 5 DM for medium and 7 DM for large packages.[40] The BeitrEntlG 1996 raised all co-payments by 1 DM (Art. 2 No. 8a). The 2.GKV–NOG then further increased co-payments to 9 DM, 11 DM and 13 DM respectively (Art. 1 No. 8b).

The introduction, in 1989, of a reference pricing system for drugs (§ 12 (2) SGB V) had an even greater impact on cost coverage. The joint self-administration was tasked with defining maximum prices for pharmaceuticals sharing the same or similar active ingredients (§ 35 SGB V). Reimbursement was limited to that maximum price (§ 31 SGB V). If the patient wanted a drug more expensive than the defined price, s/he had to bear the additional costs. Initially, no co-payments applied for drugs without a reference price, but this exception was eliminated by the GSG which imposed co-payments on these pharmaceuticals, too.

Similar to the reform plans for drugs, the GRG restructured charges for remedies: the co-payment of 4 DM per prescription was replaced by a charge of 10 per cent of costs (§ 32 SGB V). In this case, the reform was put into effect. The 2.GKV–NOG later raised co-payments to 15 per cent of costs (Art. 1 No. 9).

Medical aids and appliances: A reference pricing system was also implemented for medical aids and appliances through the GRG (§36 SGB V). Hence, only the agreed upon reference price was reimbursed. In addition, the 2.GKV–NOG introduced a co-payment for bandages, orthotics and medical aids for compression therapy of 20 per cent of costs (Art. 1 No. 10).[41]

Dental care and appliances: As had its predecessor, the Kohl government further aligned cost coverage of dentures between funds. The national associations of SHI funds were assigned to determine the cost coverage of dental appliances in 1989. § 30 SGB V stipulated that they were to establish categories of cost coverage ranging between 40 and 60 per cent, whereby complex appliances should receive lower subsidies. According to the explanatory memorandum, subsidies for more complex appliances were set lower than those for less complex ones in order to encourage personal dental hygiene (BT–Drs. 11/2237, p. 172). For the same purpose, the GRG determined that subsidies for dental appliances were to be increased by 10 and 15 per cent respectively if the patient had regularly attended preventive dental examination (§ 30 (5) SGB V).

In 1996, after the BeitrEntlG had excluded dental appliances almost entirely for individuals born after 1978 (see above), the subsidies for those born before 1978 were changed from a percentage to fixed sum payments which were to be defined by the BAZÄK (Art. 1 No. 6 2.GKV–NOG). As part of the same reform, the subsidy reward for good dental hygiene was increased to 20 per cent (Art. 1 No. 6d).

Contrary to the general retrenchment policies, the 2.SGBVÄndG determined that people not exempted from co-payments, but who earned just above the income ceiling established in § 61 (2) SGB V, would pay a smaller share of costs for dental appliances (Art. 1 No. 20).

SHI orthodontic treatment had been provided as benefit in kind in the past. The GRG introduced a reimbursement system instead, which was a break with one of the core principals of the SHI (Döhler 1990, p. 490). In principle, 80 per cent of costs were reimbursed (§ 29 SGB V); but if two or more children from one family underwent orthodontic treatment, coverage for the second as well as any additional child was increased to 90 per cent of costs. The remaining costs were covered by SHI only if patients fully completed treatment.

Ophthalmic care and optical appliances: The reference pricing system for medical aids and appliances implemented by the GRG also applied to glasses. Thus, patients were only reimbursed the reference price. The same was true for frames. Here, patients could choose between frames for which a reference price was established, or a 20 DM subsidy if no reference prices applied (§ 33 (4) and § 36 SGB V). This already minimal subsidy for frames was abolished in 1996, and frames were totally removed from the SHI benefits package (Art.2 No. 9 BeitrEntlG).

Summary

During their 16 years in office, the Christian Democrats and Liberals retrenched generosity of and access to healthcare entitlement as no other government had done before. Yet reforms differed in intensity and focus over time. The first six years were characterised by low reform activity, and with regard to healthcare entitlement, the Kohl government merely realised the plans of its predecessor. Then, in 1988, the government passed the most comprehensive and incisive entitlement reform of its term with the GRG. The next big reform, the GSG cut entitlement, too, but its focus was on structural reforms and hence, healthcare entitlement cuts were less comprehensive and severe than those of the GRG. Between the GRG and the GSG one small reform stood out: the 2.SGBV-ÄndG attenuated cost coverage reforms in order to lower the cost burden for the ill and low income earners. After the GSG, six years passed without any entitlement reform, but then three incisive reforms followed: the BeitrEntlG, the first and the second GKV–NOG.

With regard to *population coverage*, the CDU/CSU/FDP government followed the path of its predecessor, at least during its first decade in office. It further restricted access to SHI membership for pensioners and the voluntarily insured. Based on an understanding of solidarity which implies reciprocity, its policies followed the principle of consideration: only those who have done their bit (i.e. those who have paid contributions) were entitled to receive benefits in the case of need. Contrary to this notion of solidarity, family members were granted almost full rights without being required to contribute. Interestingly, population coverage was no longer the focus of the Christian Democratic–Liberal government after 1992, and no further limitations or expansions were made.

With regard to *generosity*, reforms followed a piecemeal strategy, often inter-linking service coverage and cost coverage measures.[42] Again, mainly non-core areas such as dental and optical appliances, and medical aids and appliances were subject to reform. This time, however, core service areas (ambulatory and hospital care) were also under attack. Furthermore, restrictions of drug coverage were severe and affected more than just a particular type of drug. A new mode of retrenchment was to restrict *service coverage* by tightening service criteria. The GRG required all services provided by SHI to be 'economic', and the joint self-administration was tasked with assessing services and applying these criteria. In a similar vein, clear limits of SHI coverage were set out through applying the principle of self-responsibility and through restricting the provision of services falling within the 'personal sphere' of the insured. Although on average, reforms massively cut generosity of SHI, almost all reforms included measures that broadened coverage. Most were designed for future savings (e.g. dental prevention, hospice services). *Co-payments* were continuously increased, with the effect that the share of co-payments in SHI expenditures rose from 3.1 per cent in 1982 to 4.9 in 1985 (Döhler 1990, p. 414). These numbers, however, do not reveal the whole picture.

Reference pricing schemes were a clever instrument for politicians to increase the cost burden for patients without risking too much blame: patients could get treatment for free, but choices between different treatments became costly.

3.5 Social Democratic–Green healthcare entitlement reforms 1998–2005

What had happened in the UK in 1997 occurred in Germany one year later: long-term conservative rule ended, and the centre-left assumed power. Contrary to the situation in the UK, however, the Social Democrats were forced to share power with the Greens. Furthermore, the renewal of the SPD was not yet as advanced as it was by their counterparts in the UK. Nonetheless, the change of government was triggered by the same desire for policy change. This section describes to what degree these wishes were fulfilled in health policy generally, and healthcare entitlement policies in particular. Similarly as in the previous sections, first an overview of the general political and economic situation is given, and then major health policies of the new government are presented. Most of the section is dedicated to the description and analysis of healthcare entitlement reforms under the Red–Green government. Results are summarised at the end of the section.

Political and economic background

After 16 years at the helm of government, Kohl was forced to step down in 1998. He stood for reelection, but the CDU and CSU saw the worst poll results since 1949. The Social Democrats, with their charismatic leader Gerhard Schröder, drew in 40.9 per cent of the vote and decided to form a coalition with the Green Party. In its first year, the government was lacking a coherent vision, and policies resembled a trial and error process (Egle, Ostheim and Zohlnhöfer 2003, p. 17). With regard to social policies, it delivered on its election pledges and otherwise remained rather inactive. Especially between late 1999 and 2001, reform activity was low as unexpected growth, falling unemployment and good poll results lowered the pressure to make reforms (Egle, Ostheim and Zohlnhöfer 2003, p. 18; Seeleib-Kaiser 2003, p. 348). Substantial reforms would have been hard to realise, because the governing coalition parties had lost their majority in the *Bundesrat* in April 1999. Unemployment and subsequent reform activity increased again in late 2001 (Egle, Ostheim and Zohlnhöfer 2003, p. 18; Seeleib-Kaiser 2003, p. 348).

In 2002, polls indicated a coming change of government with the next *Bundestag* elections, but several clever moves on the part of the ruling coalition, a major flood in East Germany and the possibility of war in Iraq, all helped to turn the tide (Egle, Ostheim and Zohlnhöfer 2003, p. 20). Nevertheless, the second Red–Green coalition was forced to govern with a weak majority of four seats in the *Bundestag* and no majority in the *Bundesrat*. Furthermore, it experienced a rough start as the economy was weaker than expected and the public budget faced a large deficit. At first, the government seemed to have no answers and lacked any strategy to solve the problems (Zohlnhöfer and Egle 2007, p. 12). But this changed with

Schröder's government statement of March 2003, in which he outlined the Agenda 2010 strategy (Zohlnhöfer and Egle 2007, p. 13). The Agenda 2010 redefined the basic principles of the Social Democrats: The welfare state was no longer seen as a means to granting the working population a fair share of society's wealth; instead, the primary goal of social policy was to increase employment in order to enable people to take part in the market (Hegelich, Knollmann and Kuhlmann 2011, pp. 12f.). With this radical reform of social democratic principles, the 'Agenda 2010' is analogous to New Labour in the UK (Hegelich, Knollmann and Kuhlmann 2011, p. 12). The most famous and radical elements of the Agenda 2010 were the pension reform of 2001[43] and the Hartz reforms[44] of 2002/2003. With this pension reform, the Red–Green government moved away from the German social insurance model and introduced a publicly subsidised private pension (*Riester-Rente*), reduced the average pension and adopted a tax-financed and means-tested basic public pension (Hegelich, Knollmann and Kuhlmann 2011, pp. 28ff.; Schmidt 2003, pp. 247ff.). The Hartz reforms introduced the principles of 'promoting and demanding' (*Fördern und Fordern*), the German equivalent to Blair's 'rights and responsibilities', into the German labour and unemployment system. The reforms were comprised of various measures ranging from organisational restructuring of the public employment agency to the tightening of eligibility criteria for unemployment benefits. The core element of the Hartz reforms was the amalgamation of unemployment aid[45] and social assistance for Unemployment Benefit II (*Arbeitslosengeld II*), a basic benefit for all persons able to work.

The Agenda 2010 reforms were not uncontested. They met staunch resistance from the unions which mobilised thousands of people to demonstrate against the reforms in 2003 (Zohlnhöfer and Egle 2007, p. 15). The reforms also led to a major dispute within the governing coalition parties, which caused an unstable majority: several SPD and Green members of the *Bundestag* threatened to (and some did) vote against reforms (Zohlnhöfer and Egle 2007, pp. 14f.). In the wake of the Agenda 2010, the SPD and Greens lost several *Länder* elections, with the result that all state governments were either held by the opposition or by coalitions formed of governing and opposition parties. In response, Chancellor Schröder called snap elections in May 2005.

Social Democratic–Green health policy

Directly after entering office, the new government delivered on their election pledges by withdrawing several competition elements and cost burden increases introduced by the previous government through an interim law (*Vorschaltgesetz*).[46] This reform sought to further remedy the precarious financial situation of SHI by enforcing several budgetary restrictions (Deppe 2005, pp. 100ff.; Reiners and Müller 2012, p. 37). In 1999, the Red–Green government drafted a comprehensive structural reform, the SHI Reform Act 2000 (*GKV–Gesundheitsreformgesetz 2000*, GKVRefG). Amongst others, this reform contained measures to further integrate the ambulatory and stationary sectors, strengthen primary care, enhance patient information and counselling, tighten sectoral budgets, expand quality assurance and quality management measures, and introduce a flat rate hospital reimbursement system based on diagnosis related groups (Deppe 2005, pp. 120ff.; Reiners and Müller 2012, pp. 44f.). Once again, core elements, such as the introduction of a global budget and the reform of hospital financing, could not be realised due to the broad opposition of the *Länder* (Brandhorst 2003, pp. 215f.; Deppe 2005, p. 120).[47]

After its reelection, the government once again took up with an interim law[48] to confine SHI expenditures and to stabilise contribution rates, which in 2001, for the first time, reached 14 per cent of gross income (Hartmann 2003, p. 266). The reform again had to be split in order to evade being blocked by the *Bundesrat*. Most measures requiring approval of the *Bundesrat* could not be passed. The part of the reform not requiring approval was mainly comprised of cost-containment measures affecting providers (Bandelow and Hartmann 2007, pp. 336f.).

In his policy statement on the Agenda 2010, Chancellor Schröder presented the framework for a comprehensive health reform. The presented plans already included concessions to the opposition, which Schröder knew he needed since opposition parties had been holding the majority in the *Bundesrat* since May 2002 (Blank 2011, p. 122). In close cooperation with the CDU/CSU, the government worked out a comprehensive health reform with the biggest retrenchment in the history of the SHI (Deppe 2005, p. 143). This health reform – the SHI Modernisation Act (*Gesundheitsmodernisierungsgesetz*, GMG) – can be seen as the litmus test for the Agenda 2010 retrenchment which followed in other social areas. Core retrenchment elements of the reform included the reduction of cost coverage (see below) and the suspension of parity financing of SHI for sick pay financed exclusively from contributions of the insured. Moreover, the GMG implemented various competition elements, but unlike the competition policies of the Christian Democrats and Liberals, these aimed at increasing competition between providers instead of between SHI funds (Brandhorst 2003, pp. 220ff.).[49]

Social Democratic–Green healthcare entitlement reforms

Both major health reforms of the Red–Green government strongly affected healthcare entitlement. Also extremely relevant was the first health law from the Red–Green government – the Act on the Promotion of Solidarity in Statutory Health Insurance (GKV–SolG) – which fulfilled election promises and strove to consolidate SHI expenditures. Moreover, several smaller reforms effected single amendments of healthcare entitlement (see Table 3.4). Additionally, modifications of SHI population coverage often resulted from reforms conducted in other social programmes.

Germany incorporated European case law concerning treatment abroad[50] into its social security law in 2004 (§ 13 (4) and (5) SGB V as introduced by the GMG). German SHI members were granted the right, in addition to that of the E112 scheme, to go abroad to EEA countries for treatment (see Chapter 2.7). This right was subject to several restrictions more or less resembling the criteria established by the ECJ. First, choice of providers was limited to 'approved providers',

Table 3.4 Reforms affecting healthcare entitlement, Germany 1998–2005[51]

Law German short title	Adoption Commencement	Abbreviation
Act on the Promotion of Solidarity in SHI *GKV–Solidaritätsstärkungsgesetz*	19.12.1998 *01.01.1999*	GKVSolG
SHI Reform Act 2000 *GKV–Gesundheitsreformgesetz 2000*	22.12.1999 *01.01.2000*	GKVRefG
Law to end the Discrimination of same-sex couples *Gesetz zur Beendigung der Diskriminierung* *gleichgeschlechtlicher Gemeinschaften*	16.02.2001 *01.08.2001*	/
Tenth SGB V Amendment Act *Zehntes SGB V Änderungsgesetz*	23.03.2002 *29.03.2002*	10.SGBVÄndG
Contribution Rate Stabilisation Act *Beitragssatzsicherungsgesetz*	23.12.2002 *01.01.2003*	BSSichG
SHI-Modernisation Act *GKV–Modernisierungsgesetz*	14.11.2003 *01.01.2004*	GMG
Fourth Act for Modern Services on the Labour Market *Viertes Gesetz für moderne Dienstleistungen am* *Arbeitsmarkt*	24.12.2003 *01.01.2004*	/
Act to Adjust the Financing of Dentures *Gesetz zur Anpassung der Finanzierung von* *Zahnersatz*	15.12.2004 *21.12.2004*	/

i.e. providers providing services for the public health system of the foreign country or whose profession is regulated by EU law. Second, costs were reimbursed only up to the level of those that would have been incurred in Germany, and patients were responsible for paying administrative costs and German co-payments. If treatment was not possible in Germany, the insurance fund could incur any costs. Third, for hospital treatment, patients had to obtain prior approval from their health fund. However, the fund was not to deny allowance if an equivalent treatment was not available in Germany in a timely manner.

Being 'instruments of private insurance', and as such being foreign to the system of social health insurance (BT–Drs. 14/24, p. 18), the possibility of service differentiation between health funds, as well as the possibility for health funds to extend their benefits package beyond the general SHI level (formerly § 56 SGB V), were abolished by the GKVSolG (Art. 1 No. 7).

Governance – who decides about healthcare entitlement?

The GKVGRefG once again expanded the regulatory tasks of the joint self-administration.[52] Besides other new tasks, it was responsible for the definition of SHI coverage of hospital services (see below). For this new duty, a Hospital Committee (*Ausschuss Krankenhaus*) was established. This was staffed by representatives of the national associations of SHI funds and SHI Physicians, as well as by representatives of the German Hospital Federation (*Deutsche Krankenhausge-sellschaft*) (§ 137c (2) SGB V).

In 2004, the legislature restructured the joint self-administration: its committees – the Federal Committee of Physicians and Sickness Funds, the Federal Committee of Dentists and Sickness Funds, the Hospital Committee and the Coordination Committee[53] – were merged into a joint committee called the Federal Joint Committee (FJC). The FJC consisted of three independent members, of whom one was the chairman of the FJC, nine representatives of the SHI funds and nine representatives of providers' associations. Altogether, the FJC had six sub-committees, each responsible for a different service area. Coverage decisions were taken in these sub-committees. The inclusion of patients into decision-making was new to the joint self-administration system, although they were without voting rights. As part of the same reform, the role of the FJC in defining the health benefits package was once again specified. This had become necessary due to several decisions of the Federal Social Court challenging the legal basis of coverage decisions made by the BAÄK. In the course of the reform, the power of the FJC to exclude services was enacted into law. According to the amended § 92 (1) SGB V, the FJC may 'restrict or exclude the provision and prescription of services and benefits if the diagnostic or therapeutic benefit, the medical necessity or the efficiency according to the generally accepted state of the art of medical knowledge is not proven' (author's translation).

Furthermore, the GMG established a new body, the Institute for Quality and Efficiency in healthcare (*Institut für Qualität und Wirtschaftlichkeit im Gesundheitswesen*, IQWiG). The IQWiG is comprised of independent experts and tasked with conducting health technology assessments, on the basis of which the FJC takes its coverage decisions. IQWiG recommendations strongly influence FJC coverage decisions, but final decision-making power remains with the FJC. For this reason, reforms concerning IQWIG are not considered in the further course of this study.

Access – population coverage

Following the policies of its precursors, the Red–Green government further tightened access to SHI membership. With the GKVRefG, the possibility of returning to SHI after having held a private insurance was abolished for people over the age of 54 if they had not been insured with SHI for at least the last five years (§ 6 (3a) SGB V, introduced by Art. 1 No. 3 GKVRefG). In addition, the possibility to voluntarily insure with SHI after having been insured as a family member of an SHI insurant was limited by introducing a minimum membership period of 24 months within the last five years, or 12 months within the last 12 months (Art. 1 No. 5 GKVRefG). At the same time, the criteria for family insurance were tightened as to abolish the possibility of SHI coverage for spouses during maternal and parental leave who had not been insured with SHI before the child was born (Art. 1 No. 6 GKVRefG).

In 2000, the Federal Constitutional Court declared the tightening of coverage criteria for pensioners (implemented with the GSG in 1992) unconstitutional.

Because the government did not reregulate the coverage conditions of pensioners, the old status (before the GSG reform) was reconstituted in 2002. This meant that all voluntarily insured pensioners meeting the old minimum compulsory membership period became compulsorily insured. In order to avoid contribution increases for this group, the 10th SGB V Reform Act gave those people the right to join SHI. Thus, pensioners could decide if they wanted to join SHI and pay pensioner contributions, or if they wanted to remain voluntarily insured. This was a generous regulation costing roughly 40 million DM (explanatory memorandum BT–Drs. 14/8099, p. 3).

Between 2001 and 2003, population coverage was amended by several reforms not primarily aimed at changing SHI membership. With the introduction of civil partnerships[54] in 2001, most social rights formerly granted to married partners only were conferred to spouses living in a civil (same-sex) partnership. With regard to healthcare rights (and responsibilities), these partnerships received almost the same status as married couples. Thus, partners of SHI members became entitled to family coverage, i.e. they became insured by SHI if they were not insured themselves.

In the course of the restructuring of unemployment benefits and social assistance (see above), SHI membership of recipients was amended. Beneficiaries of Unemployment Benefit II became compulsorily insured,[55] while beneficiaries of social assistance remained excluded from SHI membership.[56] This meant a huge expansion of SHI coverage, as roughly 90 per cent of social assistance beneficiaries were transferred from social assistance to Unemployment Benefit II (Eekhoff 2008, p. 20) and hence became covered by SHI. Remaining recipients of social assistance who had never held a private health insurance before and who had never been insured with SHI got the one-time possibility to join SHI as voluntary members between 1 January and 30 June 2005 (§ 9 (1) No. 8 SGB V, introduced by Art. 5 No. 3a Fourth Act for Modern Services on the Labour Market, see also Kruse and Hänlein 2004, p. 33). Beneficiaries of Unemployment Benefit I remained compulsorily insured.

Generosity – service coverage

Prevention: The GKVRefG extended primary prevention, yet most measures fell under the voluntary provision of the SHI funds. SHI funds were again allowed to provide primary prevention as statutory services,[57] and they were asked to provide occupational health promotion. In addition, the promotion of self-help groups and organisations was expanded by instructing SHI funds to spend 1 DM per member per year for the advancement of self-help groups and by changing the wording of the regulation from 'may' to 'shall' (Art. 1 No. 8 GKVRefG). The obligation of SHI funds to promote and fund dental prophylaxis for children at schools and kindergartens, where the risk for dental diseases is especially high, was extended to cover children up to the age of 15 (Art. 1 No. 9 GKVRefG). The age limit for schools with 'normal' risk remained 12 years. Arguing that individual prophylactic dental services for adults were 'unspecific' and thus 'ineffective' and 'inefficient', the government omitted these services from coverage with the same reform (explanatory memorandum BT–Drs. 14/1245, p. 64).

Primary care and specialised ambulatory care: In 2000, supportive social care for mentally ill people (*Soziotherapie*) was added to the SHI benefits package (§ 37a SGB V introduced by Art. 1 No. 18 GKVRefG). This type of treatment focuses on mentally ill persons having a low compliance with treatment due to their disease. It was hoped that hospital treatment could be avoided if ambulatory treatment were coordinated. For this reason, the prevention of hospital treatment was made a precondition for the receipt of supportive social care. The services were limited to 120 hours within three years, and the BAÄK was tasked with defining further eligibility criteria.

Sterilisation was eliminated from the SHI benefits package in 2003. It was now covered only if necessary due to a disease (Art. 1 No. 11 GMG). The GMG also greatly restricted reimbursement for artificial insemination (Art. 1 No. 14 GMG). Service coverage was reduced from four to three trials. Furthermore, the law tightened eligibility criteria by introducing an age limit which ranged between 25 and 40 years for women, and between 25 and 50 years for men. This age limit was much more restrictive than the age limit set by the Fertility Directive of the FJC. The deepest cut, however, was the reduction of cost coverage from 100 to 50 per cent of costs.

Hospital care: The GKVRefG, for the first time in SHI history, introduced the possibility for exclusion of hospital services from the SHI benefits package. At the request of one of the national associations of SHI funds, the newly established Hospital Committee of the joint self-administration had to assess if a particular diagnosis or treatment method complied with the criteria of appropriateness, sufficiency and efficiency as demanded by the SGB V. If the result was negative, it had to be removed from SHI coverage. Compared to ambulatory services, the default for hospital services is reversed: as long as the joint self-administration does not take a decision, any method is covered.

Pharmaceuticals: The health reform of 1999 again attempted to introduce a positive list for drugs, i.e. a list of all active ingredients being reimbursed by SHI. The positive list was drawn up by the ministry, but the corresponding law[58] was rejected by the *Bundesrat*, where the opposition held the majority.

Over-the-counter (OTC) drugs were almost completely excluded from coverage in 2003 (Art. 1 No. 22 GMG).[59] Only children younger than 12 years and young adults with a developmental disorder remained eligible. OTC drugs belonging to the standard treatment of severe diseases also continued to be covered. The FJC was tasked with defining these exemptions in its Pharmaceutical Directive.

Pharmaceuticals 'primarily aiming at improving the quality of life', such as drugs for the treatment of erectile dysfunction, smoking cessation or weight reduction, were prohibited for provision (§ 35b SGB V introduced by Art. 1 No. 22 GMG). These so called 'lifestyle drugs' had already been excluded from coverage by the Pharmaceutical Directive of the FJC, but the legal status of this type of directive was contested (Orlowski and Wasem 2003, p. 53).

The GMG provided for the testing of an 'additional benefit' (*Zusatznutzen*) of pharmaceuticals with a new active ingredient (Art. 1 No. 25). For this task, the joint self-administration was commissioned to found an institute for the assessment of new drugs and treatments (IQWIG, see above). On the basis of IQWIG assessments, the FJC issues compulsory recommendations in its Pharmaceutical Directive about the scope of application, or it excludes the drug from SHI coverage.

The ministerial order listing 'inefficient' pharmaceuticals not covered by SHI was amended twice.[60] In 2000, the first amendment shortened the list of non-reimbursed drugs combining two or more active agents, from 22 to 12. Furthermore, the list of active ingredients for which effectiveness was not proven was extended from 264 substances (mainly homeopathic or herbal substances) to 828, of which 331 were homeopathic substances, 126 herbal substances and 73 baths and bath additives. The second amendment, in 2002, made only minor changes. In 2003, the ministerial order was updated and integrated into the Pharmaceutical Directive of FJC. Since then, it has rarely been updated.

Dental care and appliances: The GKVSolG withdrew the exclusion of dental appliances for people born after 1978. It furthermore re-introduced the principle of benefits in kind for dental appliances (see section on cost coverage). The GKVRefG went on to retract the general exclusion of dental prostheses based on implants (called 'super-constructions'). These super-constructions could be provided in exceptional cases, which had to be specified by the BAZÄK (Art. 1 No. 17 GKVRefG). The GMG again intended to almost completely ban dental appliances from SHI coverage (Art. 1 No. 17). This plan, however, was rejected by the Red–Green government before it could take effect in 2004.[61]

Similar to the reform of dental appliances, orthodontic treatment for children once again became a benefit in kind. However, the patient's contribution of 20 per cent of costs until treatment was completely finished was maintained (Reiners and Müller 2012, p. 43).

Ophthalmic care and optical appliances: Visual aids were almost completely eliminated from the SHI benefits package in 2003. Only children and young adults below the age of 18, people with very severe visual impairment and people needing a therapeutic visual aid in the course of a treatment of an injury or optical disease remained eligible (Art. 1 No. 20 GMG).

Generosity – cost coverage

The GKVSolG withdrew or softened several reforms affecting cost coverage that had been implemented by the former government: patients suffering from chronic disease were fully exempted from co-payments if they had spent at least one per cent of their income on co-payments the previous year (Art. 1 No. 9a), and the linkage between contribution rates and co-payment increases was abolished (Art. 1 No. 25) before any such case ever occurred, as was the automatic increase of co-payments for preventive and other regimens, pharmaceuticals, stationary rehabilitative services and traveling expenses (Art. 1 No.10). The possibility of varying co-payments between health funds was also eliminated (Art. 1 No. 7).

Co-payments were completely reformed by the GMG in 2003. All co-payments became centrally regulated in § 61 SGB V and most co-payments were equal to

10 per cent of costs with a minimum of 5 Euro and a maximum of 10 Euro. Only hospital treatment and other stationary treatment had charges of 10 Euro per day. This alignment meant a decrease in cost coverage for most service areas (for details, see below). In the course of the same reform, total exemption from charges was abolished, and the new co-payment limit was applied to all insured. This means that persons formerly not having had to make any co-payments (e.g. people receiving unemployment benefits or low income earners), now had to pay one or two per cent of their income, no matter how high this income was. In return, all co-payments counted towards the maximum charge amount, while formerly only co-payments for drugs, dressings and remedies had been taken into account (Orlowski and Wasem 2003, p. 67). The limit remained more or less the same: one per cent of the yearly gross income for the chronically ill, and two per cent for all other patients.

The GMG introduced a flat co-payment, called 'practice charge' (*Praxisgebühr*) of 10 Euro. The charge was incurred with every first visit of an ambulatory doctor within a quarter year (§ 28 (4) SGB V introduced by Art. 1 No. 15 GMG). The fee was charged for medical, dental and psychotherapeutic treatments separately, which means patients had to pay 30 Euro if they had all three categories of treatments within a quarter. The charge did not apply to preventive services.

Primary care and specialised ambulatory care: The GKVSolG completely abolished co-payments for ambulatory psychotherapy (Art. 2 No. 1). The GMG was less generous, cutting coverage for artificial insemination to half of costs (Art. 1 No. 14), and introducing a co-payment for supportive social care of 10 per cent of costs per day, with a 5 Euro minimum and 10 Euro maximum (Art. 1 No. 28).

Hospital care: The GMG increased co-payments for hospital treatment from 9 to 10 Euro per day, and prolonged the maximum time for which co-payments have to be paid from 14 to 28 days (Art. 1 No. 30).

Pharmaceuticals: The SPD–Green government reduced co-payments for pharmaceuticals in 1998 from 9 to 8 DM for small, from 11 to 9 DM for medium and from 13 to 10 DM for large packages (Art. 1 No. 5b GKVSolG). With the GMG (Art. 1 No. 31), co-payments were increased again from 4 Euro for small, 4.50 Euro for medium and 5 Euro for large packages, to 10 per cent of costs with a 5 Euro minimum and a 10 Euro maximum per drug. The same reform extended the reference pricing system to cover pharmaceuticals with patent protection, with the exception of drugs containing new active ingredients bringing about a therapeutic improvement, or for which no similar treatment exists (§ 35 SGB V as amended by the GMG). Co-payments for remedies were decreased by the GMG from 15 per cent of costs to 10 per cent of costs (Art. 1 No. 19). However, patients had to pay an additional 10 Euro per prescription.

Medical aids and appliances: Co-payments were reduced by the GMG from 20 per cent to 10 per cent with a 5 Euro minimum and a 10 Euro maximum. Furthermore, co-payments for medical aids with a high application rate, like stoma pouches for example, were capped at 10 Euro per month per indication (Art. 1 No. 20). At the same time, however, co-payments were extended from bandages, insoles and medical aids for compression therapy to apply to all medical aids (Orlowski and Wasem 2003, p. 63).

For many of the medical aids and appliances (e.g. visual aids, mobility aids, toilet aids) the regional associations of health funds had set a fixed price valid for their particular federal state. With the GMG reform (Art. 1 No. 90), price definition was moved to the national level, and health funds were allowed to negotiate cheaper prices with manufacturers. If they did so, cost coverage was lowered to the average price of the cheapest third of negotiated prices. As a result, patients had to either get their medical aids and appliances from a producer with whom their health fund had negotiated a price, or pay additional costs.

Dental care and appliances: With the reintegration of dental appliances into the public health benefits package, the principle of reimbursement of costs, along with the reference pricing system, were abolished, and dental appliances were once again provided as benefits in kind. These changes to the system did not affect generosity: co-payments came to equal what they had before.

In 2003, the CDU/CSU and the government negotiated to exclude dental appliances from coverage again. Unlike the previous reform, SHI funds were this time obligated to provide for cost coverage of dental appliances in their statutes (Art. 1 No. 36 GMG affecting §§ 56–59 SGB V). The crux of the reform was that SHI funds were to levy additional contributions to be borne solely by employees. The insured were given the choice of being insured through their health fund or taking out private insurance covering at least the same amount of treatment costs as their SHI fund. The FJC was commissioned with defining diagnoses and standard treatments fulfilling conditions of medical necessity, i.e. those to be reimbursed by the SHI funds. In addition, the FJC was to determine costs for standard treatments. From this fixed amount, the SHI funds had to cover 50 per cent (*Festzuschüsse*), irrespective of the actual costs of treatment. The percentage of reimbursed costs increased if the patient had taken care of their teeth and had regularly undergone preventive treatment. The law provided for several exemptions (mainly people with low income or benefit receipts) for which SHI funds were to cover the entire cost of treatment, but no more than the fixed sum determined by the FJC. However, before this reform could come into effect, it was abolished by the Act to Adjust the Financing of Dentures, and thus, dental appliances remained covered. The choice between SHI and private funds for obligatory insurance of dental appliances was not introduced. But not all reforms were reversed. The fixed reimbursement remained, i.e. patients received only a fixed sum equal to 50 per cent of standard costs. Furthermore, the additional contribution was still required, and even increased to 0.9 per cent of income.

Summary

The electorate had high hopes that the Greens, and in particular the Social Democrats, would alter the course of social policy towards more social justice and less retrenchment. At first, it seemed as if the new government would meet these expectations as it withdrew the previous government's retrenchment measures right away. But everything that came afterwards – at least with regard to healthcare entitlement – followed the old retrenchment path of their predecessors. The

GKVRefG further restricted access to SHI membership; it lowered service coverage by introducing a positive list of drugs; and it opened up the exclusion of coverage for hospital treatment. However, it did not touch cost coverage, and it slightly expanded prevention. The big bang retrenchment came four years later: in joint cooperation with the opposition, the SPD and Greens excluded various services and massively limited cost coverage.[62] Service coverage cuts focused particularly on services for which medical need was low or contested (e.g. OTC drugs, sterilisation, lifestyle drugs).

The Red–Greens followed their predecessors in another aspect: they further expanded the role of the joint self-administration in defining SHI healthcare entitlement. For this purpose, they diversified decision-making processes and restructured the relevant bodies (see Chapter 3.8 for further discussion).

Interestingly, amendments to population coverage followed two directions. First, the GKVRefG again tightened access to SHI membership for non-compulsory members. Contrary to this trend, membership access was then broadened the following years. The inclusion of recipients of social assistance and of civil partners, however, did not originate from health policy but was the 'by-product' of other policies, and easier access for pensioners resulted from an FCC judgement.

3.6 Grand coalition healthcare entitlement reforms 2005–2009

The snap elections of 2005 unexpectedly resulted in a joint government of CDU/CSU and SPD. Although health policy was one of the core themes of the Grand Coalition, reforms of healthcare entitlement could nearly be counted on the fingers of one hand. Nevertheless, with regard to population coverage, the coalition government fundamentally altered the health system. In this section, all relevant healthcare entitlement reforms are described. Beforehand, a short outline of the election results and of the general economic conditions, as well as an overview of important reforms in the health sector are given. A short summary is provided at the end.

Political and economic background

The outcome of the snap elections in 2005 was as unexpected as the elections themselves. Compared to the 2002 elections, the Social Democrats lost votes, but the CDU/CSU opposition did too. The Christian Democrats could not convince the electorate it would improve things (Kornelius and Roth 2007, p. 37) and drew in only one per cent more votes than the SPD.[63] Winners of the 2005 elections were the small parties: the Greens captured 8.1 per cent, the FDP 9.8 per cent and the new left alliance of PDS[64] and the Electoral Alternative for Labour and Social Justice, The Left Party.PDS[65] took 8.7 per cent. With these results, neither a CDU/CSU/FDP nor an SPD/Green government was possible, and hence, 'out of necessity' (Egle and Zohlnhöfer 2010, p. 11), the CDU/CSU and SPD formed a grand coalition.

A grand coalition provides the opportunity to realise far-reaching reforms because it commands a comfortable majority of the *Bundestag* and vetoes by the

Bundesrat are not to be feared. At the same time, however, a grand coalition also runs the risk of postponing reforms to the next legislative period and of implementing only small compromises (Egle and Zohlnhöfer 2010, pp. 18ff.). With regard to social policy, the Grand Coalition pursued the path of the Agenda 2010, but less radically than the former government had (Schmidt 2010). The retirement age, for example, was increased to 67, and simultaneously, cuts in public pensions made by the Red–Green government were reduced. The welfare state was even expanded in areas such as elderly care and family policies (Schmidt 2010, pp. 305ff.). The coalition could afford these generous policies as economic conditions were good during their first three years in office. The economy grew by more than three per cent in 2006 and 2007, and unemployment decreased from 13 per cent in 2005 to 8.7 in 2008 (Statistisches Bundesamt 2014). When the global financial crisis hit Germany in the fall of 2008, GDP growth fell to 1.1 per cent, and to negative 5.1 per cent in 2009 (OECD 2014a). In response to the crisis, the government implemented various demand-side measures and expanded short-time work (Schmidt 2010, p. 314). The crisis coincided with election campaigns, and thus crisis management was laced with election year bonuses such as pension and child benefit increases, and decreases in health insurance contributions (Schmidt 2010, p. 315).

Grand coalition health policy

Unlike during the previous elections, health policy played an important role in the 2005 campaigns. Social Democrats and Christian Democrats developed opposing reform models for the future financing of SHI. The SPD promoted a 'citizens' insurance' (*Bürgerversicherung*) covering all German residents – which resolved the dualism of private and public health insurance – and financed from contributions based on total as opposed to earned income. The CDU/CSU proposed a 'capitation fee' (*Kopfpauschale*) consisting of two parts: a contribution paid by the employer as a percentage of income, and a flat rate premium paid by the employee (see Reiners and Müller 2012). The employer's contribution was to be fixed, meaning that future cost increases would be borne by employees alone. Furthermore, this model adhered to the dual system of private and public health insurances. Since both parties formed the government, they had to find a compromise integrating the antagonistic concepts. The result was a reformed financial SHI architecture that contained elements of both models, but allowed for future developments in both directions. Contributions remained based on income paid by the employer and employee. The power to define the contribution rate was taken from the funds; instead the government[66] determined a general contribution rate that applied to all funds. The contributions are pooled together with money from the state budget within a central fund (*Gesundheitsfonds*), and the money is then distributed amongst SHI funds according to gender, age and health status of the insured. If health funds need more resources than they get from the central fund, they must levy an 'additional premium' (*Zusatzbeitrag*). The dual system of private and public insurances was retained, but a general obligation to insure was introduced (see below).

The reforms just described were implemented with the Act to Strengthen Competition in Statutory Health Insurance (*Gesetz zur Stärkung des Wettbewerbs in der gesetzlichen Krankenversicherung*, GKV–WSG), the only major healthcare reform of the Grand Coalition. Apart from the financial reforms, it also implemented various measures to increase competition between SHI funds (e.g. optional tariffs), reformed the ambulatory reimbursement system, and replaced the national associations of SHI funds by the National Association of SHI Funds (*GKV-Spitzenverband*), to name only the most important measures.[67]

Compared to previous reforms, providers, health funds and other lobbyists had only weak influence on reform outcomes because of the strong political coalition and the fact that most core decisions were taken by the heads of government parties (Hartmann 2010, pp. 338ff.; Paquet and Schroeder 2009, p. 21). This might explain why the government now succeeded in disempowering the provider organisations, and in particular the health funds (Paquet and Schroeder 2009, p. 24).

Grand coalition healthcare entitlement reforms

Most reforms of healthcare entitlement under the Grand Coalition were affected by the GKV–WSG in 2007. All other reforms listed in Table 3.5 made only smaller amendments. In addition, a seminal judgement of the Federal Constitutional Court found healthcare entitlement regulation in conflict with the German Basic Law and claimed almost unlimited benefits for morbidly ill patients.

Governance – Who decides about healthcare entitlement?

The organisational structure of the Federal Joint Committee was changed once again by the GKV–WSG. As of 1 July 2008, all decisions had to be taken in the

Table 3.5 Reforms affecting healthcare entitlement, Germany 2005–2009

Law German short title	Adoption Commencement	Abbreviation
Act to Improve the Efficiency of Pharmaceutical Services *Gesetz zur Verbesserung der Wirtschaftlichkeit in der Arzneimittelversorgung*	26.04.2006 *01.05.2006*	/
Act to Strengthen Competition in SHI *GKV–Wettbewerbstärkungsgesetz*	26.03.2007 *01.04.2007*	GKV–WSG
Act for the Further Development of Organisational Structures in SHI *Gesetz zur Weiterentwicklung der Organisationsstrukturen in der GKV*	15.12.2008 *01.01.2009*	GKV–OrgWG
Pharmaceutical Law and Other Regulations Amendment Act *Gesetz zur Änderung arzneimittelrechtlicher und anderer Vorschriften*	17.07.2009 *22.07.2009*	/

FJC plenum. This reform had an important effect on coverage decision-making as decisions now had to be taken by all providers (ambulatory and stationary) together. Furthermore, committee meetings were open to the public.

Access – population coverage

The GKV–WSG implemented one of the most fundamental reforms in the history of the German welfare state: it obliged every resident to have health insurance. Due to historic reasons (see Chapter 3.1), SHI covered only around 90 per cent of the population. The remaining 10 per cent were free to insure privately, or not at all. In 2003, around 188,000 people were neither with SHI nor privately insured (explanatory memorandum BT–Drs. 16/3100, p. 94). Although this was less than one per cent of the population, the governing parties perceived the situation as unacceptable because the main reason people were uninsured was that they could not afford private insurance premiums. In order to produce relief, the coalition introduced a general obligation to insure in 2007, which took effect in 2009. All those so far not insured had to either insure with SHI or to take out private health insurance. All persons previously not insured and who had never held an insurance, or who had been insured with SHI before being uninsured, had to join SHI. Persons formerly not having been obligated to insure with SHI, and persons previously not insured but who had been privately insured in the past, had to take out private insurance.[68] Private health funds were obligated to admit everyone not ineligible for SHI and to provide them a basic tariff. The service coverage of this tariff equals the service coverage of SHI, and the maximum premium is defined by law.

In the course of the 2007 reform, the insurance coverage of those receiving Unemployment Benefit II was modified. Formerly, recipients of Unemployment Benefit II were automatically insured with SHI and their contributions were paid by the Federal Employment Agency (*Bundesagentur für Arbeit*, BA). After the reform, recipients who had been privately insured before they became entitled to Unemployment Benefit II, or who had been freed from obligatory insurance and had not taken out private insurance, had to insure with a private health insurance fund. The BA, however, incurred premiums only up to the general SHI contribution rate and the unemployed had to bear the rest. As most private insurance premiums are much higher than the standard SHI rate,[69] the reform worsened the situation of many of the unemployed. Only after a judgement of the FSC in 2011[70] was the whole premium borne by the BA.

Generosity – service coverage

In 2005, the Federal Constitutional Court took a leading decision[71] concerning the service coverage of SHI. In its judgement, which is called 'St. Nicholas judgement' because it was delivered on 6 December 2005, the FCC revoked almost all restrictions on service coverage for morbidly ill patients. It found that service restrictions in these cases are incompatible with the fundamental rights of Article 2 (1) (right to free development), in conjunction with Article 20 (welfare state principle), and

Article 2 (2) (right to life and physical integrity) of the Basic Law. In detail, the finding stated that in the case of life threatening disease or diseases that 'regularly result in death for which a standard therapy does not exist', SHI funds have to pay for every treatment that promises a 'barely remote chance for cure or improvements in the course of disease' (marginal No. 64, author's translation). The court recognised that there is no constitutional right to particular health services, but – as SHI is obligatory and contributions and service coverage cannot be influenced by the individual – decisions on service exclusions must take into account personal freedom rights. The decision was incorporated into law by the GKV–VStG in 2011 which introduced § 2 (1a) SGB V.

Prevention: The GKV–WSG completely restructured and reformed the chapter on prevention of the SGB V (Art. 1 No. 12). Occupational health promotion was extended and is now regulated by a separate paragraph. In addition, the sponsoring of self-help groups became an obligatory task for every SHI fund. Furthermore, vaccinations were made a statutory service of SHI and the FJC was tasked with defining which vaccinations would be obligatorily covered (new § 20d SGB V).[72] Vaccinations that are needed for private holidays remain excluded.

Primary care and ambulatory specialised care: The GKV–WSG introduced an entitlement to ambulatory palliative care and assigned the FJC to decide on the particulars of entitlement (Art. 1 No. 23 introduced § 37b SGB V).

Pharmaceuticals: The GKV–WSG extended service coverage to include the off-label use of pharmaceuticals if those are provided in the course of a clinical study and if several conditions (e.g. potential additional medical benefit, appropriate costs) are met (§ 35c SGB V as introduced by Art. 1 No. 20a GKV–WSG).

At the same time, however, the GKV–WSG almost completely abolished the choice amongst different drugs with the same active ingredient. Patients could get merely the brand for which their health fund had negotiated a rebate contract. Patients could get the drug of their (or their doctor's) choice only if their doctor had forbidden a substitute pharmaceutical on the prescription (§ 129 (1) SGB V).

The GKV–OrgWG extended coverage of dietetic products from formerly four product groups[73] to all 'medically necessary, appropriate and efficient' diets not being normal edibles (§ 31 (5) SGB V as introduced by Art. 1 No. 1a GKV–OrgWG). It tasked the FJC with defining covered diets and eligibility criteria for their reimbursement.

Generosity – cost coverage

The GKV–WSG (Art. 1 No. 37) contained several measures that sanctioned health misconduct. It increased the maximum co-payment limit from one to two per cent of gross income for the chronically ill born after 1972 if they had not regularly scheduled preventive health check-ups. The limit was also increased for patients suffering from cancer for which early detection tests were available, if the patient had not regularly obtained such examinations during the last years.[74] The GKV–WSG also required the chronically ill to demonstrate 'compliant behaviour' in order to become eligible for co-payment reduction. Moreover, the reform committed patients to bear part of the treatment costs if treatment became necessary as a 'result of a medically not indicated procedure' such as tattoos, piercings or plastic surgery (Art. 1 No. 31 GKV–WSG introduced § 52 (2) SGB V).

Pharmaceuticals: As an incentive for the use of lower cost drugs, the Act to Improve the Efficiency of Pharmaceutical Services allowed the Association of SHI funds to remit co-payments for drugs if the drug price was at least 30 per cent lower than the reference price. The GKV–WSG further extended this possibility by allowing SHI funds to reduce or remit co-payments for drugs for which they had negotiated a discount with the producer (Art. 1 No. 16b amended § 31 (3) SGB V).

Hospital care: Cost coverage of stationary and semi-stationary hospice services was set at 90 per cent of costs for adults and 95 per cent for children at all SHI funds (§ 39a SGB V as amended by the Pharmaceutical Law and Other Regulations Amendment Act). Formerly, each SHI fund had to individually specify the amount of cost coverage within its statutes.

Summary

With regard to healthcare entitlement, the Grand Coalition departed from the traditional path of cost and service coverage retrenchment. It neither increased co-payments nor excluded services from SHI coverage. However, it introduced several conditions of conduct that financially sanction 'poor' health behaviour. The Grand Coalition even expanded service coverage. In doing so, it followed the policies of its precursors by almost exclusively admitting new services in the area of prevention and palliative care. In summary, healthcare entitlement policies played only a minor role under the CDU/CSU and SPD government, at least with regard to service and cost coverage. This is not true for population coverage, where the Grand Coalition set a milestone by introducing an obligation to insure for every German resident. Another exceptional incident was the judgement of the FCC that constituted almost unlimited service coverage for the terminally ill. This was the first time in SHI history that the FCC ruled SHI entitlement to infringe on German Basic Law.

3.7   Christian Democratic–Liberal healthcare entitlement reforms 2009–2013

With the change of government in 2009, the health ministry was consigned to the hands of the Liberals for the first time in German history. What this meant for healthcare entitlement policies is described in the following chapter. Following the structure of the preceding chapters, an overview of the political and economic situation, as well as a brief summary of Christian Democratic–Liberal health policy, are given before healthcare entitlement reforms are analysed in detail. A short section at the end summarises the findings.

Political and economic background

The Grand Coalition was voted out in 2009. While the Christian Democrats could more or less sustain voter's support, the SPD suffered a landslide loss of

11.2 per cent and captured only 23.0 per cent of total votes. Social Democratic voters were displeased with their party, in particular with its social policy, and hence voted for the new left alternative, the Left (*Die Linke*)[75] which managed to draw 11.9 per cent of total votes (Niedermayer 2011, p. 13). Nevertheless, the Liberals were the winners in the 2009 elections. They achieved 14.6 per cent of the vote – the best result in their history – and went into coalition with the CDU/CSU. The dominance of CDU/CSU and FDP in the *Bundestag* was not mirrored in the *Bundesrat*. The government parties lost their majority in the *Bundesrat* right after the first federal state elections in July 2010. They lost even more votes during the following years, and thus always needed the support of the opposition to realise reforms requiring approval of the *Bundesrat*.

Germany recovered quickly from the global financial crisis, and after only one year of negative growth in 2009, the economy grew again and kept a moderate growth during the whole legislative period. Since 2010, unemployment has steadily declined, reaching an historic low since unification of 7.7 per cent for 2013 (Statistisches Bundesamt 2014).

Social policy was not high on the agenda of the Christian Democratic–Liberal coalition. All three parties had witnessed what the Agenda 2010 had done to the Social Democrats and hence tried to avoid radical reforms. Apart from the expansion of long-term care and a much contested child care subsidy, social policy of the CDU/CSU/FDP coalition was rather characterised by stalemate. The political agenda was dominated by other themes, such as the 'Energiewende' (the transition from nuclear and non-renewable energies to sustainable, renewable energy sources), abolition of compulsory military service and the Euro crisis.

Christian Democratic–Liberal health policy

The change in government saw the first Liberal health minister since the founding of the Federal Republic. The minister had great plans regarding a financial reform of SHI, but given a very tight state budget and a negative SHI budget in the beginning, he was unable to realise them (Reiners and Müller 2012, pp. 74f.). The government tried to balance the SHI budget with two reforms, the Act for Sustainable and Socially Balanced Financing of SHI (*GKV–Finanzierungsgesetz*, GKV–FinG) and the Act on the Reform of the Market for Medicinal Products (*Arzneimittelmarktneuordnungsgesetz*, AMNOG). The latter induced various measures aimed at reducing SHI drug expenditures in the short and long run. One of its most important instruments was a value-based pricing system for new drugs (see below). For Germany, this was a revolutionary reform because until now, attempts to limit SHI drug provision always failed due to the resistance of the pharmaceutical lobby. Even more remarkably, the pharmaceutical industry was disempowered by the Liberals who were usually quite receptive to the interests of the pharmaceutical lobby.

The GKV–FinG abstained from short-term measures increasing the cost burden of patients, such as co-payment increases. Instead, it froze the share of the employer's contribution and amended the additional contribution to become unlimited and flat-rate, with the effect that contribution increases in the future were to be borne by the insured alone (Rosenbrock and Gerlinger 2014, p. 460).

The budgetary situation relaxed markedly in 2011, and SHI encountered the best financial conditions in more than 30 years. Hence, there was no urgent need for reform, and problems were widely solved by throwing money at them. For example, the shortage of doctors in rural areas was dealt with by rewarding doctors – one of the most important supporters of the Liberals – a rich fee increase.

Christian Democratic–Liberal healthcare entitlement reforms

Healthcare entitlement reforms played only a minor role under the CDU/CSU/FDP government. Table 3.6 lists all relevant reforms affecting healthcare entitlement. Most of these reforms involved only one or two amendments.

After the Red–Green government had abolished most service and cost coverage differences between SHI funds 12 years ago, the CSU/CSU/FDP government again increased variation in service coverage between funds in 2011. They allowed funds to provide services not included as part of the SHI general benefits package, given the condition that they are not explicitly excluded by the FJC (§ 11 (6) SGB V introduced by Art. 1 No. 2 GKV–VStG).[76]

Table 3.6 Reforms affecting healthcare entitlement, Germany 2009–2013

Law German short title	Adoption Commencement	Abbreviation
Act on the Reform of the Market for Medicinal Products *Arzneimittelmarktneuordnungsgesetz*	22.12.2010 *01.01.2011*	AMNOG
Act to Improve the Provision of SHI Services *GKV–Versorgungsstrukturgesetz*	22.12.2011 *01.01.2012*	GKV–VStG
Act to Adjust Long-Term Care *Pflege-Neuausrichtungs-Gesetz*	23.10.2012 *30.10.2012*	PNG
Act to Regulate the Additional Care Needs in Stationary Prevention or Rehabilitation Hospitals *Gesetz zur Regelung des Assistenzpflegebedarfs in stationären Vorsorge- oder Rehabilitationseinrichtungen*	20.12.20012 *01.0.1.2013*	AssPflStatRG
Act on Cancer Screening and Clinical Cancer Registry *Krebsfrüherkennungs- und – registergesetz*	03.04.2013 *09.04.2013*	KFRG
Act to Reduce the Excessive Burden of Contribution Debts in Health Insurance *Gesetz zur Beseitigung sozialer Überforderung bei Beitragsschulden in der Krankenversicherung*	15.07.2013 *01.08.2013*	BeitrSchuldG

Governance – who decides about healthcare entitlement?

The AMNOG confined the power of the ministry to exclude services from the SHI benefits package (Art. 1 No. 3). First, the power of the ministry to exclude 'non-economic drugs', as well as those for the treatment of minor diseases, was abolished. This task is now exclusively performed by the FJC. Second, the ministry's right to exclude medical aids and appliances with low or contested medical benefit via ministerial order was eliminated from the SGB V. According to the explanatory memorandum, this option was abolished because the ministry had never employed the instrument in the past (explanatory memorandum BT–Drs. 17/2413, p. 19).

In 2011, the *Bundestag* decided to increase the requisite for service exclusions. Decisions of the FJC aiming to exclude services provided in both sectors (ambulatory and hospital) from SHI coverage now need nine out of 13 votes to pass (Art. 1 No. 29f GKV–VStG). Formerly, a simple majority was sufficient.

Access – population coverage

Some people did not follow the obligation to take out health insurance because they could not afford to re-margin their contribution debts. Others were insured with SHI but had not paid contributions and thus were entitled to a very limited scope of benefits. Attempting to remedy that problem, the BeitrSchuldG implemented several measures to lower the debt burden of contribution defaulters. The most important measures included a late payment fine reduction, a debt relief for persons obligated to insure with SHI who had failed to do so, and the introduction of a 'distress tariff' (*Notlagentarif*) in private health insurance for all insured not having paid premiums.

Generosity – service and cost coverage

Given low levels of budget pressure, there was no need to cut generosity. Hence, only few reforms addressed service and cost coverage at all. Only two reforms affected *cost coverage* of SHI. First, in the forefront of the next *Bundestag* poll, the unpopular and ineffective practice charge was abolished by the AssPflStatRG, taking effect on 1 January 2013. Second, the KFRG eliminated the increased co-payment limit for patients suffering from cancer and not having regularly attended available check-ups (Art. 1 No. 3 KFRG). It furthermore softened the requirements concerning the yearly attestation of chronic illnesses. With regard to *service coverage*, reforms mainly aimed at amending the decision-making procedures or criteria of coverage decisions:

Prevention: The KFRG introduced so called 'organised cancer screenings' (*organisierte Früherkennungsprogramme*) and tasked the FJC with developing similar population programmes for diseases for which European Commission best-practice guidelines exist (§ 25a SGB V introduced by Art. 1 No. 2). Core content of these programmes is the regular scheduling of adults for screenings, the provision of information about risks and benefits of the screening, and the establishment of a national cancer registry.

Hospital care: With the GKV–VStG, the criteria for the exclusion of hospital services were tightened. While formerly all services not meeting the standard conditions of SHI coverage (sufficient, appropriate, efficient) could be excluded, the SGB V now specifies that the benefit of a treatment or diagnosis method is 'not sufficiently proven and that it does not possess the potential to become a necessary treatment alternative, notably because it is harmful or ineffective' (§ 137c (1) SGB V as amended by Art. 1 No. 54 GKV–VStG, author's translation).

Pharmaceuticals: The AMNOG weakened the strict limitations of entitlement for drugs for which health funds had negotiated rebate contracts. Patients may now receive other drugs but have to bear the additional costs.

Furthermore, the AMNOG introduced an 'early benefit assessment' (*Frühe Nutzenbewertung*) for all newly licensed drugs with a new active ingredient (§ 35a SGB V introduced by Art. 1 No. 5 AMNOG). The FJC was tasked with assessing the drug's additional benefit compared to the existing standard therapy. If there is no additional benefit, the FJC has three options: it can put the drug into an adequate reference pricing category, exclude it from coverage or restrict eligibility (explanatory memorandum BT–Drs. 17/3698, p. 52). If the drug improves treatment, the assessment serves as basis for price negotiations between SHI funds and manufacturers (new § 130d SGB V). The early benefit assessment is a revolutionary reform in a system that so far failed to restrict pharmaceutical supply at all. The new system requires every new drug to be assessed with regard to its benefits for SHI patients, and only real innovations are remunerated. However, it remains to be seen if this new system will limit access to new drugs or increase the cost burden of patients, and if it is a successful instrument for keeping the prices of less and non-innovative new drugs low.

In addition, the AMNOG reversed the requirements for the exclusion of drugs and changed the criteria for exclusion. Formerly, it was possible to exclude drugs if their medical necessity or efficiency was not proven. After the changes made by the AMNOG, the SGB V required that 'the inappropriateness is proven' (§ 92 (1) SGB V as amended by Art. 1 No. 13b AMNOG). This does not only shift the burden of proof, but also eliminates the efficiency criteria as appropriateness refers to the quality and effectiveness of a treatment but not to its costs.[77] With these reverses in requirements, the exclusion of drugs became far more difficult as von Stackelberg, the head of the Association of SHI Funds, as well as Hess, the former head of FJC have pointed out (gpk 2011a, p. 3; 2011b, p. 19).

Summary

Given the very good financial conditions of SHI (at least since 2011), the need for cutting generosity was low, and thus the CDU/CSU/FDP government avoided any such reform. Interestingly, the government did not only refrain from excluding benefits, but even modified the regulatory framework as to impede service exclusions in the future. With respect to governance, it continued delegating coverage decision-making to the joint self-administration and diminished the role of the ministry in day-to-day coverage decisions. Finally, the Christian Democrats and Liberals advanced the realisation of universal population coverage.

3.8 The role of the joint self-administration in defining SHI healthcare entitlement

The joint self-administration has played an ever increasing role in specifying SHI healthcare entitlement, as the analysis above has shown. In order to get a full picture of healthcare entitlement in Germany, it is therefore necessary to examine the work of the Federal Joint Committee and its precursors. Aiming to trace the stepwise delegation of decision-making powers, this chapter first provides an overview of the directives issued by the joint self-administration. In a second step, three of the most important directives are investigated in more detail.

Table 3.7 lists all healthcare entitlement relevant directives having been passed by the FJC and its precursor committees since the 1970s.[78] This overview demonstrates the impressive expansion of its tasks over the years: while in 1977 the joint-self administration had issued 10 directives on healthcare entitlement, that number had almost tripled to 27 in 2013. However, the increase in numbers does not always mean an increase in delegation. The BAÄK had long been tasked with preparing directives on the prescription of hospital treatment and the prescription of remedies and medical aids, but did not meet these obligations before 1982. Eight of the newer directives result from an expansion of service coverage (marked with an E in Table 3.7), and five primarily aim at regulating restrictions in either cost or service coverage (marked with an L in Table 3.7).[79]

The FJC more or less updates its directives on a regular basis. The year given before the name of the directive indicates the date of the last general revision of the directive. The frequency of general revisions does not suggest the real relevance of the directive. Directives are amended (but not revised) with every decision taken. The Maternity Directive, for example, dates from 1985, but the FJC usually amends it several times per year. However, there are major differences between directives. Some directives have never been amended (e.g. the Supportive Social Care Directive), and many are only rarely updated. On the contrary, the FJC has taken more than 130 decisions concerning the Pharmaceutical Directive in 2013 alone. These differences indicate that directives differ in their scope, as well as with regard to their relevance for healthcare coverage. A complete analysis of the content of directives and their amendments would require a separate book. In order to give at least partial insight into the regulatory content of directives and changes over time, three directives – one for each of the three biggest healthcare sectors according to SHI expenditure – are presented and analysed in the following sections.

In the ambulatory sector, new diagnosis and treatment methods are allowed to be provided only after the joint self-administration had evaluated their therapeutic benefits (since 1990) and their efficiency (since 1997), and positively recommended the new method in its Directive on Ambulatory Diagnosis and Treatment

Table 3.7 Healthcare entitlement directives of the joint self-administration 1977, 1990, 2000 and 2013

1977	1990	2000	2013
1972 Dental Care Directive *Behandlungs-Richtlinie*	1972 Dental Care Directive *Behandlungs-Richtlinie*	1993 Dental Care Directive *Behandlungs-Richtlinie*	2003 Dental Care Directive *Behandlungs-Richtlinie*
1973 Orthodontics Directive *Kieferorthopädie-Richtlinie*	1973 Orthodontics Directive *Kieferorthopädie-Richtlinie*	1993 Orthodontics Directive *Kieferorthopädie-Richtlinie*	2003 Orthodontics Directive *Kieferorthopädie-Richtlinie*
1974 Pharmaceutical Directive *Arzneimittel-Richtlinie*	1978 Pharmaceutical Directive *Arzneimittel-Richtlinie*	1993 Pharmaceutical Directive *Arzneimittel-Richtlinie*	2008/2009 Pharmaceutical Directive *Arzneimittel-Richtlinie*
1974 Maternity Directive *Mutterschafts-Richtlinie*	1985 Maternity Directive *Mutterschafts-Richtlinie*	1985 Maternity Directive *Mutterschafts-Richtlinie*	1985 Maternity Directive *Mutterschafts-Richtlinie*
1975 Fertility Regulation and Termination of Pregnancy Directive *Richtlinie über Sonstige Hilfen*	1985 Fertility Regulation and Termination of Pregnancy Directive *Richtlinie über Sonstige Hilfen*	1985 Fertility Regulation and Termination of Pregnancy Directive *Richtlinie zur Empfängnisregelung und zum Schwangerschaftsabbruch*	1985 Fertility Regulation and Termination of Pregnancy Directive *Richtlinie zur Empfängnisregelung und zum Schwangerschaftsabbruch*
1975 Rehabilitation Directive *Rehablilitations-Richtlinie*	1975 Rehabilitation Directive *Rehablilitations-Richtlinie*	1975 Rehabilitation Directive *Rehablilitations-Richtlinie*	2004 Rehabilitation Directive *Rehablilitations-Richtlinie*
1976 Pediatric Directive *Kinder-Richtlinie*	1976 Pediatric Directive *Kinder-Richtlinie*	1976 Pediatric Directive *Kinder-Richtlinie*	1976 Pediatric Directive *Kinder-Richtlinie*
1976 Cancer Screening Directive *Krebsfrüherkennungs-Richtlinie*	1976 Cancer Screening Directive *Krebsfrüherkennungs-Richtlinie*	1976 Cancer Screening Directive *Krebsfrüherkennungs-Richtlinie*	2009 Cancer Screening Directive *Krebsfrüherkennungs-Richtlinie*
1976 Psychotherapy Directive *Psychotherapie-Richtlinie*	1987 Psychotherapy Directive *Psychotherapie-Richtlinie*	1998 Psychotherapy Directive *Psychotherapie-Richtlinie*	2009 Psychotherapy Directive *Psychotherapie-Richtlinie*
1977 Dental Prostheses Directive *Zahnersatz-Richtlinie*	1985 Dental Prostheses Directive *Zahnersatz-Richtlinie*	1977 Dental Prostheses Directive *Zahnersatz-Richtlinie*	2004 Dental Prostheses Directive *Zahnersatz-Richtlinie*

	1982 Patient Transportation Directive *Krankentransport-Richtlinie*	1992 Patient Transportation Directive *Krankentransport-Richtlinie*	2004 Patient Transportation Directive *Krankentransport-Richtlinie*
	1982 Prescription of Hospital Treatment D. *Krankenhausbehandlungs-Richtlinie*	1982 Prescription of Hospital Treatment D. *Krankenhausbehandlungs-Richtlinie*	2003 Prescription of Hospital Treatment D. *Krankenhausbehandlungs-Richtlinie*
	1982 Remedies and Medical Aids Directive *Heil- und Hilfsmittel-Richtlinie*	1992 Medical Aids Directive *Hilfsmittel-Richtlinie*	2011 Medical Aids Directive *Hilfsmittel-Richtlinie*
		2000 Remedies Directive *Heilmittel-Richtlinie*	2011 Remedies Directive *Heilmittel-Richtlinie*
E	1989 Health Check Directive *Gesundheitsuntersuchungs-Richtlinie*	1989 Health Check Directive *Gesundheitsuntersuchungs-Richtlinie*	1989 Health Check Directive *Gesundheitsuntersuchungs-Richtlinie*
E	1990 Directive on Artificial Insemination *Richtlinie künstliche Befruchtung*	1990 Directive on Artificial Insemination *Richtlinie künstliche Befruchtung*	1990 Directive on Artificial Insemination *Richtlinie künstliche Befruchtung*
L	1990 Directive on the Introduction of New Diagnosis and Treatment Methods *Richtlinie Einführung neuer Unter-suchungs- u. Behandlungsmethoden*	1999 Directive on the Evaluation of Ambulatory Diagnoses and Treatments *Richtlinie Bewertung ärztlicher Unter-suchungs- u. Behandlungsmethoden*	2006 Directive on Ambulatory Diagnosis and Treatment Methods *Richtlinie Methoden vertragsärztliche Versorgung*
E	1990 Directive on Measures for the Prevention of Dental Diseases *Richtlinie über Maßnahmen zur Verhütung von Zahnerkrankungen*	1990 Directive on Measures for the Prevention of Dental Diseases *Richtlinie über Maßnahmen zur Verhütung von Zahnerkrankungen*	2003 Directive on Measures for the Prevention of Dental Diseases *Richtlinie über Maßnahmen zur Verhütung von Zahnerkrankungen*
E		1998 Youth Health Check Directive *Jugendgesundheitsuntersuchungs-Richtlinie.*	1998 Youth Health Check Directive *Jugendgesundheitsuntersuchungs-Richtlinie.*

(*Continued*)

Table 3.7 (Continued)

1977	1990	2000	2013
		L 1999 New Dental Diagnosis and Treatment Directive (*repealed 2006*) *NUB-Richtlinie*	E 2001 Supportive Social Care Directive *Soziotherapie-Richtlinie*
		2000 Home Care Directive *Häusliche Krankenpflege-Richtlinie*	2009 Home Care Directive *Häusliche Krankenpflege-Richtlinie*
			E 2003 Early Diagnosis of Dental Diseases *Zahnärztliche Früherkennungs-Richtlinie.*
			L 2004 Dental Care Fixed Reimbursement Directive *Festzuschuss-Richtlinie*
			L 2004 Chronic Patients Directive *Chroniker-Richtlinie*
			L 2006 Directive on Hospital Diagnosis and Treatment Methods *Richtlinie Methoden Krankenhaus*
			E 2007 Vaccination Directive *Schutzimpfungs-Richtlinie*
			E 2007 Directive on the Prescription of Specialised Outpatient Palliative Care *Spezialisierte ambulante Palliativversorgungs-Richtlinie*

Note: The table displays all directives issued by the joint self-administration with relevance for healthcare entitlement at four points in time. The dates given before the name of the directive either indicate the year of adoption, or the year of the last general revision. The table does not show amendments between two points in time. Directives marked with an E result from expansion of service coverage; directives marked with an L became necessary due to a limitation of service or cost coverage.

Methods.[80] Since 1999, services already covered under SHI may also be evaluated by the FJC/BAÄK with regard to their therapeutic benefits and efficiency and, as the case may be, either be excluded from coverage or restricted to the treatment of particular diseases. The current directive adheres to general matters such as the legal basis (which is § 135 (1) SGB V), the scope of application and the evaluation process. The content of single decisions is given in the annexes of the directive: annex I (formerly A) contains all methods for which the FJC/BAÄK decided positively, and were thus included into the benefits package; annex II (formerly B) comprises all methods for which the FJC/BAÄK decided against, and were hence excluded or not admitted; and annex III (formerly C) lists all methods for which evaluation was suspended. As of 2013, annex I encompassed 19 items including such methods as positron emission tomography, testing of genotypic HIV-resistance or neuropsychological therapy, for example. The concrete content of decisions varies widely: detailed regulations concerning the indications are given for each method; in addition the directive may provide regulations concerning the diagnosis and treatment process, necessary documentation, quality assurance measures and sometimes sets licensing requirements. Annex II comprised 48 methods, including, for example, autologous chondrocyte implantation, hyperbaric oxygen therapy and acupuncture other than for patients suffering from chronic pain. In 2013, 10 decisions were deferred until better knowledge on the methods could be obtained. Usually, the FJC/BAÄK takes between one and four decisions per year concerning this directive.

For the hospital sector, the relevant directive is the Directive on Hospital Diagnosis and Treatment Methods.[81] Contrary to the ambulatory sector, all methods provided as inpatient services are covered by SHI. Only if the joint self-administration evaluates a diagnosis or treatment method and draws the conclusion that it is not sufficient, appropriate or efficient, may a method be excluded. In 2011 (taking effect in 2012), these criteria were changed. Now, a method may be excluded only if its benefit is 'not sufficiently proven and it does not possess the potential to become a necessary treatment alternative, notably because it is harmful or ineffective' (§ 137c (1) SGB V). After a short reference to the legal basis (which is § 137c (1) SGB V), the binding character of the directive, and the evaluation process, the directive lists in § 4 (formerly annex B) the methods not allowed to be provided as SHI hospital services. As of 2013, there were 15 methods (36 condition-treatment pairs), of which nine are for the treatment of benign prostatic hyperplasia. Most methods are not completely excluded; they are only excluded for particular indications. All methods prohibited for inpatient treatment are also not approved for the outpatient sector.[82] Annex I (formerly A) includes all methods that have been assessed but not excluded from coverage. As of 2013, annex 1 contained six methods. These six were also listed in § 4, but for different indications. Annex II contains diagnosis and treatment methods for which decisions have temporarily been suspended. Between 2003 and 2011, the FJC/BAÄK had taken 4.6 coverage decisions on average per year (own calculation).[83] In 2012, the FJC took only one, and in 2013 three decisions, of which only one was an exclusion from coverage. These low numbers might be the result of the changed criteria for coverage exclusions.

The Pharmaceutical Directive is one of the oldest directives, and by far the most comprehensive. It regulates various issues, ranging from coverage of off-label use, to the classification of drugs within the reference pricing scheme. The regulatory tasks of the FJC/BAÄK have been massively expanded over time, which is mirrored in the length of the directive: while the 1978 Pharmaceutical Directive was two and a half pages long plus one annex, its 2013 version covered almost 30 pages and 14 annexes. The body of the current directive is divided into a general and a special section. The general section defines the purpose of the directive and its scope of application, denotes the legal basis regarding the scope and limits of SHI entitlement to pharmaceuticals, and it sets requirements with regard to prescription, documentation and other matters. The special section sets out in detail the regulations specifying pharmaceutical entitlement. In addition, the Pharmaceutical Directive has 14 annexes, many of which list pharmaceuticals that fulfil or do not fulfil entitlement criteria and hence are in- or excluded from coverage. Table 3.8 provides an overview of the content of the special section and the annexes of the Pharmaceutical Directive as of 2013. The broad content of the Pharmaceutical Directive reflects the different tasks the FJC/BAÄK was assigned by legislators, and the diversity of regulatory instruments used to influence pharmaceutical coverage. Regulatory tasks of the FJC range from the determination of exceptional coverage of OTC drugs, to decisions about the off-label use of drugs in clinical studies. Instruments include explicit coverage decisions (in- and exclusions), as well as price setting measures.

Table 3.8 Content of the pharmaceutical directive – overview

Part	Legal Basis SGB V	Content
		Special Section
F	§ 34 (1) s. 2, s. 6 and s. 7	Exclusion of drugs from coverage by law and allowed exemptions
G	§ 34 (2) and (3)	Exclusion of drugs from coverage by ministerial order
H	§ 92 (1) s. 1 cl. 3, §92 (2) s. 7	Exclusions from and limitations of drug coverage by the Pharmaceutical Directive
I	§ 31 (1) s. 2	Legal exemptions regarding the coverage of amino acid mixtures, albumenhydrolyzates, elemental diets and diets for tube feeding
J	diverse	Coverage of medical products
K	§ 35c (1) i.c.w. § 92 (1) s. 2 No. 6	Coverage of off-label use
L	§ 35c (2) i.c.w. § 92 (1) s. 2 No. 6	Coverage of off-label use in clinical studies
M	diverse	Further regulations concerning the economic provision of drugs
N		(repealed)
O	§ 35a	Early benefit assessment of drugs with new active ingredients

Part	Legal Basis SGB V	Content
		Annexes
I	§ 34 (1) s. 2	List of OTC drugs which are covered in specified, exceptional cases
II	§ 34 (1) s. 7	List of lifestyle drugs that are excluded from coverage
III	§ 34 (1) s. 6, § 34 (3), § 92 (1) s. 1 cl. 3	List of drugs that are excluded from coverage or for which prescription is restricted due to inappropriateness, due to lower efficiency compared to equivalent drugs, or due to other reasons; OTC drugs that are not even covered for children and young adults
IV	§ 92 (2) s. 7	Therapeutic advice for high-cost drugs that specify the 'economic prescription' of these drugs
V	§ 31 (1) s. 2 and s. 3	List of medical products (e.g. irrigations, laxatives) with indications for which products are covered
VI	§ 35c (1) i.c.w. § 92 (1) s. 2 No. 6	List of drugs that are covered for defined off-label use (part A) and drugs not covered for off-label uses (part B)
VII	§ 129 (1a)	Advice regarding the commutability of pharmaceutical forms
VIII	§ 92 (2)	Prescription advice regarding drugs that are comparable with regard to their pharmacological active substance or with regard to their therapeutic effect
IX	§ 35 (1)	Assignment of drugs to the reference pricing scheme
X	§ 35 (3)	List of drugs for which the daily or single dose was actualised changing their classification within the reference pricing system
XI		(repealed)
XII	§ 35a	Results of the early benefit assessments (see Chapter 3.7)
Negative List	§ 34 (3)	Negative list of drugs excluded from coverage via ministerial order
Clinical Studies	§ 35c (2)	Decisions about exceptional coverage of drugs used off-label in the course of clinical studies

The aim of the short presentation of the three directives was to provide a more detailed picture of the work of the FJC/BAÄK and to illustrate the massive regulatory power the joint self-administration possesses. In addition, the description revealed the vast differences between the three sectors. In the ambulatory sector, healthcare coverage is fixed, and only if the FJC takes a positive decision, coverage is expanded. In the hospital sector, however, healthcare coverage is almost unlimited, i.e. everything may be provided unless expressly excluded in a decision of the FJC. Thus, a decision of the FJC has an opposite effect in the two sectors. In the pharmaceutical sector, the tasks of the FJC are manifold and the explicit ex- and inclusion of drugs from coverage is only one of several instruments the FJC has to influence healthcare entitlement. Apart from the broad exclusion of OTC drugs, lifestyle drugs and the old negative list, pharmaceutical entitlement is rarely regulated through direct coverage decisions, but rather indirectly through pricing policies. These differences reveal how the impact of the joint self-administration on healthcare entitlement is heavily determined by the statutory provisions of its tasks.

From a governance perspective, the transference of regulatory power to the joint self-administration has some advantages over hierarchical state regulation. First, given the huge number of specific entitlement decisions to be taken, and given the specific knowledge required to take them, the delegation of decision-making to experts and stakeholders improves the quality of decisions and saves state resources. Second, the compliance of providers and funds with decisions is enhanced as it is 'their' decisions which must be followed. Third, in particular, when decisions aim at restricting generosity of entitlement, blame is shifted to the joint self-administration and does not impact politicians. The joint self-administration, however, was not given full autonomy, but rather must act 'with a concrete mandate and under permanent control of the state' (Bandelow 1998, p. 161, my translation). The parliament can amend or withdraw this mandate at any time and has often done so in the past. Another possibility of influencing the decision-making of the joint self-administration is through adjustment of the institutional framework of the decision-making process, for example the composition of the committee, or the decision rule.[84] What the ministry once tried in the past but failed to do is to influence single decisions of the FJC. All directives are subject to ministerial supervision. The ministry, however, may only reject a decision of the FJC if the decision-making process was unlawful; it has no power to judge the content of the directive as the FSC ruled in 2009.[85]

In conclusion, the role of the joint self-administration in coverage decision-making in Germany is immense. The FJC specifies entitlement in all healthcare sectors. In doing so, it is free to decide the particulars of coverage. However, the joint self-administration must act within the framework determined by parliament, which not only decides on coverage criteria and the institutional setting of decision-making, but also on the powers of the FJC.

3.9   Discussion

The 37 years of healthcare entitlement reforms in Germany can roughly be divided into two phases: a retrenchment era lasting from 1977 until 2003, and a rather generous phase afterwards. The two phases differ not only in the level of generosity, but also in the way healthcare entitlement was regulated. The first phase was dominated by classic measures such as explicit service exclusions, often via ministerial order or by law, and new or increased co-payments. Since the late 1990s, co-payments and explicit service exclusions have lost their importance. Instead various new instruments were applied to restrict entitlement. First are the pricing instruments, notably the reference pricing schemes (e.g. for drugs and medical aids), the value-based pricing system for new drugs and the rebate contracts between health funds and pharmaceutical manufacturers, all three of which restrict entitlement to the cheapest or most economic treatment option. Patients may choose alternative products, but must bear the additional costs. Second, the joint self-administration was tasked with taking explicit coverage decisions for almost all service areas. Other than the broad service exclusions of the 1980s and 1990s, the coverage decisions of the joint self-administration concern only single treatments. Moreover, the assessments do not always lead to a complete exclusion of the treatment, but often a particular subgroup of patients (or particular diseases) that benefit (most) from treatment is identified, and eligibility is tailored accordingly.

What might have caused this gradual but persistent conversion of instruments in the regulation of healthcare entitlement? One answer to this question is provided by the functional arguments brought forward in Chapter 3.8. The delegation of decision-making to the joint self-administration offers several benefits for policy makers: the state budget is unburdened, quality of decisions increased, compliance of stakeholders improved, and last, and maybe most importantly, blame for unpopular decisions can be shifted to actors not subject to sanctioning by the electorate. The decreased importance of co-payments can be explained by similar functional arguments. During the 1980s and 1990s, it was hoped that co-payments could help to avoid overconsumption of medical goods and services[86] and, furthermore, generate additional income (e.g. Breyer and Haufler 2000; Newhouse 1993). However, it soon became clear that co-payments cannot fulfil this task, at least, not without endangering access of the most vulnerable members of society to healthcare (see Sachverständigenrat für die Konzertierte Aktion im Gesundheitswesen 1994).

The last argument directs us towards a more fundamental reason for the changes in regulatory instruments. The new instruments do not limit generosity (service and cost coverage) to the same extent as the old ones did, and thus do not, in the long run, threaten the legitimacy of the statutory health insurance system. Co-payments could not be expanded much further if universal access was to be obtained. Similarly, further exclusions would sooner or later have reached to core service areas, after almost all non-core services had been excluded from SHI coverage during the 1980s and 1990s. This, however, would have challenged the legitimacy of SHI, which promises to provide all medically necessary treatments (§ 12 SGB V). Further retrenchment would have called the SHI system into question, in particular because an alternative system existed. Cuts would have been hard to justify against the backdrop of a private system providing more generous benefits at lower costs, but for which access was restricted to an elite minority. Yet without an alternative to SHI, high co-payments and reduced benefits would have cast obligatory insurance into question: people already paid plenty of money for SHI, so why should they do so when forced to pay a major portion of costs out of pocket anyway? The advantage of the new instruments is that they do not endanger the pretensions of SHI to provide every medically necessary treatment. The pricing instruments named above limit the number of drugs from which the patient and his/her doctor can choose; yet, their only bearing on entitlement is that they reduce choice amongst different brands, while access to treatment is not restricted. In a similar vein, the tailored entitlement of the FJC directives helps to avoid unnecessary and ineffective treatment, but guarantees that everyone with a medical health need receives necessary and effective treatment. I leave it to the reader to judge if these new instruments represent a new form of retrenchment, or if they provide a good solution for maintaining the provision of necessary treatment under constrained budgets.

A second remarkable transformation of the German social right to healthcare is the universalisation of population coverage. Traditionally, the SHI system had provided coverage for particular groups of the population only. This segregation, however, contradicts the formal equality of citizenship. Why should people with an equal status not be equal with regard to healthcare rights? In response to this contradiction, SHI rights of blue-collar and white-collar workers were stepwise equated between 1989 and 1992. The integration of the better off into SHI, however, could not be accomplished against the broad resistance of stakeholders (privately insured, private insurance companies and providers). However, the exclusion of the better off is a lesser problem because this group can afford private insurance and hence often enjoys better service and cost coverage. Morally problematic was the group of people not having enough money to insure privately, but also not eligible for SHI coverage. Their exclusion from public health insurance coverage contradicted not only the formal equality of citizenship, but also violated basic human rights, and was thus perceived as 'not acceptable [for a] modern welfare state' (explanatory memorandum BT–Drs. 16/3100, p. 94, author's translation). The problem of uninsured members of society was solved with the introduction of an obligation to insure. Since 2009, every German resident is bound to either insure with SHI or, if s/he is not entitled to SHI membership, to take out private insurance. Private insurance companies must provide a basic tariff offering the same benefits as SHI and for which the maximum premium is determined by the state. Furthermore, they are obliged to accept everyone who cannot insure with SHI. Thus, every German resident now has (at least de jure)[87] access to health insurance.

Contrary to the general expansion of population coverage, access to SHI was severely restricted for several population groups over the decades, in particular for pensioners, the voluntarily insured, students and the unemployed. This contradiction of policies results from the different normative principles guiding healthcare policy-making in Germany. The expansion of health insurance coverage was driven on the one hand by the normative idea of access to healthcare as a fundamental right that legitimately cannot be denied to any member of society. The exclusion of particular members of society from SHI membership, on the other hand, followed the principle of reciprocal solidarity upon which SHI was built. Originating from mutual societies, SHI funds traditionally granted benefits only to those who previously had contributed their share to the community. These principles, however, are contradictory: universal coverage requires unconditional access, while SHI demands previous contributions. This conflict is solved in the German system through recourse to the private health insurance system. Everyone not meeting the requirements of SHI must be covered by the private system. Hence, the dual system of private and public healthcare systems allows Germany to grant its residents universal access without having to forgo SHI's fundamental principle of reciprocal solidarity.

Notes

1 With the exemption of substitute funds (*Ersatzkassen*). Traditionally, these were governed exclusively by representatives of the insured.

2 The FJC has been in existence since 2004. Its precursor committees were named 'Federal Committee of Physicians and Sickness Funds' and 'Federal Committee of Dentists and Sickness Funds' respectively; see Chapter 3.5.

3 Contributions for pensioners are shared between pensioners and statutory pension insurance, while contributions of unemployed are paid by the unemployment insurance.

4 The additional premium was introduced with the GKV–WSG, which was decided in 2007, but the relevant regulations took effect in 2009.

5 If funds achieve a surplus, they may refund premiums to the insured.

6 In 1977, special regulations existed for farmers, servants, pedlars, seamen, home workers, apprentices, discontinuous employed, certain self-employed (§§ 416ff. RVO), mineworkers and disabled persons. The variety of special regulations has been reduced during the period under investigation. Today, only statutory health insurance of farmers and artists deviates from general regulations.

7 In this book, the term 'economic', in relation to the German case, is exclusively used to refer to the economic imperative.

8 Doctors' decisions are strongly influenced by the fee schedule because only treatments listed there are reimbursed.

9 Ambulatory care includes: certain preventive examinations, primary care, specialised ambulatory care, dental care and appliances, medical aids and appliances, and ophthalmic care and appliances.

10 Additional benefits are usually called *Mehrleistungen* or *Satzungsleistungen* (statute benefits) because they must be specified within the fund's statutes.

11 In 1977, additional benefits encompassed convalescent care (§ 187 No. 2), individual preventive measures (§ 187 No. 4), the promotion of disabled sport (§ 193 No. 1), substitutive rehabilitation for the disabled (§ 193 No. 2), the payment of travelling expenses of one family visit per month during long hospital stays (§ 194 (2)), an increased burial allowance (§ 204 RVO), family allowance for other family members than spouses and children (§ 205 (3) RVO) and a burial allowance for still births (§ 205b s. 3 RVO).

12 Differences in service coverage of substitute funds are also disregarded. While the so-called 'RVO funds' (general regional funds, company-based sickness funds, guild funds, the Federal Miners' Insurance, the Seamen's Health Insurance Fund and farmers' funds) were obligated to provide the benefits defined in the RVO, the substitute funds were free to define service coverage within their statutes. They were obliged to provide at least the amount of benefits included in the benefits package of the RVO funds for their compulsory insured members (Reiners et al. 1977, p. 54; § 507 RVO). They were almost completely free to define the services for the voluntarily insured (Stolt 1973, p. 92). In fact, the difference between the service coverage of the two types of funds concerning their compulsory insured members was minimal (Reiners et al. 1977, p. 54). Today, the regulation of service coverage is the same for all funds.

13 *Richtlinien des Bundesausschusses der Zahnärzte und Krankenkassen für eine ausreichende, zweckmäßige und wirtschaftliche kassenzahnärztliche Versorgung mit Zahnersatz und Zahnkronen*, dated 25.10.1977 (Bundesanzeiger No. 230, pp. 1f.).

14 SPD, *Sozialdemokratische Partei Deutschlands*.

15 FDP, *Freie Demokratische Partei*.

16 All election data in this section is drawn from Ritter (1991).

17 This condition was slightly changed to 9/10 of the second half of working life by the GRG in 1988.

18 The description here is limited to the two main groups of pensioners, compulsorily and voluntarily insured SHI members. The KVKG completely renewed SHI coverage of pensioners and hence contained various regulations for all kinds of special cases. For a detailed explication of the reform, see Zipperer (1978).

19 Children insured via family allowance already had been exempted in the past (§ 205 (1) RVO).

20 See explanatory memorandum BT–Drs. 09/845, p. 13.

21 Retrenchment could also be observed in areas not covered by this thesis, for example treatment in health resorts and household help. Service coverage was expanded, however, to cover home care.

22 CDU, *Christlich Demokratische Union Deutschlands* (Christian Democratic Union of Germany); CSU, *Christlich Soziale Union Deutschlands* (Christian Social Union of Germany). The CSU is the sister party of the CDU in Bavaria. It is present in Bavaria only, while the CDU represents the Christian Democrats in all other federal states. Both parties always form a coalition at the national level.

23 All election data is taken from the *Official Election Statistics* (2014).

24 The CDU/CSU got 47.3 per cent of the vote, the FDP 10.6 per cent, the SPD again lost votes and achieved only 37.0 per cent, while the Greens were further able to expand their share from 5.6 in 1983 to 8.3 per cent (*Official Election Statistics* 2014).

25 In December 1990, the first general elections in unified Germany were held. The CDU/CSU got 43.8 per cent of the vote and the FDP achieved a very high result of 11 per cent. The SPD was not very successful in winning votes in the east, and again had to take its seats on the opposition benches next to the *Bündnis' 90/Die Grünen* (the eastern offshoot of the Green Party) along with the successor of the GDR Socialist Unity Party, the Party of Democratic Socialism (PDS). In the general elections of 1994, the CDU/CSU won 41.5 per cent and the FDP 6.9 per cent of the vote. The SPD vote increased from 33.5 in 1990 to 36.4 per cent in 1994. The Greens merged their eastern and western parties and thereby captured 7.3 per cent of the vote. The PDS got 19.8 per cent in Eastern Germany, but only 4.4 per cent overall. Nevertheless, they entered the *Bundestag* by winning four direct mandates (*Official Election Statistics* 2014).

26 The opposition parties had held a majority in the *Bundesrat* since June 1990, but with the elections of the state parliaments in the new five federal states in October 1990, the Christian Democrats and Liberals recaptured the majority in the *Bundesrat* until March 1991 (Ritter 2007, pp. 25f.).

27 Since 1992, yearly pension amendments were calculated on general net income and thus contribution increases in other social insurance branches let pension growth decline (Wasem, Greß and Hessel 2007, p. 671).

28 The 'Programme for More Growth and Employment' (*Programm für mehr Wachstum und Beschäftigung*) encompassed various retrenchment laws. These, for example, cut job protection, increased the retirement age of women and reduced unemployment benefits (Deppe 2000, p. 131). The law affecting healthcare was named 'The Health Insurance Contribution Rate Exoneration Act 1996' (*Beitragssatzentlastungsgesetz*, BeitrEntlG).

29 In 1989, the gross income limit was 54,900 DM per year (Beckmann and Kuhn 1989, p. 128).

30 This regulation was declared unconstitutional by the FCC in 2000. See Chapter 3.5 for further details.

31 Healthcare for people receiving social assistance was, and still is, paid for by the beneficiary's municipal social service department. See Chapter 3.5 for more details.

32 Formerly, such a therapy was covered only if it had been provided by a medical doctor or by a psychotherapist acting on behalf of the doctor.

33 See Chapter 3.2 for a definition of 'economic'.

34 *Verordnung über unwirtschaftliche Arzneimittel in der GKV* (Order on Inefficient Drugs in SHI), dated 21.2.1990 (BGBl. I, No. 8, p. 301).

35 *Verordnung über Hilfsmittel von geringem therapeutischen Nutzen oder geringem Abgabepreis in der gesetzlichen Krankenversicherung* (Order on Medical Aids with Little Therapeutic Benefits or Low Price), dated 13.12.1989 (BGBl. I, No. 59, p. 2237).

36 Apart from the negative list released by the ministry, there exists also (indirectly) a positive list of medical aids prepared by the joint self-administration. From a legal point of view, this list is not exhaustive, meaning that entitlement to medical aids is not restricted to those listed, yet it influences decisions about SHI provision of medical aids in practice (Kamps 2009, p. 135; Krauskopf 1997, no. 11).

37 *Erste Verordnung zur Änderung der Verordnung über Hilfsmittel von geringem therapeutischen Nutzen oder geringem Abgabepreis in der gesetzlichen Krankenversicherung* (First Amendment of the Order on Medical Aids with Little Therapeutic Benefits or Low Price), dated 17.01.1995 (BGBl. I, No. 3, p. 44).

38 Details of the reimbursement reform of orthodontic treatment and dental appliances are described below in the section on cost coverage.

39 The introduction of hospital co-payments was the idea of the Liberals and had already been accepted by the previous government (Huster 1982, p. 699), but could not be implemented before the changeover.

40 The package size was determined by ministerial order: *Verordnung über die Zuzahlung bei der Abgabe von Arznei- und Verbandmitteln in der vertragsärztlichen Versorgung* (Order on Co-Payments for Pharmaceuticals and Bandages in SHI), dated 9.9.1993 (BGBl. I, No. 48, p. 1557).

41 Initially, it was planned to completely exclude these medical aids from reimbursement (see first draft of the 2.GKV–NOG, BT–Drs. 13/6087, p. 6).

42 A very good example is drugs. First, drugs for the treatment of minor diseases were excluded. In a second step, 'non-economic' drugs were ruled out as well. At the same time, a reference pricing system was introduced and co-payments were restructured. In a third step, a positive list was planned (but never created). Accompanying all of these reforms were continual increases in co-payments.

43 The term *Agenda 2010* was first used by Schröder in March 2003. However, several reforms from the first legislative period already followed the new Leitmotives of the Social Democrats and thus belong to the *Agenda 2010* as well (Hegelich, Knollmann and Kuhlmann 2011, p. 25).

44 The name of the reform goes back to Peter Hartz, chairman of the non-parliamentary expert commission tasked with developing reform strategies for restructuring the German employment agency, who in the end brought about far-reaching labour market reform.

45 Unemployment Aid (*Arbeitslosenhilfe*) was a contribution-based unemployment benefit paid to members of the statutory unemployment insurance after their eligibility to Unemployment Benefit I (*Arbeitslosengeld I*) expired after 32 months.

46 Act on the Promotion of Solidarity in Statutory Health Insurance 1998 (*GKV–Solidaritätsstärkungsgesetz*, GKV–SolG).

47 The ruling coalition parties had lost the majority in the *Bundesrat* in February 1999. However, not only *Länder* governed by the opposition, but all 16 of them, voted against this bill (Deppe 2005, p. 120).

48 Contribution Rate Stabilisation Act 2002 (*Beitragssatzsicherungsgesetz 2002*, BSSichG).

49 Further important reform measures of the GMG included the increase of patient sovereignty, the implementation of new provider structures, the further development and strengthening of integrated medical care, a reimbursement reform of the ambulatory sector, the inclusion of particular drugs into the reference pricing scheme, reforms of the organisational structures of SHI funds and additional money from taxes. For more details see Kruse and Hänlein (2004), Orlowski and Wasem (2003), and Reiners and Müller (2012).

50 In particular the cases 'Kohll' (C-158/96), 'Decker' (C-120/95), 'Smits and Peerbooms' (C-157/99) and 'Müller-Fauré/van Riet' (C-385/99), see Chapter 2.7.

51 Reforms affecting only small sub-groups of the population (e.g. artists, farmers), as well as reforms affecting cash payments and regimen, have not been considered for analysis and hence are not included in this table.
52 For tasks concerning the definition of SHI entitlement, see below; and for a general overview, see Urban (2001, pp. 31ff.).
53 The Coordination Committee was founded by the GKVGRefG and was assigned the development of guidelines and administrative tasks (§ 137e SGB V 2000).
54 Civil partnerships are similar to marriages but apply to persons of the same sex only, for whom marriage is forbidden in Germany. Rights of civil partners are similar to those of married partners but less far-reaching. Concerning social rights (and responsibilities), the rights of civil partners are almost equal to those of married partners.
55 Beneficiaries of Unemployment Aid had been compulsorily insured, hence nothing changed for them with the replacement of Unemployment Aid with Unemployment Benefit II.
56 The GMG later included recipients of social assistance into SHI but only with regard to organisational matters. Beneficiaries did not become members of SHI and did not pay contributions. SHI merely organised health services for them and costs of treatment were paid for by the municipal social services department. For a detailed description of reforms, see Kruse and Hänlein (2004, pp. 31ff.).
57 The possibility of providing preventive services as statutory services had already existed since 1988, but was abolished with the BeitrEntlG in 1996.
58 *Gesetz über die Verordnungsfähigkeit von Arzneimitteln in der vertragsärztlichen Versorgung* (BT–Drs. 15/800 and 15/1071).
59 Germany was the only country in which public health insurance paid for OTC drugs (Orlowski and Wasem 2003, p. 116).
60 *Verordnung zur Veränderung der Verordnung über unwirtschaftliche Arzneimittel in der gesetzlichen Krankenversicherung* (Order on Inefficient Drugs in Social Health Insurance Amendment Order), dated 16.11.2000 (BGBl. I, No. 8, p. 30); *Zweite Verordnung zur Veränderung der Verordnung über unwirtschaftliche Arzneimittel in der gesetzlichen Krankenversicherung* (Order on Inefficient Drugs in Social Health Insurance Second Amendment Order), dated 9.12.2002 (BGBl. I, No. 51, p. 1593).
61 For details, see the section on cost coverage below.
62 The GMG also abolished SHI cash benefits such as the burial and the childbirth allowances.
63 The CDU/CSU won 35.2, and the SPD 34.2 per cent of votes (*Official Election Statistics* 2014).
64 PDS, *Partei des Demokratischen Sozialismus* (Party of Democratic Socialism).
65 The Electoral Alternative for Labour and Social Justice (*Arbeit und soziale Gerechtigkeit – Die Wahlalternative*, WASG) was founded in 2005 by leftist Social Democrats who were dissatisfied with the Agenda 2010 policies of the SPD together with unionists with the goal of providing an alternative left to the SPD. For the federal elections of 2005, the PDS and WASG decided to form an electoral alliance. The PDS therefore changed its name into The Left Party.PDS and opened to candidates from the WASG and other leftists. In 2007, PDS and WASG then merged into one party, called The Left (*Die Linke*).
66 Since 2014, the general contribution rate is determined by the *Bundestag*.
67 For a detailed description of reforms, see Orlowski and Wasem (2007), Paquet and Schroeder (2009) and Wille and Koch (2007).
68 The obligation to insure applied to all persons resident in Germany without adequate health insurance or other equal coverage. It did not apply to beneficiaries of social assistance and asylum seekers. Persons moving to Germany in order to receive treatment were not allowed to become members of SHI (§ 52a SGB V as introduced by Art. 1 No. 32 GKV–WSG).
69 Unemployed in the private basic tariff can apply for a reduction of half their premium, but this is in many cases still more than the general SHI contribution rate.

70 Decision B 4 AS 108/10 R of the Federal Social Court, dated 18.1.2011.

71 Decision 1 BvR 347/98 of the Federal Constitutional Court, dated 6.12.2005.

72 In the past, each health fund could decide on its own if it reimbursed vaccinations for adults.

73 Service coverage was restricted to amino acid mixtures, albumen hydrolyzates, elemental diets and diets for sip and tube feeding.

74 The condition applied to women born after 1 April 1987 and men born after 1 April 1962.

75 The Left evolved from the merger of the PDS and the WASG in 2007. See above, note 65.

76 In detail, SHI funds may expand their scope of benefits in the following areas: prevention and rehabilitation, artificial insemination, dental care but not dental appliances, OTC drugs only available in pharmacies, remedies, medical aids, care at home, home help and services provided by unregistered providers. Since 2013, SHI funds are also allowed to provide additional midwife services (Art. 3 No. 1 PNG).

77 Drugs can still be excluded if there exists a drug with similar diagnostic or therapeutic benefits which is more economic (§ 92 (1) s. 1 SGB V).

78 The specification of healthcare entitlement is only one of several tasks of the joint self-administration. For example, the FJC also issues directives on quality assurance and quality measures, and capacity planning. § 92 SGB V (formerly § 368p RVO) lists all matters for which the FJC must establish directives. All current directives (as well as previous versions at least up to 2004) are provided on the webpage of the FJC http://www.g-ba.de/informationen/richtlinien/ (17.11.2014).

79 In fact, the joint self-administration was and still is commissioned with restricting service coverage in several more cases. In 1977, the BAÄK was to issue a negative list of drugs, but this directive never took effect because it was not accepted by the ministry. Since 2003, the FJC is responsible for determining lifestyle drugs that are excluded from coverage (annex II of the Pharmaceutical Directive) and for defining exemptions regarding the exclusion of OTC drugs (annex I of the Pharmaceutical Directive). Since 1989, new remedies are allowed to be provided only after an evaluation by the BAÄK/FJC (Remedies Directive).

80 The German name of the directive is *Richtlinie zu Untersuchungs- und Behandlungsmethoden der vertragsärztlichen Versorgun*, passed 17.01.2006 (Bundesanzeiger No. 48, 2006). The previous version from 1997 was called the Directive on the Evaluation of Ambulatory Diagnosis and Treatment Methods (*Richtlinie über die Bewertung ärztlicher Untersuchungs- und Behandlungsmethoden gemäß § 135 Abs. 1 SGB V und Änderungen*, short BUB–Richtlinie), issued 01.10.1997 (Bundesanzeiger No. 243, 1997); the version from 1990 was called the Directive on the Introduction of New Diagnosis and Treatment Methods (*Richtlinie über die Einführung neuer Untersuchungs- und Behandlungsmethoden*, short NUB–Richtlinie), issued 04.12.1990 (Bundesarbeitsblatt No. 2, 1991).

81 The German name of the directive is *Richtlinie zu Untersuchungs- und Behandlungsmethoden im Krankenhaus*, short *Richtlinie Methoden Krankenhaus*, passed 21.03.2006 (Bundesanzeiger No. 111, 2006). Formerly, the decisions were part of the Rules of Procedure of the Hospital Committee (*Verfahrensregeln des Ausschusses Krankenhaus*), passed 28.01.2002 (Bundesanzeiger No. 77, 2002). Passed in 2002, the Hospital Directive is quite new compared to the directive for the ambulatory sector. Historically, the joint self-administration was exclusively responsible for the ambulatory sector. Only since the late 1970s was their sphere of influence gradually expanded by legislators to also include the hospital sector (Böhm 2008; Döhler and Manow-Borgwardt 1992b).

82 With the exemption of proton therapy, hematopoietic stem cell transplantation and stents (which are only inserted at a hospital anyway), all methods are explicitly excluded by the ambulatory directive.

83 The year 2006 was not considered for the calculation because in that year the directive was generally revised and no single decision was taken. Decisions concerning

    quality measures and/or amendments to the decision-making process were not taken into account.

84 See the governance sections of the chapters above for examples.

85 Decision B 6 A 1/08 R of the Federal Social Court, dated 6.5.2009. See also Landwehr and Böhm (2014).

86 According to neo-classical economic theory, demand for medical goods is indefinite. Hence, because patients in public healthcare systems are not required to pay for medical treatment, they consume more goods and services than they would under market conditions, which leads to a welfare loss (e.g. Breyer and Haufler 2000).

87 There are still some people without health insurance because administrative hurdles and costs are too high. But there are attempts to lower these barriers. The BeitrSchuldG, for example, implemented several measures reducing the debt burden of contribution defaulters. However, there will always be some people without health insurance because the German system requires the beneficiary to take action, to get insured and to pay contributions or premiums.

4   The transformation of the social right to healthcare

This chapter is dedicated to the study's first research question: it describes how the social right to healthcare has been altered over the last 35 years. Based on the analytical categories developed in Chapter 1, Section 4.1 analyses the extent and mode of retrenchment. Section 4.2 identifies similar patterns of governance reforms in both countries and discusses their implications. More interesting than the quantitative modifications of healthcare entitlement, however, are the qualitative transformations of the social right to healthcare that took place in the two countries, i.e. the universalisation of access in Germany, and the individualisation of the collective social right in England. These processes are portrayed and discussed in section 4.3 and 4.4, respectively. Because the individualisation process has profound implications for the social right to healthcare in England (see Chapter 5), and because it may be paradigmatic for collective social rights in other countries, this process is more thoroughly analysed.

4.1   Healthcare entitlement retrenchment

In this section, I assess the degree to which access to and generosity of public healthcare have been restrained by entitlement reforms over the last 35 years. Summarising and comparing the results of Chapters 2 and 3, the detailed research questions presented in Chapter 1, section 1.4 are answered. First, amendments to population coverage, and then those to service and cost coverage, are evaluated, followed by a discussion of the impact of these changes on access and generosity.[1] Finally, conclusions about the extent of retrenchment are drawn for both countries.

Access – population coverage

The German SHI and the English NHS fundamentally differ with regard to population coverage. The English NHS provides universal coverage of all residents, while German SHI membership is selective and excludes certain parts of the population. Universal coverage is a founding principle of the NHS and has not been touched by any reform. Contrastingly, access in Germany was severely restricted from the 1970s to the 1990s by increasing the conditionality of SHI membership. Population coverage criteria were tightened so as to exclude persons who had not (or not sufficiently) contributed to SHI (e.g. pensioners not having been insured with SHI during active participation in the workforce). On the contrary, access to SHI has been expanded for some population groups (beneficiaries of Unemployment Benefit II, same-sex couples and pensioners) since the new millennium. This expansion of access, however, mainly resulted from reforms in other social sectors or from an FJC judgement. In 2009, a general obligation to insure was established. Since then, Germany has been offering health insurance coverage to all its residents, albeit not exclusively within the SHI system, but by utilising the private system. This universalisation of access signifies a fundamental transformation and is further discussed in Chapter 4.3.

Generosity – service coverage and cost coverage

The services and goods covered by the English NHS are mostly not specified by law, which allows providers and health authorities the flexibility to adapt entitlement to medical need and financial resources.[2] Hence, it is not surprising that explicit service exclusions in England have been few: the limited lists of drugs and the exclusion of optical appliances, both realised during the 1980s, are the only noteworthy examples. In Germany, on the contrary, exclusions of services and goods were broader and affected almost all service areas. Legal reforms directly limited coverage of drugs, as well as of medical, optical and dental appliances (including orthodontics). Service coverage retrenchment in Germany reached its peak during the late 1980s and the 1990s. After 2003, no service coverage reforms were implemented. Reforms in England and Germany not only restricted service coverage, but also expanded coverage for preventive healthcare measures. Preventive services were extended almost throughout the whole period under investigation. In addition, Germany enhanced entitlement in other areas (e.g. psychiatric services, palliative and hospice care), thereby primarily intending to avoid further, more expensive treatments.

In both countries, the explicit exclusions of broad categories of services by law were replaced by evaluation processes of single or small groups of treatments carried out by independent agencies. In Germany, the Federal Joint Committee (FJC) was stepwise tasked with establishing assessment processes for all service areas, and in England, NICE was assigned the assessment of most kinds of technologies within its Technology Appraisal Process (see also Chapter 4.2). To what degree these assessments may be characterised as retrenchment depends on the particular processes and the definition of retrenchment applied. For example, since 1989, new treatments and diagnostic methods may be provided under German SHI only if the FJC has given a positive recommendation. The implementation of this hurdle for ambulatory care can be clearly categorised as retrenchment because entitlement to ambulatory care was previously nearly unrestricted. Now, however, each positive decision of the FJC in ambulatory care expands entitlement. Positive recommendations of NICE also enlarge entitlement but do not necessarily increase generosity: the health budget is limited, and hence, explicit entitlement to treatments recommended by NICE means less money available for other treatments.

In terms of the criteria applied for the ex- and inclusion of services, the two countries differ widely. German SHI is bound by law to cover all services that are *sufficient*, *appropriate*, *efficient* and *necessary*.[3] Efficiency is an important criterion, but it is considered only in cases where treatment alternatives exist because of the patient's right to have all medical needs met. Referring to the criterion of efficiency, Germany excluded treatments for which cheaper alternatives existed (e.g. through the drug negative list) and established processes for the exclusion of 'uneconomic' treatments.[4] Under the principle of personal responsibility, established in SHI law in 1989, services and goods serving less critical medical needs (e.g. drugs for the treatment of minor diseases), or for which medical need was disavowed (e.g. 'lifestyle' drugs) or contested (e.g. dental appliances) were banned from SHI coverage. England has not specified any service coverage criteria by law, but most drugs appearing on the black list are for the treatment of minor diseases, or drugs classified in Germany as 'lifestyle drugs'. When NICE assesses technologies, it takes into account clinical need, clinical benefit and the technology's innovation potential, but its main decision criterion is the cost effectiveness of a treatment measured as cost per QALY.[5]

One aim of this study was to determine if generosity had been restricted by tightening the conditionality of benefit receipt. Eligibility criteria referring to a particular characteristic of the individual patient or a characteristic of his/her disease are relevant primarily for service coverage decisions concerning single treatments. NICE and FJC often target eligibility for patient groups that gain most from treatment. Otherwise, eligibility criteria are applied in special cases (e.g. drugs and medical aids for the treatment of erectile dysfunction in England and artificial insemination in Germany), or for optical appliances. In sum, conditionality was not notably increased by tightening eligibility criteria. However, criteria for service coverage became stricter, and beneficiaries were thus entitled to fewer goods and services.

Regarding cost coverage, England and Germany had similar starting points at the end of the 1970s. Both countries levied charges for drugs, medical aids and appliances, as well as dental appliances. England also charged co-payments for dental care and optical appliances. None of the English governments introduced new charges during the period of investigation. However, co-payments were drastically increased under the Conservatives. Germany imposed new co-payments for a variety of goods and services (e.g. glasses, hospital stays, artificial insemination), and it levied a so called 'practice charge' for ambulatory consultation. Yet charge increases were less far-reaching than in England. Thus, retrenchment of cost coverage was more far-reaching than retrenchment in service coverage in both countries.

Eligibility for exemption from co-payments was more generous in England than in Germany during the 1970s and was even expanded during the period under investigation. In England, the elderly, children, low income earners and recipients of particular social benefits are generally exempted from paying charges. Eligibility criteria defining these groups were broadened stepwise during the late 1980s and 1990s, until by 1996, only 15 per cent of the population had to pay charges at all (Hockley 2012, p. 152). In 2009, all patients suffering from cancer additionally became exempted from paying charges. In Germany, pensioners, children, persons with a reduced capability to work of at least 50 per cent and persons who received sick pay were generally exempted from paying charges for pharmaceuticals, remedies, dressings and dental appliances until 1977.[6] Then exemptions were severely limited to hardship cases until exemption policies became more generous in 1989. That year, a partial exemption was additionally introduced in which charges were remitted if one (for low income earners) or two (for high income earners) per cent of available income had already been spent on co-payments. In 1998, all chronically ill patients also became fully exempted. In 2004, however, total exemption was abolished: the chronically ill had to pay up to one per cent of their income and all other patients up to two per cent before becoming exempted. Furthermore, Germany increased conditionality by implementing conditions of conduct: the limit of the maximum co-payment for chronic patients and cancer patients, for example, became contingent upon prior attendance of preventive health checks. Similar instruments are applied in the area of dental appliances and orthodontic treatment. Summing up, England became even more generous regarding exemption from co-payments while Germany massively tightened eligibility criteria for exemption during the period of investigation.

Co-payments played an important role in both countries during the late 1970s, 1980s and early 1990s, but eventually became less important. During the 1970s and 1980s, it was hoped that co-payments would deter patients from consuming unnecessary services, but this was shown not to be the case. Co-payments were also introduced to generate additional income for public healthcare systems. This income, however, remained rather limited under the intention that needy patients should not be deterred from seeking treatment through high costs. Thus, alternative cost-containment instruments were implemented with varying degrees of impact on cost coverage. Germany introduced a reference pricing system for drugs and visual aids in 1989, a price negotiation scheme for drugs in 2001, and the same for medical appliances in 2004. These schemes have a direct impact on cost coverage for patients because they must pay additional (or full) costs if they do not want the cheapest brands. England, in contrast, directly controls profits of drug manufacturers and this does not impact cost coverage for patients. England, however, implemented a voucher system for glasses in 1986 which has a very similar effect on cost coverage for patients as reference prices: patients are reimbursed for the lowest cost treatments and must assume all costs exceeding the minimum.

Conclusion

In general, healthcare entitlement is more generous in Germany than in England. The German SHI covers all services that are sufficient, appropriate, efficient and necessary. A denial of necessary treatment on mere financial grounds is illegal in Germany. This is the fundamental difference to England, where available resources determine entitlement, and if resources are not sufficient (which proved to be the rule rather than exception), not all medical needs must be met. Explicit healthcare entitlement cuts in Germany were limited by the fundamental requirement that SHI services must be appropriate and sufficient. Hence, if core principles were not to be abandoned, the scope for retrenchment in Germany was very narrow. Reforms addressing service coverage could thus exclude only services that did not fulfil the above named conditions. Cost coverage could be reduced only up to a limit that did not deter patients from seeking necessary treatment. England was more flexible (as it does not provide absolute rights) and could adapt service provision to financial resources, which meant implicit rationing without cuts to explicit entitlement. It is nearly impossible to estimate the actual extent of indirect cuts inflicted on NHS entitlement because budget changes do not necessarily have an impact on entitlement. In real terms, the NHS budget was raised every year, with the exception of 1982, 2010 and 2011 (see Table 5.1 to Table 5.3). But demand also grew, so it is not clear if budget increases were sufficient to retain entitlement. During the early 1980s and mid-1990s in particular, budget growth was so limited that we can assume real retrenchment of entitlement during these years.

By and large, however, the retrenchment of healthcare entitlement in both countries remained within limits. Generosity was cut, but did not reach core benefits or endanger access through overly high co-payments. The findings of this study confirm the results obtained through entitlement studies of other welfare areas: retrenchment of healthcare entitlement reached its peak during the late 1970s up to the 1990s, and afterwards notable restrictions of entitlement were not carried out. Quite to the contrary, generosity was slightly increased in England (up to 2009) and to a remarkable extent in Germany.

4.2   Governance reforms

The regulation maps (Table 2.2 and Table 3.2) reveal the differences in healthcare entitlement regulation between the two countries. In England, entitlement is only vaguely defined by primary legislation; concrete entitlement can only be found in statutory instruments. This is unlike Germany, where statutory orders play almost no role in the definition of healthcare entitlement. Instead, entitlement is defined by public law and specified through directives of the joint self-administration. Hence, most amendments to healthcare entitlement are made by the Secretary of State via statutory instrument in England; while in Germany, primary legislation must be amended by the *Bundestag*. This has strong implications for the feasibility of reform, as is shown in Chapter 5.

Despite these structural differences, the governance of healthcare entitlement definition developed similarly in both countries: the role of state actors (parliament, ministry) in explicit entitlement definition diminished, while the role of non-governmental bodies increased. In England, entitlement definition at the national level was delegated to NICE, an independent expert body. In Germany, the joint self-administration, namely the FJC, was tasked with ever more entitlement decisions over the years. Although the institutional characteristics of the two committees are dissimilar,[7] they are assigned similar tasks and possess similar competencies. Both committees primarily decide on the coverage of single treatments while basing their decisions on health technology assessments. All decisions of the FJC are binding, while only positive recommendations of NICE must be fol-lowed by PCTs (now CCGs). Recommendations against the funding of a particular treatment are not binding, although most PCTs did not provide these services due to tight budgets.

The delegation of governmental tasks to non-majoritarian, independent bod-ies mirrors a general trend in the governance of advanced democracies (Majone 1997). Delegation to independent agencies has become popular for several rea-sons: the complexity of policy decision-making requires specific knowledge and expertise which is not held by politicians, and thus it is more efficient to delegate decision-making to experts, relieving politicians of the work. Furthermore, delega-tion allows politicians to avoid blame for unpopular decisions. Last, delegation may increase the credibility of policies (Majone 1999, pp. 3ff.). However, delega-tion implies a loss of legitimacy because relevant policy decisions are taken by non-elected actors, and thus are not subject to democratic control (Majone 1999). The low legitimacy of these bodies is particularly problematic for healthcare enti-tlement. These bodies decide about the (re)distribution of a substantial share of societal resources, and moreover, they determine entitlement to vitally important goods while citizens are unable to influence their decision-making. Reacting to these criticisms, NICE, and to some extent also the FJC, have increased public participation in decision-making over the last years. However, this participation remains selective and does not make up for the lack of democratic legitimacy. The deficit in legitimacy exists only with regard to single decisions. Macro-regulation of healthcare entitlement (e.g. the institutional design of decision-making), and other more general coverage decisions remained largely in the hands of the parlia-ment or ministry in both countries (Landwehr 2013).

4.3   The universalisation of access in Germany

When Germany introduced its obligation to insure in 2009, the majority of welfare states had already provided universal coverage for their populations. Germany is a latecomer not only regarding the universalisation of healthcare rights. With its special solution for granting universal access to healthcare through SHI and the private health insurance sector, the German case reveals the inherent contradiction of a universal right being based on insurance membership.

State and social insurance healthcare systems fundamentally differ in their con-ception of social rights with regard to population coverage. In most state healthcare systems, population coverage is based on status, i.e. every citizen or resident is granted access to public healthcare without having to fulfil any further conditions. In a social health insurance system, on the contrary, access to public healthcare is provided for insurance members only, and insurance membership is typically contingent upon the fulfilment of particular conditions (e.g. paid employment, maximum income). Persons not qualifying for insurance membership are usually not entitled to receive healthcare from the social health insurance system and must rely on either private insurances or pay healthcare costs out of pocket. Yet people lacking adequate resources for private insurance or for paying healthcare out of pocket do not have access to healthcare. However, access to at least basic health-care is a human right, and no welfare state can afford to infringe on something so fundamental. Hence, welfare states with a social insurance system must somehow provide their uninsured members with healthcare. In principle, they could resort to one of two solutions: they could either establish a second, alternative public healthcare scheme for all non-insured, or they could broaden access to the extant system. Broadening access, however, inevitably requires reducing the condition-ality of membership. Even if all population coverage criteria are repealed, there remains the requirement of contribution payments and with it, the problem of the insured being unable or unwilling to fulfil this obligation.

This problem has not been solved by the German reform of 2007. Germany obliged private health insurers to insure all those not eligible for SHI membership. In doing so, they could maintain reciprocal solidarity within SHI and at the same time, secure access to healthcare for all other residents not eligible for SHI membership. However, private insurance, just as SHI membership, is acquired through contribu-tion payments. Thus, this does not solve the problem of people not being able to pay contributions or premiums. Those who have not paid their SHI contributions or private premiums are only entitled to emergency and preventive care. Furthermore, the bureaucratic exigencies of becoming a private or SHI insurance member deter many from claiming their rights, and thus universality is not yet fully realised.

Understood as a universal human right, access to healthcare should be uncon-ditional. The inherent conditionality of social insurance systems, however, contra-dicts universality. This contradiction was not solved by the obligatory insurance introduced in Germany in 2009. Nevertheless, obligatory insurance improved the situation for many formerly uninsured and thus signifies an important step towards full universality.

4.4   The individualisation of the collective social right to healthcare

One of the fundamental transformations uncovered by this study is the individu-alisation of the collective social right to healthcare in England (see Chapter 2 for details). The aim of this chapter is to better understand and evaluate this process. For this purpose, the central characteristics of the English collective social right and the German individual social right to healthcare are elaborated in a first step.[8][9] As a second step, these characteristics are then used to identify the patterns of individualisation in England. In a third step, the individualisation process is evalu-ated by comparing the characteristics of the 'new' English social right to healthcare with those of the 'old' and the German individual rights to healthcare.

England and Germany: collective and individual social rights compared

Following Jost (2003, pp. 265ff.), who analysed healthcare entitlement in the US, England and Germany, my categorisation of healthcare rights is based on the following dimensions: conceptual basis, population coverage and legal enforce-ability. In addition to Jost, I also consider the reference point of social rights (i.e. society or the individual), the equality of rights and the degree of specification.

English healthcare rights closely resemble T. H. Marshall's model of social citi-zenship rights. They are based on status, i.e. they are granted every English resident irrespective of any personal characteristic or condition. This equality of status is mirrored in the equality of rights: all English residents are equally entitled to be provided with NHS healthcare.[10] At the core of Marshall's approach is the welfare of society which, when necessary, takes precedence over individual claims. This is also the case with NHS healthcare rights, and why I term them *collective social rights*. There is no individual entitlement to healthcare in England. Instead, the SoS and NHS bodies decide on a day-to-day basis about how to best meet the health needs of the English population with the given resources. Hence, entitlements depend on the availability of resources and thus are not absolute. Instead of granting individual rights, NHS law imposes obligations on public authorities to provide services. These obligations are formulated in a rather general way and do not specify entitlements. As no absolute right to healthcare exists, claims cannot be enforced by legal action. However, this does not mean that it is impossible to challenge decisions of the public health administration. Substantive appeals directed against the result of a decision are not possible, but procedural challenges may be made.[11]

The German social right to healthcare differs in all of the above named aspects from its English counterpart. First, German healthcare rights result from an insur-ance contract and are based on an exchange relationship where entitlements are acquired through contribution payments (Jost 2003, p. 266).[12] Second, population coverage is selective, i.e. only those who fulfil the conditions of SHI membership may receive coverage. Third, several healthcare entitlements are left to the discre-tion of health funds and thus entitlement, at least to some degree, differs between funds. Fourth, healthcare rights in Germany are individual rights. SHI law grants individual SHI members a right to treatment (and prevention) and thus clearly focuses on the individual. This also becomes apparent by the fact that healthcare rights in Germany are absolute rights granted to the individual irrespective of the rights of others, and almost irrespective of current financial resources.[13] In some aspects, entitlements are conditional (e.g. based on the existence of certain needs or illness), but they are absolute in the sense that claims must always be ful-filled if the requisite conditions are met.[14] Fifth, as rights are absolute, they can be legally enforced either through the courts or administrative proceedings. Sixth, the level of specification of entitlements is much more detailed compared to England. Table 4.1 provides an overview of the differences between the English collective and the German individual social right to healthcare as described above.

The course and patterns of individualisation

During the period of investigation, the English collective social right to healthcare gradually transformed towards a more individualistic right. A first tentative step was taken with the Patient's Charter in 1991. The transformation then intensified

Table 4.1 Collective and individual social rights to healthcare in comparison

	The English collective social right	The German individual social right
Conceptual basis	*Status (residency)*	*Contract*
Population coverage	*Universal*	*Selective*
Reference point	*Society*	*Individual*
Equality of rights	*Yes (formal)*	*Small differences between health funds*
Absolute entitlement and legal enforceability	*No, only procedural claims possible*	*Yes*
Level of specification	*General*	*Detailed*

under New Labour with the introduction of NICE technology appraisals and the launch of the NHS Constitution. In addition, decisions of the European Court of Justice (ECJ) on patient mobility, as well as the courts at home, contributed to individualisation.

The Patient's Charter was the first document to explicitly reference the rights of patients. This was a novelty in the NHS and signified a groundbreaking shift considering that NHS law does not even recognise patients as subjects. However, the rights catalogued in the Charter were minimal. They included, for example, the right to receive healthcare on the basis of clinical need, the right to be registered with a GP and the right to access hospital treatment within two years. The Charter did not grant new rights, but merely reformulated the legal duties of NHS bodies as the rights of patients. Moreover, the Charter was not a legal document and thus did not improve enforceability of rights.

The establishment of the NICE Technology Appraisal Process, for the first time in NHS history, allowed for a specification of entitlement to concrete treatments and drugs, thus making (at least part of) NHS healthcare entitlement explicit. The more important step, however, was the obligation of PCTs to fund the technologies positively recommended by NICE, introduced in 2002. With it, entitlement to these treatments and drugs became an absolute right because the recommended technologies must be provided irrespective of the financial situation of PCTs (and now CCGs). Thus, two characteristics of individual social rights – a more detailed level of specification, and absolute and enforceable entitlement – were implemented, albeit only for a fraction of total NHS services.

Another step towards a more individualistic social right was made with the NHS Constitution in 2009. Until its publication, healthcare entitlement could only be derived from NHS administrative law defining the rights and responsibilities of NHS bodies concerning the provision of services. The Constitution frames these responsibilities of NHS bodies as the rights of individuals in relation to the NHS. In this regard, it is similar to the Patient's Charter, but its rights have greater scope. Next to anti-discrimination rights (e.g. the right to be treated with dignity and respect), personal freedom rights (e.g. consent to treatment), rights to information and choice (e.g. the right to choose a GP), rights to quality services (e.g. the right to monitoring of quality) and rights that help to enforce patients' rights (e.g. the right to lodge a complaint), the Constitution established a right to receive services free of charge, a right to treatment in other European countries, rights to be treated within defined waiting time limits, a right to all drugs and treatments recommended by NICE and to vaccinations recommended by the Joint Committee on Vaccination and Immunisation. The Constitution has no direct legal effect, but health authorities and healthcare providers are bound by law to respect the rights listed by the Constitution (s. 2 Health Act 2009).

Individualisation was also triggered by the ECJ through its judgements on patient mobility (see Chapter 2.7). Applying an 'individualistic conception of rights to healthcare' (Newdick 2009, p. 846),[15] the ECJ constituted an absolute right to treatment abroad for individual patients. This right encompasses all treatments provided by the particular Member State. Only hospital and special treatment require prior approval, but denial is not permitted if the treatment cannot be provided by the Member State's public healthcare system within a medically acceptable timeframe. With this absolute, individual right to treatment abroad, the ECJ created an exit option for English patients: now they can travel to any European country for treatment if NHS waiting times are too long.

With the Patient's Charter and the NHS Constitution, patients have been provided an individual rights perspective by the NHS. It seems that they have adopted this perspective and now claim their rights: ever more patients take legal action if they are denied funding. These claims are increasingly accepted by judges who are also more willing to intervene in allocative decisions of health authorities (see Chapter 2.6). So far, however, courts have only overturned funding decisions (based on procedural grounds), and have referred the decision back to the relevant health authority for reconsideration.

Discussion

I have argued strongly that the social right to healthcare in England is shifting towards an individual social right. Having brought forward the points supporting my thesis, I also want to bring up the limitations of my argument. The NHS is far from providing individual rights as the overview below shows (Table 4.2). Population coverage has always been based on residency and hence population coverage has been universal. There is no evidence that this will change in the future. Although the individual has become an important reference point for NHS rights, the importance of general societal welfare still looms much larger than in the German healthcare system. Moreover, individual rights still are not enshrined in NHS law, but constituted in quasi-law only.

The obligation to fund treatments positively recommended by NICE technology appraisals established an absolute right to these treatments. However, the technologies assessed make up only a very small percentage of overall NHS benefits. Furthermore, absolute entitlement to technologies positively recommended by NICE negatively impact on other entitlements: given that resources are fixed, the funding of treatments and drugs recommended by NICE means that fewer

Table 4.2 Classification of NHS healthcare rights today

	Collective social right	NHS healthcare rights today	Individual social right
Conceptual basis	Status (citizenship)	*Status (residency)*	Contract
Coverage	Universal	*Universal*	Selective
Reference point	Society	*Society and the individual*	Individual
Equality of rights	Yes (formal)	*Yes (formal)*	Small differences between health funds
Absolute entitlement and legal enforceability	No, only procedural claims possible	*Yes, for treatments recommended by NICE, no, for other services; Only procedural claims possible but EU exit option*	Yes
Level of specification	General	*General: NHS law; Detailed: NICE recommendations*	Detailed

resources are available for services not assessed by NICE. Hence, while on the one hand NICE recommendations grant an absolute entitlement to few services, on the other they reduce entitlement to the bulk of non-assessed benefits, thus making the relationship between entitlement and available resources even more obvious.[16] Apart from NICE recommended treatments, UK law does not grant absolute rights, and patients cannot enforce them by taking legal action. Yet EU law assigns patients the absolute right to treatment abroad and thus provides them with an exit option if their demands are not met at home. However, an absolute right resulting from EU law is difficult for patients to enforce. EU law implicitly assumes that national public healthcare systems have a defined health service package specifying the goods and services citizens or the insured are entitled to, which, however, the NHS does not possess. Hence, patients who go abroad risk reimbursement if the treatment received there is not also provided by their CCG. In addition to the risk of having to assume the costs, there are many other factors making treatment abroad an unattractive option (e.g. time loss, language and cultural barriers, a lack of trust). Thus it is not to be expected that many patients will realise their rights by going abroad. And last, specification of healthcare entitlement has become more detailed only for treatments considered by NICE technology appraisals.

To summarise, during the last two decades, the collective social right to healthcare granted by the English NHS underwent a considerable transformation. Yet it is still far from being an individual social right as provided in Germany. However, individualisation has various routes, and is at least a partly self-enforcing process. Chapter 5 more deeply analyses the causes of the individualisation process and furthermore discusses its long-run implications for the NHS.

Notes

1 Determining the extent of retrenchment is difficult and is done here by comparing reforms to the situations in 1977 and 1979 respectively, as well as by comparing reforms between the two countries. In Chapter 5.1 a different approach is followed by assessing relative retrenchment, i.e. reforms are compared to all other retrenchment reforms within one country.

2 Yet precisely because legal regulations have usually not been used to alter NHS service provisions, modifications of the legal regulation of service coverage can be assumed to have been of particular importance for political actors.

3 Until 1988, these criteria had applied to ambulatory care only, but since then they apply to all goods and services provided under SHI.

4 'Economic' has a particular meaning within the German SHI system. For a detailed description, see the section on generosity in Chapter 3.2.

5 See Chapter 2.4 for a detailed description.

6 Cost sharing for dental prostheses and crowns differed between SHI funds and was defined within the statutes of the funds. Other charges did not apply in 1977.

7 The particulars of the committees are described in the country chapters. For a detailed discussion of both committees, see Landwehr and Böhm (2014).

8 Newdick (2009) uses a similar dual distinction between collective and individual rights in his analysis of the impact of the ECJ rulings on the social right to healthcare. He calls the two models 'communitarian conception of rights' and 'individualistic conception of rights to healthcare' (p. 846).

9 Also Trägårdh and Svedberg (2013) distinguish between collective and individual rights. Their distinction, however, is one between collective social rights and individual civil rights (freedom rights), although the distinction is not always made clear in their description of the changing relationship between the state and the individual in the Swedish welfare state. Trägårdh and Svedberg contend that there is an inherent contradiction between collective social rights and individual freedom rights ('iron law of rights'). As a solution to this conflict, they propose individual social rights such as care vouchers, however, without conceptualising these as individual social rights.

10 Entitlement is concretised on the local or regional level and depends on available resources. Thus, actual entitlement often varies widely between local areas.

11 Furthermore, patients do have the possibility to submit their case for review to their public health authority, which usually has an appeals procedure in place.

12 In contrast to private health insurance, however, there is only an indirect linkage between contribution payments and rights in social health insurance systems, i.e. the content of entitlement is de-linked from the amount of contributions, and entitlements may be assigned to specified groups that do not have to pay contributions (e.g. conferred entitlement for spouses or children).

13 If financial resources are not sufficient to meet all eligible claims, contributions must be increased.

14 For the sake of clarity, it should be noted that claims can be directed only towards the public healthcare system, not towards other individuals. Furthermore, rights are absolute only insofar as they have a valid legal basis, which may be altered at any time by legitimate, democratically elected actors.

15 In his paper, Newdick argues that the ECJ rulings endanger the social right to healthcare provided by Member States because the ECJ recognises only individual rights to healthcare being absolute and enforceable 'irrespective of their impact on others' (p. 848). Due to his exclusive focus on the UK, Newdick neglects to acknowledge that the individualistic conception of the social right to healthcare is not unique to the ECJ, but is shared by many European countries. For their social rights, the impact of ECJ is less relevant.

16 I thank Katharina Kieslich for raising the argument regarding the negative effects of NICE recommendations on other entitlements to me.

5 Explaining healthcare entitlement reforms

In this chapter, I address the second research question and illuminate the causes of reforms triggering the transformation of the social right to healthcare. Concentrating on the two main findings of the study[1] – the retrenchment of healthcare entitlement in both countries during the 1980s and 1990s, and the individualisation of the social right to healthcare in England – the driving causes behind the reforms are explored. The analysis of the causes of retrenchment, which is provided in the first part of this chapter, resorts to the hypotheses compiled from welfare state theories in Chapter 1. The analysis of the causes of individualisation, which makes up the second part of this chapter, cannot be drawn from classic welfare state theories. Instead, it is based on alternative approaches, such as consumerism and Europeanisation theories.

5.1 Explaining healthcare entitlement retrenchment

It is not surprising that England and Germany did not drastically cut healthcare entitlement given the general arguments against radical welfare state retrenchment, as well as the particularities of public healthcare systems which make such retrenchments highly unlikely (see Chapter 1). Yet it is not that healthcare entitlement went untouched. Both countries implemented various reforms during the last three and a half decades that restricted the social right to healthcare. It is the task of this chapter to explain these retrenchments. For this purpose, the periods of retrenchment are identified based on the detailed analyses in Chapters 2 and 3. Next, the conditions potentially favouring extensive cuts (hypothesis 1) are analysed. In addition, it is considered whether partisan politics can explain the outcome of reforms (hypothesis 2). Both these steps are carried out for each country separately. Finally, the results for the two countries are compared and the role of institutional factors in explaining welfare state reform are discussed

England

Periods of retrenchment

Most retrenchment reforms were enacted under Conservative rule. During the late 1970s and 1980s, the focus of reforms was on charges; they were massively increased in 1979 and 1980, and to a smaller extent during the later 1980s. In 1984 and 1985, charge increases were accompanied by service exclusions (visual aids, limited lists of drugs). Conservative retrenchment reached another peak during the early and mid-1990s with double-digit charge increases and the expansion of the drug limited list in 1992. Under Labour, retrenchment was moderate, but not absent. In 1998, 2000 and 2004, charges were raised more than the rate of inflation. In contrast, the current coalition government has, to the date of this writing, completely abstained from any retrenchment of legal healthcare entitlement.

For the analysis, all reforms for each year have been grouped and categorised as minor, medium or extensive retrenchment.[2] For a year categorised as having *minor* retrenchment, the charge increases[3] surmounted the inflation rate by a maximum of 50 per cent, or several smaller services were excluded. A year in which retrenchment was categorised as *medium* indicates that charge increases were between three and five times higher than the inflation rate, or that charges were increased more than 1.5 times the inflation rate, and in addition, one relevant service was excluded that year. (A service is defined as relevant if it is needed by a large group of patients.) For a year of *extensive* retrenchment, charges were raised more than five times the inflation rate, or increases exceeded the inflation rate more than three times, and in addition, one or more relevant services were explicitly excluded from the NHS benefits package. The retrenchment grade is given for each year between 1979 and 2013 in Table 5.1 to Table 5.3. Table A.9 of the appendix provides further details of the classification system.

The constrained budget argument

Pierson's constrained budget argument (hypothesis 1a) is confirmed by the English case: all medium and extensive retrenchments of healthcare entitlement were carried out under negative state budgets (see Table 5.1). However, it must be mentioned that during the entire period of investigation, only seven of the years had a positive budget at all. In the past, this was not the case. Between 1946 and 1974, the budget shrank only once. Thus the relatively minor budget shortfalls of the late 1970s and 1980s represented an exceptional situation for those times and hence provided a good justification for cuts. During the mid-1990s, budget deficits reached unknown heights which led to increased legitimacy of retrenchment reforms. During the 2000s, deficits were rather moderate and did not result in any noteworthy cuts. Since 2009, budget deficits have been exceptionally high, but interestingly, healthcare entitlement has not been subject to cuts, and generosity was even slightly expanded in 2009. Hence, a budgetary crisis was a necessary but not sufficient condition for medium and extensive retrenchments in the English case.

The electoral slack argument

Another argument of Pierson's 'new politics' thesis is that radical cuts are more likely if politicians do not fear being voted out of office by the electorate (hypotheses 1b). The British first past the post electoral system commonly brings about

Table 5.1 Healthcare entitlement retrenchment in England and its explanatory factors – the Conservative years

Year	1979	1980	1981	1982	1983	1984	1985	1986	1987	1988	1989	1990	1991	1992	1993	1994	1995	1996	1997
Retrenchment[a]	XXX	XXX	–	XX	X	XX	XXX	X	X	X	X	–	X	XX	XXX	XXX	XX	X	X
State budget[b] (% of GDP)	-1.81	-2.94	-1.27	-1.42	-1.92	-2.08	-1.2	-1.36	-0.42	1.62	1.41	0.33	-1.94	-5.53	-6.16	-4.67	-3.24	-2.69	-0.05
NHS budget increase[c]	0.06	0.05	0.01	0.00	0.02	0.01	0.01	0.05	0.11	0.07	0.03	0.04	0.06	0.05	0.01	0.06	0.02	0.01	0.03
Electoral slack	–	–	–	ES	ES	ES	–	–	ES	ES	–	–	–	–	–	–	–	–	–
Elections	E	–	–	–	E	–	–	–	E	–	–	–	–	E	–	–	–	–	E

a X minor retrenchment, XX medium retrenchment, XXX extensive retrenchment of healthcare entitlement.

b Sources: Public Sector Current Budget, Office for National Statistics (2014).

c NHS Budget increase in real terms. Own calculation based on NHS budget data from the Office of Health Economics (2013) and the annual inflation rate as provided by OECD (2014a). There exists a controversial debate about how to calculate NHS budget development in real terms (Appleby 2013; Le Grand, Winter & Wooley 1991). In order to keep the analysis within limits, the general price inflation was used here. For alternative data see Appleby (2013).

Table 5.2 Healthcare entitlement retrenchment in England and its explanatory factors – the Labour years

Year	1997	1998	1999	2000	2001	2002	2003	2004	2005	2006	2007	2008	2009
Retrenchment[a]	–	X	–	X	–	–	–	X	–	–	–	–	–
State budget[b] (% of GDP)	1.2	2.27	2.32	1.13	-1.06	-1.46	-1.6	-1.03	-0.49	-0.44	-2.57	-5.96	-4.95
NHS budget increase[c]	0.03	0.04	0.08	0.08	0.09	0.15	0.09	0.08	0.08	0.03	0.07	0.01	0.05
Electoral slack	–	ES	ES	ES	ES	ES	ES	–	ES	–	–	–	–
Elections	–	–	–	–	E	–	–	–	E	–	–	–	–

a X minor retrenchment, XX medium retrenchment, XXX extensive retrenchment of healthcare entitlement.
b Sources: Public Sector Current Budget, Office for National Statistics (2014).
c NHS Budget increase in real terms. Own calculation based on NHS budget data from the Office of Health Economics (2013) and the annual inflation rate as provided by OECD (2014a).

Table 5.3 Healthcare entitlement retrenchment in England and its explanatory factors – the Coalition years

Year	2010	2011	2012	2013
Retrenchment	–	–	–	–
State budget[b] (% of GDP)	–3.94	–4.47	–3.76	1.2
NHS budget increase[c]	–0.01	–0.03	–[d]	–[d]
Electoral slack	–	–	–	–
Elections	E	–	–	–

b Sources: Public Sector Current Budget, Office for National Statistics (2014).
c NHS Budget increase in real terms. Own calculation based on NHS budget data from the Office of Health Economics (2013) and the annual inflation rate as provided by OECD (2014a).
d Data not available.

a one-party government, and usually, Conservatives and Labour compete for government. The likelihood of electoral slack is thus higher than in Germany, where two or more parties typically form a coalition. In England, the chance of the government party to be voted out of office is low if the only opposition party is weak. This was the case, for example, during the first two Thatcher governments when Labour was a feeble opponent due to its split. However, it is not easy for politicians to determine ex ante if their position is strong enough to risk imposing radical retrenchment (Pierson 1996, p. 177). Opinion polls help politicians to estimate the strength or weakness of opponents. Polls are regularly produced and published by diverse institutes in the UK.[4] For the sake of simplicity, I assumed that politicians estimate their current standings only from polling data, and based the determination whether an electoral slack existed for the respective year exclusively on polling data.

According to polling data, the Conservatives enjoyed a three-year electoral slack lasting from April 1982 until the beginning of 1985, with only a short break in the middle of 1984. The position of the Conservatives was again very good from February 1987 until February 1989. After that, polls showed several peaks for the Conservatives, but the periods were too short to be considered an electoral slack. Labour met broad approval from the electorate throughout its first legislative period and during the beginning of its second period.[5] Labour's lead, however, became unstable and often decreased below five per cent during the period of mid-2003 to September 2004. The polls improved again until Labour lost its lead in December 2005. The acceptance of the coalition government has never been strong enough to bring about an electoral slack. During their first months, the Conservatives had a lead over Labour, but then Labour grew stronger and several times could gather even more approval than Conservatives and Liberal Democrats together.

Table 5.1 shows that there is no positive correlation between the existence of an electoral slack and retrenchment reforms. Hence hypothesis 1b must be rejected for the English case. The most severe retrenchment reforms were even conducted under unstable or adverse conditions. This does not, however, mean that politicians did not consider the electoral consequences of their policies. Every British government during the time of observation abstained from medium or extensive retrenchment the year before an election. Furthermore, it must be noted that polling data mirror the current mood of the electorate, and thus are very sensitive to topical reform debates. For example, the Conservatives held a lead over Labour in 1984, and then lost it from June until August, the time during which the Health and Social Care Act 1984 was discussed and passed. But only major health reforms influence the polls; regular amendments and other changes being implemented via statutory instruments are less visible to the electorate (see below), and thus have no (or only minimal) impact on polling data. Hence, it seems that politicians either expected their reforms to have no negative effect on electorate opinions, or they accepted the negative effects of retrenchment reforms in order to achieve other goals. In fact, the DH and the Treasury regularly fought over the NHS budget, and the DH often had to accept charge increases in return for an increased NHS budget.

The possibility of hiding reforms

The Westminster system with its strongly centralised power is usually perceived to be prone to retrenchment because of its few veto possibilities. However, concentrated authority means that responsibility is likewise concentrated, thus leaving government open to blame for retrenchment efforts (Pierson 1996, p. 154). According to Pierson (p. 177), such a system, on the contrary, provides better opportunities to hide reforms. A good example is the low visibility of charge increases in England. Unlike the situation in Germany, charge increases are not decided by Parliament. Instead, the NHS Act confers power to the Secretary of State to establish regulations concerning the making and recovery of charges (e.g. s. 172 NHS Act 2006). For this purpose, the SoS issues statutory instruments which then require the approval of Parliament. However, approval is automatically granted if the regulation is not rejected within a given timeframe, and thus charge increases usually attract low parliamentary and public attention, except from those affected. This, however, is only a small group as most patients are exempted from paying charges. Hence, hypothesis 1c is confirmed for the case of co-payments in England. The ease of implementation and the low visibility of reforms may explain why charges were increased almost every year in England, while much less regularly in Germany.

Institutional amendments

Pierson (1996) assumes retrenchment to be more likely if political actors are able to change the institutional framework within which decisions are taken into a more favourable setting allowing for better justification of retrenchment and the shifting of blame (hypothesis 1d). With regard to healthcare entitlement, two relevant institutional amendments could be witnessed in England between 1979 and 2013:

the increasing relevance of the EU level and the foundation of NICE. The shift-ing of responsibility to the EU level was not intended, but is a typical example of negative integration. Furthermore, ECJ judgements increased rather than restricted healthcare rights.

With NICE, the DH established a new institution responsible for explicit cover-age decisions. Until then, explicit coverage decisions were almost unknown to the NHS. From the viewpoint of a vote-seeking politician, explicit decisions are highly delicate because they make entitlement restrictions visible. Thus, in order to avoid blame, the task was assigned to an independent body. Furthermore, the institutional decision-making process was cleverly designed: NICE was not tasked with exclud-ing services, but rather with deciding about the compulsory funding of treatment. This makes a huge difference in the public perception of the work of NICE, while not in the outcome of its recommendations.[6] With the foundation of NICE, the DH could claim credit for having established a national standard of healthcare entitle-ment, while simultaneously shifting the blame for unpopular decisions to an expert body. In order not to endanger the fragile construction of blame shifting, the DH does not interfere with NICE's decision-making (Wood 2013). But blame shifting does not work well. NICE is very well known in the public, and its decisions, in particular its negative decisions not to fund a technology, receive high media cov-erage and often lead to intense public pressure on politicians. Hence the coalition government tried to abolish the mandatory recommendations of NICE and to hand decision-making power over to the CCGs. This would have lowered the visibility of entitlement decisions yet again; but doctors, not wanting to take on the blame, opposed the reform. In sum, the establishment of NICE confirms hypothesis 1d: the exclusion of treatments became possible when decisions were transferred to an independent public agency, allowing (at least partly) for blame shifting; framing NICE decisions positively as the granting of rights allowed for favourable public perception, at least in the beginning.

The previous example of opposition from doctors is exceptional in English healthcare policy-making. In general, doctors in England have far less veto power than their counterparts in Germany, particularly since being defeated by Thatcher (Klein 2010, pp. 158ff., 238; see also Chapter 2.3). Furthermore, doctors have not had much interest in intervening in healthcare entitlement reforms. Most retrench-ment concerned cost coverage of NHS services which primarily impacted patients, not doctors. To the contrary, restriction of pharmaceutical coverage met doctors' opposition because they perceived it as weakening their professional decision-making powers. Thus in 1984, doctors strongly opposed the limited list, but with minimal success (Rivett 1998, p. 326).

Party politics

With regard to power resource theory, the English case seems clear: all medium and extensive retrenchments of healthcare entitlement were conducted by Conser-vative governments, while Labour was responsible for only few minor retrench-ments. Thus the findings support the party-politics-still-matter thesis and moreover, they prove that the traditional right-left dichotomy is still valid: the centre-right party retrenched, and the left party defended and even extended social rights. Thus, hypothesis 2 must be rejected for the English case. However, the story is not quite so simple; at least one inconsistency casts some doubt on it. The Conservatives have been in government since 2010, and to the date of this writing, they had not yet implemented any restrictions to healthcare entitlement, despite the very tight economic and budgetary situations. One could argue that their coalition partner might have opposed retrenchment, but because of the weak position of the Liberal Democrats within the government and in the polls, combined with the fact that the position of Secretary of State for Health is held by the Conservatives, this argument is not convincing. It is not that the Conservatives completely abstained from cuts: the budget they allocated to the NHS is very tight. Moreover, they undertook one of the biggest reorganisations in the history of the NHS, thus proving that they are capable of conducting reform. Hence, the question arises: why then did they not touch healthcare entitlement? There are several possible answers. One possibility may be that due to the generous expansion of eligibility criteria by the former Conservative and Labour governments, the majority of patients were already exempt from paying charges. Thus, charge increases would generate very little additional income, and therefore were not worth risking votes. Another possible reason may be that the coalition government concentrated on structural reforms (the Health and Social Care Act 2012) and did not want to endanger their ambitious plans by implementing additional unpopular reforms. Third, the Conservatives had already reached the maximum possible explicit exclusion of services during the 1980s and 1990s. Further exclusions, as well as new charges, would have cut into core service areas of the NHS (e.g. GP and hospital services) which would have caused immense outcry and broad opposition, and without doubt, been opposed by the electorate. Finally, the coalition government did not restrict entitlement explicitly, but limited the NHS budget. As entitlement depends upon the availability of resources, they thereby cut entitlements indirectly. Furthermore, the failed attempts of Conservatives and Liberal Democrats at abolishing rights granted by positive recommendations of NICE demonstrate how difficult it is to restrict already existing rights. To conclude, the healthcare entitlement policies of the coalition government are not really 'inconsistent' with the party-matters thesis, and thus, the English case study of healthcare entitlement reform does not confirm hypothesis 2.

Germany

Periods of retrenchment

healthcare entitlement was drastically cut by the Social–Liberal coalition for the first time in 1977. The same government passed another retrenchment law in 1981, which was, however, milder than the first one. The coalition of Christian Democrats and Liberals continued retrenchment policies and implemented the first notable cuts in 1983 (e.g. the exclusion of drugs for the treatment of minor diseases, the introduction of co-payments for hospital stays). A profound reform was then enacted in 1988: the GRG sharply reduced cost coverage for several treatments, and restricted service coverage of ambulatory medical and dental care, to name only the most incisive cuts. In addition, the GRG restricted access to SHI membership for the voluntarily insured and students. The next relevant retrenchment law was passed in 1992. The GSG increased several charges and excluded orthodontic treatment for adults from the SHI benefits package. After a pause of three years, cost coverage was again seriously reduced twice in 1996 and 1997. Retrenchments did not let up under the Red–Green government. In 1999, the Red–Green coalition restricted access to SHI membership for older people and for family members. In the same year, they allowed for the possibility of the exclusion of hospital services from the benefits package. Even more radical was the 2003 reform, which introduced numerous new co-payments, raised existing charges and excluded several services from coverage (e.g. OTC drugs, visual aids). The successive grand coalition of Social Democrats and Christian Democrats did not apply traditional retrenchment measures, but cut entitlement by introducing several conditions of conduct that financially sanctioned 'poor' health behaviour in 2007. Contrary to the general expansion of population coverage, the Grand Coalition furthermore restricted access to SHI for the unemployed. The coalition of Christian Democrats and Liberals did not conduct any retrenchment reform during its four years in office.

Similar to the English case, retrenchment reforms were classified as minor, medium or extensive. Yet alternative criteria guided classification in the German case because healthcare entitlement regulation, and hence reforms, differ so widely from those in England. For the German case, retrenchment reforms of one year were categorised as *minor* if they involved one relevant cut and/or several smaller cuts. A retrenchment measure was defined as relevant if it introduced a new charge in one of the core service areas; if it excluded a larger group of benefits or a treatment needed by a larger group of patients; if it tightened eligibility for a larger group of patients; or if it increased conditionality of SHI membership for a larger group of SHI members. Years with more than one relevant cut or several smaller cuts in each of the three categories (service coverage, cost coverage and population coverage) were categorised as *medium*. And finally, years with more than three relevant cuts in at least two categories were classified as *extensive*. The categorisation of retrenchment for each year is shown in Table 5.4 to Table 5.8. A full description of reforms and the rationale for classification is given in Table A.10 of the appendix.

The constrained budget argument

In Germany, the public healthcare system is financed from contributions paid by employers and employees. Only since 2004, a small (but increasing) share of the SHI resources has come from taxes. Hence, in order to determine if there was a constrained budget in a particular year, we must look at SHI finances instead of the public budget. Table 5.4 to Table 5.8 provide the net balance of the SHI budget for each year from 1976 to 2013, and reveal that almost all medium and extensive retrenchments were conducted during years with negative budgets – or the year after, as was the case in 1997. Only in 1977 and 1982 was healthcare entitlement severely restrained under seemingly slack budgetary conditions. In 1977, however, the financial situation of SHI was anything but relaxed. A negative budget could be avoided only because contribution rates had been markedly raised the year before, as shown in Table 5.4. Rising contribution rates were perceived as particularly problematic because, as contributions are paid out of earned income, they increase labour costs, and thus, it was feared, negatively impact on Germany's global competitiveness. Hence, almost all health reform debates during the last three decades in Germany centered on the problem of mounting contributions and how to avoid a further surge in labour costs. Rising social insurance contributions were also behind the 1982 reform. Similar to the 1977 reform, cost-containment measures became necessary due to a cost shift from statutory pension insurance (SPI) to SHI. The Accompanying Budget Law 1983 reduced the amount of money being paid by SPI to SHI for the pensioners' health insurance in order to relieve the budget of SPI, and to keep SPI contributions low. In order to balance the reduced revenues of SHI, cost-containment measures then had to be enacted within SHI. Hence, constrained budgets were also a necessary but not sufficient condition for healthcare entitlement cuts in Germany. Thus, hypothesis 1a also holds true for the German case.

Table 5.4 Healthcare entitlement retrenchment in Germany and its explanatory factors – the SPD/FDP years

Year	1976	1977	1978	1979	1980	1981
Retrenchment[a]	–	XXX	–	–	–	X
SHI budget[b] (net total, m. DM)	3,640	3,675	1,645	−238	−1,382	95
Percent. increase of average SHI contribution rate[c]	8.1	0.8	0.4	−1.3	1.1	3.7
Elections	E	–	–	–	E	–[d]
Majority of government parties in both chambers	–	–	–	–	–	–

a X minor retrenchment, XX medium retrenchment, XXX extensive retrenchment of healthcare entitlement.
b Sources: BMG, Daten des Gesundheitswesens, various years. Until 1990, data is given for West Germany only.
c Source: Own calculation based on BMG, Daten des Gesundheitswesens, various years. Until 1990, data is given for West Germany only.
d Government changed in September 1982 because the Liberals broke with the Social Democrats and went into coalition with the Christian Democrats.

Table 5.5 Healthcare entitlement retrenchment in Germany and its explanatory factors – the Kohl era

Year	1982	1983	1984	1985	1986	1987	1988	1989	1990	1991	1992	1993	1994	1995	1996	1997
Retrenchment[a]	XX	–	–	–	–	–	XXX	–	X	–	XX	–	–	–	XX	XX
SHI budget[b] (net total, m. DM)	4,485	2,792	–2,871	–2,277	–1,361	77	–1,737	9,755	6,099	–2,820	–9,354	10,410	2,202	–7,157	–6,947	1,683
Percent. increase of average SHI contribution rate[c]	1.5	–1.3	–3.4	3.3	3.3	3.4	2.2	0.1	–2.9	–1.4	2.8	4.0	–0.4	–0.2	2.5	0.7
Elections	–	E	–	–	–	E	–	–	E	–	–	–	E	–	–	–
Majority of government parties in both chambers	–	M	M	M	M	M	M	M	M (not June – Oct.)	M (until Apr.)	–	–	–	–	–	–

a X minor retrenchment, XX medium retrenchment, XXX extensive retrenchment of healthcare entitlement.
b Sources: BMG, Daten des Gesundheitswesens, various years. Until 1990, data is given for West Germany only.
c Source: Own calculation based on BMG, Daten des Gesundheitswesens, various years. Until 1990, data is given for West Germany only.

Table 5.6 Healthcare entitlement retrenchment in Germany and its explanatory factors – the Red–Green years

Year	1998	1999	2000	2001	2002	2003	2004
Retrenchment[a]	–	XX	–	–	–	XXX	–
SHI budget[b] (net total, m. Euro)	277	–80	103	–2,691	–3,409	–3,441	4,020
Percent. increase of average SHI contribution rate[c]	0.3	–0.1	–0.2	0.1	2.9	2.4	–0.6
Elections	E	–	–	–	E	–	–
Majority of government parties in both chambers	M	M (until Apr.)	–	–	–	–	–

a X minor retrenchment, XX medium retrenchment, XXX extensive retrenchment of healthcare entitlement.
b Sources: BMG, Daten des Gesundheitswesens, various years. Until 1990, data is given for West Germany only.
c Source: Own calculation based on BMG, Daten des Gesundheitswesens, various years. Until 1990, data is given for West Germany only.

Table 5.7 Healthcare entitlement retrenchment in Germany and its explanatory factors – the Grand Coalition

Year	2005	2006	2007	2008	2009
Retrenchment[a]	–	–	X	–	–
SHI budget[b] (net total, m. Euro)	1,424	5,459	1,744	1,430	1,418
Percent. increase of average SHI contribution rate[c]	break[e]	0.3	4.4	0.7	break[f]
Elections	E	–	–	–	E
Majority of government parties in both chambers	M (until Nov.)	M	M	M	M (not Mar – Sept.)

a X minor retrenchment, XX medium retrenchment, XXX extensive retrenchment of healthcare entitlement.
b Sources: BMG, Daten des Gesundheitswesens, various years. Until 1990, data is given for West Germany only.
c Source: Own calculation based on BMG, Daten des Gesundheitswesens, various years. Until 1990, data is given for West Germany only.
e Since 2005, the contributions are no longer equally shared between employers and employees. Employees must pay 0.9 per cent of their income in addition to half of the contribution rate. This additional contribution is not taken into account for the calculation of the average SHI contribution rate.
f Since 2009, the contribution rate is determined by the health ministry and SHI funds are allowed to levy additional contributions which are to be paid by the insured alone. Hence the average contribution rate no longer reflects the income situation of SHI and for this reason is not provided for the last years.

Table 5.8 Healthcare entitlement retrenchment in Germany and its explanatory factors – the CDU/CSU/FDP years

Year	2010	2011	2012	2013
Retrenchment	–	–	–	–
SHI budget[b] (net total, m. Euro)	–396	4,165	5,440	1,36
Elections	–	–	–	E
Majority of government parties in both chambers	M (until June)	–	–	–

b Sources: BMG, Daten des Gesundheitswesens, various years. Until 1990, data is given for West Germany only.

The electoral slack argument

Electoral slack is a rare phenomenon in Germany. Due to its multi-party system – in which three or more parties are voted into parliament and coalition strategies always change – there is usually no guarantee that a party will be elected to government. Moreover, during the long period from the mid-1980s until 2002, the share of the vote held by the two main parties remained fairly balanced, and the governing party constantly had to fear being voted out of office with the next election. Although since 2002 the CDU/CSU has consistently enjoyed greater support at the polls than the SPD, it had to fight for every vote during the period 2009–2013, due to the weakness of its liberal coalition partner and a strong Green Party.[7] The nearest Germany came to an electoral slack was the early part of the 'Kohl era' (1984–1989), when the government parties were markedly stronger than the SPD, and government participation of the Greens was highly unlikely. During these years, only a single, albeit major, healthcare entitlement retrenchment was enacted. Summing up, hypotheses 1b does not hold true for the German case.

Table 5.4 to Table 5.8 reveal that most governments were in fear of being sanctioned by the electorate for their healthcare reforms: with the exception of the Kohl government in 1982 and 1997,[8] none dared to pass major healthcare entitlement cuts in the year prior to election.

The possibility of hiding reforms

Compared to England, legal healthcare entitlement reforms are more visible in Germany. Each cost coverage amendment and fundamental service coverage decision must pass the *Bundestag*, and thus attracts broad public attention. As expected on the basis of hypothesis 1c, the frequency of cost coverage retrenchment reforms was thus lower in Germany than in England. Perhaps because cuts are highly visible in Germany, the government tried several times to disguise the real extent of cost coverage reform by restructuring the entire co-payment system. The KVKG, the GRG, the GSG and the GMG all amended the system of drug charges, thereby rendering any direct comparison of cost burden before and after reform impossible.

Institutional amendments

In order to avoid the regular and highly unpopular decisions to increase charges, the Kohl government intended to implement automatic increases for several healthcare services through the 2.GKV–NOG. More specifically, it planned to link the level of co-payments to the increase of aggregate wages. Thus, the yearly increase would not only have compensated for inflation, but charges also would have automatically risen with wage increases. This plan could be easily justified: people earning more money could afford to spend a bit more of it for their health. As part of the same reform, it was additionally planned to peg co-payments to the contribution rate: per 0.1 per cent increase of the contribution rate, all absolute co-payments would rise by 1 DM and relative co-payments by one per cent. This plan would have allowed the shifting of blame to SHI funds, while taking charge increases out of the parliamentary debate. Furthermore, with two automatic charge increases running parallel, the changes would be shrouded in complexity, and most patients would not have been able to locate the reason for charge increases. However, neither of these planned reforms was realised due to changes in government before they took effect.

Similarly as in England, the institutional framework of service coverage decision-making in Germany was amended to shift responsibilities – and thus blame – to non-governmental bodies. Over the years, more and more decision-making power was delegated to the joint self-administration. In contrast to England where decisions of NICE do not go unnoticed, decisions of the responsible joint self-administration committee (the FJC) receive very little public attention. Thus, delegation not only allows for the shifting of blame, but also the movement of relevant decision-making to the back room. However, complete exclusion of treatments by the FJC is rare (see Chapter 3.8) and thus delegation does not majorly increase retrenchment.

Party politics and veto points

At first glance, party politics seem to have no influence on healthcare entitlement policies in Germany: retrenchments were implemented by all government parties as Table 5.4 to Table 5.7 show. It is not that parties do not differ in their interests with regard to healthcare entitlement, but that the particularities of the political system, as well as strong veto power of relevant actors, often impede on the direct transfer of interests into policies. To support my argument, I present party positions regarding healthcare entitlement, describe the features of the political system which impact policy formation, and briefly discuss the genesis of each of the more significant retrenchment reforms.

The *Social Democrats*[9] more or less strictly opposed co-payments and service exclusions in the past. Their position changed in the course of the general renewal of Social Democratic social policy and the Agenda 2010 strategy (Blank 2011, pp. 122ff.). In 2003, the SPD, together with the Greens, submitted a reform draft which planned to heavily increase co-payments and exclude several treatments from the SHI benefits package (BT–Drs. 15/1170).[10] The draft allowed for broad exemptions of the chronically ill, and co-payments were restructured to incentivise a more efficient use of services (e.g. co-payments for specialist treatment in cases of no referral from the GP). It is this particular focus on efficiency (and quality) that guided SPD policy-making throughout the period of investigation, and that led them to repeatedly advocate for explicit decision-making on service coverage (e.g. the drug positive list). With regard to population coverage, policies of the 1980s and 1990s put emphasis on the equalisation of blue-collar and white-collar workers within SHI. Later, the Social Democrats fought for an inclusion of all population groups within one health insurance system.

Since the late 1970s, the primary goal of the *Christian Democrats*[11] has been to keep labour costs and thereby public insurance contributions low. Generally, service exclusions and co-payments were perceived to be legitimate instruments for achieving this goal. However, voters of CDU/CSU are traditionally heterogeneous and include all relevant interest groups (employers, unions, providers, SHI funds) (Webber 1988, p. 163). These interest groups were able, with varying success, to mobilise their interests within the party. Therefore, the Christian Democratic stance towards healthcare entitlement cuts varied over time and between issues. The Christian Democrats usually supported the concept of reciprocal solidarity as well as the dual system of private and public health insurance.

The Liberals (FDP) have traditionally represented the interests of employers, high-income earners and healthcare providers (Webber 1988, p. 164). Serving employers' interest in low contribution rates, the Liberals strongly advocated co-payments and service exclusions in the past. They promoted retrenchment policies only insofar as those did not conflict with the interests of their clientele. As the party of high-income earners, the Liberals furthermore defended and supported private health insurance.

The interest constellation of parties as described above provides only a very general picture. Interests of parties may change over time or deviate from the general path given exceptional situations. Furthermore, none of the parties during the last three and a half decades was able to fully realise its interests because all parties in government had to share government seats with another party, and thus always had to seek compromises. Compromise solutions often had to be reached not only amongst government parties, but also with opposition parties, because these were able to veto reforms if they held the majority in the *Bundesrat* (the federal council). In principle, healthcare entitlement reforms do not require approval of the *Bundesrat*, but because these were in most cases part of bigger health reform packages, they had to pass the *Bundesrat*, too. Even if government parties held majorities in both chambers (as shown in the tables above), there was no guarantee that their reforms would pass in the *Bundesrat* where the interests of the federal states sometimes outweigh party interests. Yet with regard to healthcare entitlement, the interests of the federal states usually do not deviate from party interests at the national level.

Many health policy outcomes of the past can be fully understood only if the often powerful influences of providers and other interest groups are considered. Providers and health funds have a particularly strong position in the public healthcare system – due to the system of joint self-administration – as they are responsible for implementing reforms. With regard to healthcare entitlement, the interest of providers is not yet clear. It seems that providers as well as SHI funds generally do not oppose co-payments; doctors working in the ambulatory sector, at least during the last years, voted for a slimmer SHI benefits package which would enable them to privately sell additional services; while the pharmaceutical industry fights reforms that cut into their profits.

In order to understand why the Social Democrats agreed to the Health Insurance Cost-containment Act (KVKG) of *1977*, which massively expanded co-payments, some background information on the causes of reform and the course of debate is essential. At the end of the 1970s, SPI was grappling with immense financial deficits. Tackling the problem, the government reduced the contributions paid by SPI for the insurance of pensioners to SHI. This in turn tore a hole into the budget of SHI and made cost-containment reforms necessary (Vincenti 2008, p. 526).[12] The SPD favoured saving money by restricting autonomy and reimbursement of doctors, but their coalition partner, the Liberals, opposed all reforms that too negatively affected their constituents. The Liberals accepted a slight restriction of the financial autonomy of doctors and a pharmaceutical negative list, but in turn demanded increases in co-payments (Rosewitz and Webber 1990; Vincenti 2008). The agreement of the Social Democrats to an increase in co-payments was facilitated by the fact that the unions demanded lower contribution rates and thus did not oppose cost-containment policies (Webber 1988, pp. 193ff.).

After the general elections of 1980, the power of the Liberals within the government coalition increased and the ability of the Social Democrats to co-determine health reforms diminished (Webber 1988, p. 198). Hence, it was primarily the Liberals who accounted for the retrenchment reforms of *1981* and *1982*.[13]

Given the very 'good' conditions under which the CDU/CSU and FDP had to enact a health reform in 1988, the question arises why they did not cut entitlements even more deeply. The SHI budget had been negative for several years running and the contribution rate steadily increased, thus providing a good argument for cuts. The government did not want to pass an unpopular reform directly before the elections and thus postponed the reform until after the *Bundestag* elections of 1987 (Webber 1989, pp. 269f.). In fact, the original reform plans envisaged very deep cuts to entitlement: in addition to various expansions of co-payments, it was planned to reduce SHI service coverage to the 'medically necessary' (Wasem and Greß 2005, p. 404; Webber 1989, p. 271). Opposition from unions and SHI funds was moderate, but the employees' faction of the CDU and the federal states in particular resisted reform plans and achieved at least a partial reduction in cuts (Wasem and Greß 2005, p. 406; Webber 1989, p. 275).

The 1988 reform measures did not help to contain SHI expenditures for long, and given the precarious economic situation, the CDU/CSU and FDP government deemed a new health reform necessary in *1992*. In order to be able to enact far-reaching reforms, particularly in the hospital sector, the CDU health minister was forced to request the cooperation of the Social Democratic opposition because the government parties had lost the majority in the *Bundesrat* in April 1991, thus requiring the consent of the opposition. The SPD accepted and achieved (amongst other measures) an attenuation of healthcare entitlement cuts that had been envisaged in the first government draft of the healthcare Structure Act (Wasem, Greß and Hessel 2007, p. 673). For example, the SPD achieved a reduction of drug co-payments and a positive list of drugs. Furthermore, they prevented the splitting of dental appliances and orthodontic treatment into basic and elective services.

During the negotiations of the 1992 reform, the Liberals lost bargaining power and could push through only a few of their proposals (Wasem, Greß and Hessel 2007, p. 673). In response, they attempted to prevent any cooperation between the government and the SPD prior to the next health reform in *1996* (Wasem 1998, pp. 21f.). In any case, the comprehensive cuts envisaged by CDU/CSU and Liberals precluded any compromise with the opposition, and thus, the two reform bills were not approved by the *Bundesrat* (Wasem 1998, p. 23). There was also great dissent within the government regarding the content of reform as the cuts proposed by the Liberals were too far-reaching, even for the Christian Democrats (Wasem 1998, p. 22). In 1996, however, the Liberals achieved good results in the federal state elections, which increased their bargaining power (Reiners and Müller 2012, p. 28). In the end, reforms requiring approval by the *Bundesrat* were dropped, and extensive healthcare entitlement cuts were decided by the *Bundestag*.

The *1999* reform introduced a positive list for drugs, allowed for the exclusion of hospital services, and eliminated individual prophylactic dental services for adults. These measures are characterised as retrenchment by this study. In the view of the Social Democrats, however, these measures help to improve the quality and efficiency of services (see explanatory memorandum BT–Drs. 14/1245). Indeed, explicit coverage decision-making, as established by the reform for hospital services and drugs, does not necessarily imply retrenchment. Explicit decisions to not fund a particular treatment do restrict service coverage, but as long as there remain sufficient treatment alternatives, entitlement is not limited. This is guaranteed by the Social Code Book V, which allows exclusions only if treatment alternatives are available (see Chapter 3). Thus, the positive list for drugs, as well as the option to exclude hospital services, are rather instruments to improve quality and efficiency of services than instruments of retrenchment. The reform, moreover, eliminated the possibility for older people to return to SHI after having held private insurance. This restricts access to SHI membership and thus clearly cuts population coverage. It does not contradict social democratic values, but reflects SHI's founding principle of reciprocal solidarity.

The healthcare entitlement cuts of the SHI Modernisation Act of *2003* cannot exclusively be explained by the fact that the reform resulted from a compromise between the Red–Green government and the CDU/CSU opposition (which was necessary in order to ensure that the reform could pass the *Bundesrat*). Many of the cuts had already been part of the first draft penned by the Red–Green government alone (Gerlinger 2004, p. 502). The retrenchment was rather a sign of changed health policy goals and instruments of the Social Democrats (Blank 2011, pp. 122ff.) than the result of unavoidable concessions to the opposition, even when several retrenchment measures were introduced by the opposition.

In summary, hypothesis 2 can also be rejected for the German case: party politics help greatly to explain healthcare retrenchment in Germany, but only when the complexity of party interests and the particularities of the political system are taken into account. Party interests are less clear cut in Germany compared to the English case: the Christian Democrats supported retrenchment, but within limits; the Social Democratic position towards healthcare entitlement reforms was highly differentiated (pro positive lists, contra co-payments) and changed over time; only the Liberals strongly advocated for retrenchment during nearly their entire time in government.[14] In addition: coalition governments, the strong veto power of the *Bundesrat*, and the sometimes powerful influence of relevant stakeholders impeded on the full realisation of party interests.

Discussion

The analysis above tested the hypotheses developed in Chapter 1 and found quite similar results for both cases with regard to hypotheses 1a through 1d. In England, as well as in Germany, a budgetary crisis was a necessary but not sufficient condition for medium and extensive retrenchment (hypothesis 1a). Hypothesis 1b, on the contrary, was rejected for both countries: an electoral slack did not lead to retrenchment reforms. Interestingly, however, no government, with the exception of two cases during the Kohl era in Germany, dared to carry out medium or extensive healthcare entitlement retrenchment reforms one year prior to or during an election year. Whether the possibility of hiding reforms (hypothesis 1c) enabled retrenchment or not could only be answered by comparing both countries: co-payments were increased almost every year by means of statutory instruments under Conservative rule in England; while they were raised only as part of major health reforms in Germany. In the analysis above, I ascribed this difference to the higher visibility of healthcare reform as opposed to the use of statutory instruments. However, it might also be explained by higher implementation costs: statutory instruments are subject to a less complex legislative procedure than primary legislation, and thus could more easily be implemented. Alternative explanations can also be found for the amendment of institutional rules (hypothesis 1d). In both countries, governments delegated service coverage decisions to more or less independent bodies. Despite this, it cannot be proven that the delegation of explicit coverage decision-making was intended to achieve retrenchment. According to official documents, NICE was founded with the aim of establishing a national standard of service coverage, and thus to improve equality within the NHS. On the contrary, the delegation of explicit decision-making in Germany was often driven by the hope of increasing efficiency and quality of treatment. In sum, several of Pierson's assumptions about the feasibility of retrenchment reforms showed some explanatory power for the two cases studied, but alone cannot explain the occurrence of retrenchment.

The more central aim of this analysis was to find out whether party politics still matter, since this question is highly contested in welfare state research, and has rarely been researched for the area of healthcare (see Chapter 1.5). In the case of

England, there is a clear relationship between party in government and retrenchment reforms, and the nature of the relationship proves to be as predicted by the power resource theory: retrenchment is more extensive under right-wing party rule than under left-wing governments. For Germany, this relationship is less direct, but as the above analysis has shown, party politics also help to explain retrenchment reforms. The findings thus contradict the results of quantitative studies in which no significant correlation between partisanship and public healthcare spending in times of austerity were found (Jensen 2011a; Jordan 2011). One explanation for the conflicting results could be that healthcare expenditure is not a good measure of policy output because healthcare spending is influenced by various factors (see Chapter 1). But even if a direct measure of policy output is taken as the dependent variable, as is the case for this study, the role of partisanship is often not immediately obvious. Whether party interests take effect depends on the particular constitutional system. The English first past the post voting system usually produces a one-party government able to assert, nearly unhindered, its interests in the veto-free political system. Thus, nearly all policies are directly determined by the party in government, and limits are set only by the electorate. In Germany, on the contrary, policies rarely mirror the interests of only one party. Due to its proportional voting system, multiple parties are represented in the parliament, and usually two or more parties form the government. This has two effects: first, party positions are more diversified because they must not cater to the median voter (Iversen and Soskice 2006), and second, the parties in government have to waive some of their proposals in order to reach consent. The already diluted party interests are often further watered down by the need to satisfy the often contradictory interests of the *Bundesrat*. Yet this does not mean that party interests play no role at all. Healthcare entitlement retrenchment was particularly strong under Christian Democratic and Liberal rule. Furthermore, taking the particularities of the political system into account helps to explain policy output that contradicts party interests (e.g. extensive retrenchment under the Red–Green government in 2003), and moreover, helps to explain why retrenchment during the Kohl era was not as far-reaching as expected.

The comparison of the driving forces of healthcare entitlement reforms in both countries revealed, once more, the relevance of institutional factors in explaining welfare state change. Interestingly, it is not the institutional characteristics of the particular healthcare system, but the standard political institutions that mainly account for healthcare entitlement policies. Thus, this study confirms the findings of Ellen Immergut, who identified the procedural rules of political decision-making as being the key explanatory factor for the foundation of national health insurances (see Chapter 1.5). Furthermore, the politics of retrenchment seem to differ less from the politics of expansion than Pierson claimed.

In Chapter 1, I argued that the type of financing of public healthcare might have an impact on healthcare entitlement retrenchment because entitlement cuts are a good means for decentralised funding systems to keep the budget in order, while centralised systems are able to directly adjust the budget without having to amend entitlement. After having studied the two cases, it remains unclear whether entitlement reform can be explained by funding type. The decentralised funding system in Germany provides a strong argument for the necessity of retrenchment: social insurance contributions (which are paid exclusively out of earned income) may impact negatively on the global competitiveness of the German economy. This argument was consistently used in every health reform debate, and the electorate seems to have accepted entitlement cuts as a necessary evil for the sake of over-all economic welfare. However, the difference of healthcare entitlement reforms between Germany and England is, in my view, best explained by the distinctness of social healthcare rights in the two countries (see Chapter 4). In England, with its collective social right to healthcare, healthcare entitlement is only vaguely defined, thus allowing health authorities to specify entitlement according to local need and available resources. Due to the low specification and no absolute entitlement to treatment, retrenchment required no adaptation of entitlement regulation, and entitlement could be indirectly restricted by limiting the budget. In Germany, on the contrary, entitlements are specified in more detail, and in addition, SHI members are granted absolute rights, which means any entitlement that is claimed must be met. Thus, the budget cannot be defined ex ante: how much money is spent on healthcare depends on the amount of claimed entitlements. Hence, retrenchment can be realised almost exclusively via restricting entitlements.

In conclusion, the case studies have shown that the 'old theories' have not lost their explanatory powers for times of austerity. The relationship between party in government and reform content was not always clear cut: the interests and power of parties are moderated by characteristics of the political system. Thus it was necessary to combine power resource theory with institutionalist approaches in the German case. Taken together, the two approaches account very well for major healthcare entitlement retrenchment reforms.

5.2   Explaining the individualisation of the social right to healthcare in England

During the last two decades, England's social right to healthcare underwent a partial transformation from a collective into an individual right. Individual rights had so far been unknown to NHS healthcare regulation. Instead, the Secretary of State for Health and health bodies were obliged to provide health services for the population. The reference point for public healthcare was the society and not the individual: in deciding on NHS service provision, the government and NHS bodies had to weigh claims of different groups (e.g. taxpayers, various groups of patients, other welfare beneficiaries) in order to maximise the welfare of society. Allocative decisions – who shall get what – were taken locally, subject to local need and availability of resources. Following from that, there was no absolute entitlement to NHS healthcare. However, since the 1990s, a variety of processes led to a gradual transformation of this collective right,[15] profoundly changing one of the NHS core foundations, namely, its orientation towards the general instead of the individual welfare. But what are the roots of this process? This section sug-gests three general trends having caused the transformation of the social right to healthcare in England. First is the changing role of the welfare state, in particular in public service provision. Public sector reforms following the ideals of managerialism and consumerism have, on the one hand, increased individuals' expectations towards the NHS, thus indirectly triggering individualisation. On the other hand, these processes directly generated individual rights. Second, as a prime example of negative integration, the Europeanisation of health policy spawned individual rights to healthcare in England. Third, the individualisation of the social right to healthcare also has its seeds in the general individualisation of society (e.g. Beck and Beck-Gernsheim 2002). However, it is difficult to identify discrete aspects of this general social process in the area of healthcare. Thus, the following sections focus on the first two sources – market-enhancing public sector reforms, and Europeanisation. Both processes are described in detail, and a discussion of their implications for the NHS and its patients follows.

The changing role of the state and the citizen in public services

My argument here is that the individualisation of the social right to healthcare is the direct outcome of the transformation of the welfare state, in particular of the changing role of the state in public services. As extensively described in Chapter 1, welfare states of industrial societies have undergone massive restructuring since the mid-1970s, bringing about a new type of welfare state, often labeled the 'enabling state' (Gilbert 2002). This transformation not only meant altered policies, but also reform of the state's institutional arrangements (Clarke and Newman 1997, p. 19). In addition to a retreat of the state from direct service provision, the reforms addressed the structure and organisation of public services. Referred to with the catch phrase 'new public management', these reforms included the devolution of responsibilities to lower organisational levels or to autonomous agencies, the introduction of management tools stemming from the organisation of private companies (e.g. increased autonomy for managers, design of incentives, performance measurement) and the implementation of competition and other market elements into the public sector (Christensen and Lægreid 2011, pp. 5ff.). As the core public service of the British welfare state, the NHS was also forced to undergo many of these reforms over the last 30 years. The reforms transformed the NHS from a hierarchical state body with predominantly public provision of services into a decentralised service organisation governed (at least partly) by market mechanisms and utilising a variety of providers. The task of the state thereby changed from operating to controlling the system. The role of patients was altered as well: patients were treated more and more as consumers, in the hopes that their power as consumers would help to control the quasi-market of healthcare, and better align public services with need and demand. In this section, I examine these reform processes to offer an explanation of how the steps to individualisation came to be.

The Conservatives under Thatcher were well known for their critique of an oversized government that, in their view, restricted individual freedom. They wanted to release the citizen from this burden and therefore strived to empower the individual (Needham 2007, pp. 53ff.). With regard to public services, this meant that citizens were provided consumer rights in order to increase their power vis-à-vis producers. This consumer approach was first brought into healthcare via the Griffiths report, which recommended aligning services with consumer needs and preferences (Klein 2010, p. 121). While especially Thatcher emphasised the expansion of consumer choice (which often included an exit option to private services), Major aimed at empowering service users within the public system (Clarke et al. 2007, pp. 30f.; Needham 2007, p. 57). One instrument of Major's strategy was the Citizen's Charter. Its offshoot in the healthcare sector, the Patient's Charter, spelled out for the first time in NHS history the rights of patients under the NHS. The rights listed by the Charter, however, did not grant any entitlement to particular services. Instead, they established rights, for example the right to information, or the right to be treated within a particular timeframe, to increase the sovereignty of consumers. It was the Charter's primary aim 'to empower the individual as consumer, informing choice through knowledge of various providers and products, rather than enhancing his or her rights as a citizen through new legal and political rights or social entitlements' (Taylor 1999, p. 30).

Blair took up the consumerist approach and further advanced the alignment of citizens and consumers to such an extent that Needham (2007) speaks about a 'consumerised citizenship regime' (p. 27) under New Labour. Having conducted a comprehensive content analysis of New Labour speeches and official documents, Needham found two strands running through the New Labour discourse on consumerism, one of which is of particular relevance here.[16] This is the 'standardisation narrative', 'where public services are as consistent as possible, with an emphasis on fairness and equity. Legal or procedural mechanisms are put in place to secure users' rights, and ensure that they have access to information and to services' (Needham 2007, p. 37). The establishment of NICE, the obligation of PCTs to fund treatments and drugs recommended by NICE and the NHS Constitution clearly followed this aspect of consumerism. It was the task of NICE to create national standards of service provision with the aim of limiting the variation in health service provision perceived as 'unfair' and not tenable for a national service (Department of Health 1998, pp. 1.8). The NHS Constitution set out the rights of patients and made clear what patients can expect from the NHS.

The question arises why the variation in service provision, although it had existed throughout the history of the NHS, increasingly came to be perceived as problematic in the late 1990s. The answer to this question directs us to two other aspects of NHS reform that contributed to the individualisation of healthcare entitlement, namely the decentralisation of responsibilities and the implementation of quasi-markets. A collective social right requires a legitimate authority to define the public good. In the past, this was the government, or more precisely the DH and the SoS. These determined the allocation of resources and defined priorities at the macro and meso levels. At the micro level, the allocative decisions were taken by individual doctors. In the course of decentralisation, responsibilities were devolved from the DH and the SoS to various (and changing) national, regional and local actors. It is now their task to define the public good and to make allocative decisions.[17] The problem with these fragmented responsibilities is that they necessarily result in regional variations with regard to generosity of and access to healthcare services. Besides local variations in morbidity rates, treatment patterns and medical infrastructure, allocative decisions are also influenced by normative value judgements (Littlejohns et al. 2012). In allocating scarce healthcare resources, decision-makers have to weigh competing and often equally legitimate claims. For example, they have to decide between an increase in life quality from one drug and a prolongation of life from another, between young and old patients, between prevention and acute treatment, etc. There is no 'right' answer since these decisions involve normative principles, and hence, outcomes depend on normative judgements of the decision-makers. The varying outcomes of allocative decisions, however, are problematic in a national healthcare system that formally grants every resident an equal right to healthcare.[18] The granting of individual rights to treatment at the national level can be seen as an attempt to solve this problem: local decision-makers are free to decide on the allocation of resources, but are bound to respect the individual rights of patients in order to guarantee equality (McCarvill 2010, p. 6).

The devolution of powers went hand in hand with the installation of quasi-markets (see Chapters 2.3 and 2.4). In the course of the introduction of the payer-provider split, the variety of providers was increased, competition was introduced and conditions of provision were determined by individual contracts between purchasers (health authorities) and single providers. This more market-like provision of healthcare has two implications. First, the greater variation in provision and the single-provider contract make it necessary to specify in more detail the concrete content of services to be provided and the money providers receive for service provision. It is not a coincidence that countries with mainly private provision possess the most detailed health service catalogues (e.g. Germany). Second, a more market-like provision of healthcare bears the risk of unintended and unwanted outcomes: provider competition might bring about low-quality services, for example. In order to avoid such outcomes, a strict quality assurance system was established and patients were empowered to assert control as consumers. For this purpose, their consumer rights (e.g. choice, information) were heavily expanded (see above). Consumer rights, however, are individual rights (Needham 2007, p. 35) and hence contradict the collectivistic notion of public healthcare, or as Clarke and Newman (1997) have put it: 'The increasing adoption of consumerist discourse involves the dismantling of notions of a collective public in favour of individualised users of services' (p. 128). This shift of focus from the collective to the individual has severe implications for the NHS as well as for the broader society, as will be discussed below.

The Europeanisation of the social right to healthcare

The impact of European integration on national healthcare[19] has been widely discussed (e.g. Böhm and Landwehr 2014; Gerlinger, Mosebach and Schmucker 2010; Greer 2006; Hervey and McHale 2004; Mossialos et al. 2010b; Steffen 2005). The tenor of all these publications is that negative integration, i.e. market enhancing policies, have restricted Member States' sovereignty to organise their public healthcare systems. EU primary law (Art. 168 No. 7 TFEU) grants Member States the autonomy to freely organise public healthcare, but in doing so, they must respect market freedoms for almost all components necessary to run a healthcare system such as medical goods, services, professionals and patients, for example.

The core driver of the Europeanisation processes in healthcare is the European Court of Justice (Mossialos et al. 2010a, p. 18). In applying free market rules to the area of healthcare – a sphere that was perceived by many as a public and hence non-market domain – the Court stepwise extended the influence of the EU to national healthcare systems. During the late 1990s and early 2000s, the ECJ delivered several seminal judgements concerning patient mobility within the EU.[20] Arguing that medical services are subject to Articles 28 and 49 EC – the free movement of goods and services – the ECJ established a right of patients to seek treatment in another Member State at the expense of their home public healthcare system. According to these judgements, patients are generally free to move to other Member States for medical treatment (or to get medical goods), and costs of medical treatment and goods must be reimbursed by the public healthcare system of the country of affiliation, at least at the rate that applies in the home country. The freedom to travel abroad for medical treatment may be restricted only if there exist 'overriding reasons in the general interest', for example, if the financial balance of the public healthcare system would be endangered. For this reason, Member States are allowed to operate a system of prior approval for hospital care and some other special treatments. Approval, however, may only be denied if the treatment cannot be provided in the home country without 'undue delay', and provided that the treatment is part of the national healthcare benefits package.

These judgements had consequences for all European public healthcare systems, but particularly for the English NHS, because neither its legal nor its institutional settings were compatible with new EU law. Before the ECJ rulings on patient mobility, the NHS had applied a very tight territorial restriction. On principle, the NHS did not provide care outside the UK,[21] and exemptions (also treatment based on the E112 scheme) had to be directly authorised by the DH (Obermaier 2009, p. 122). Furthermore, there is neither a defined healthcare benefits package, nor are the costs of treatment always clear, because there exist no tariffs for most NHS services (Zanon 2011, p. 35). Hence, it would be difficult to determine if an English patient travelling abroad is entitled to the treatment s/he receives there as well as the exact amount s/he will be reimbursed. In addition, the long NHS waiting lists added to the likelihood of people travelling abroad to seek faster treatment (Obermaier 2009, p. 123). Finally, and most importantly for this study, the English NHS does not recognise an individual right to treatment as established by the ECJ. With its collective social right to healthcare, the NHS acknowledges the right of the English population to receive healthcare, but it does not grant individuals a right to healthcare (for a detailed discussion see Chapter 2).

In attempting to explain the individualistic approach of the ECJ to healthcare, Newdick (2009) refers to Scharpf's concept of 'constitutional asymmetry' and states that the 'more individualistic and less communitarian conception of rights reflect an institutional "asymmetry" within the EU, in which the ECJ favors private "economic" interests over the public "welfare" policies identified by national governments' (Newdick 2009, p. 864). In my view, Newdick mistakenly accuses the ECJ of 'favoring' economic interests over public social policies. It is only due to the EU constitutional asymmetry that the ECJ has no other choice than to decide in favour of economic rights. Market enhancing policies are extensively anchored in the European treaties, while, due to the resistance of Member States, social policies and other market correcting policies rarely find their way into European law (Scharpf 2002). Hence, when confronted with the task of deciding healthcare cases, the ECJ could not refer to any European social security guarantees (because they do not exist), but had to base its decisions on economic freedom rights and competition rules that are firmly constituted within EU primary law (Mossialos and Palm 2003, p. 4).

The ECJ rulings established a general right to treatment abroad, but left many details open (Palm and Glinos 2010, pp. 551f.). The Commission thus sought to clarify open issues and passed a Patients' Rights Directive in 2011. The Directive, to a greater or lesser extent, reflects the content of the ECJ rulings concerning patient mobility and, in addition, establishes several 'new' patients' rights (Sauter 2011).[22] In detail, the new rights are: the right to information necessary to make an informed choice (e.g. information about treatment alternatives, the availability and costs of treatment, quality and safety standards), the right to lodge complaints, the right to privacy of personal data, the right to receive a medical record of treatment and the right to equal treatment and non-discrimination (Art. 4 2011/24/EU). With these new rights, the Directive, however, did not outweigh the constitutional asymmetry between market and social rights. The Directive indeed expanded the regulatory competencies of the EU in healthcare, thus advancing positive integration; but the rights cited above clearly follow a consumerist approach (Palm and Baeten 2011),[23] and hence represent market rather than social rights.[24]

It is the EU's focus on market integration that leads to an increased individualisation of social rights. On the one hand, the EU directly constitutes individual healthcare rights, i.e. the right to treatment abroad and the new consumer rights of patients. On the other hand, the individual rights established at the EU level are incompatible with collective rights at the national level. At the moment, there is an absolute right to treatment abroad, but only a relative right to treatment at home. This difference is hard to justify, in particular because entitlement to treatment abroad might negatively affect NHS entitlement. Both are financed from the same budget, which means, due to the dependence of NHS entitlement on the availability of resources, treatment consumed abroad reduces entitlement to NHS services. Even more problematic for the legitimacy of the collective social right (at least if many people start travelling abroad for treatment), is that the allocation of scarce healthcare resources is no longer decided by legitimate public actors, but by individual patients.

Implications of the individualisation process

It is striking how the developments at the EU level resemble the developments at the national level in England. Patients are increasingly treated as consumers and are provided with individual market rights from both the EU as well as the NHS. As a result, the collective social right to healthcare transforms into a more individual right. This process has serious implications for the preservation of equality and solidarity within the English NHS.

It has been noted by many authors that EU patient mobility will divert resources from the needy to those travelling abroad, who are often the better off (McHale 2011, p. 261; Mossialos et al. 2010a, p. 27; Newdick 2006, p. 1646; Palm and Glinos 2010, p. 513; Veitch 2012, pp. 380f.). I assert that the unequal distribution of resources is not just a problem of patient mobility, but a problem of individual, absolute social rights per se. Absolute rights must be met, irrespective of their effects on others. Within a system of finite resources, this means that resources are directed towards those who claim their rights (Newdick 2006, pp. 1650f.). Voice and power to demand entitlement, however, vary between patients. Hence, already disadvantaged population groups such as the old, migrants or homeless receive fewer resources.[25] Similarly, particular patient groups such as the mentally ill or people suffering from sexually transmitted diseases, for example, are not able or do not dare to claim their rights. Furthermore, individual rights cause a shift of resources towards curative care at the expense of public health and group preventive measures. Public health policies are targeted towards groups and the general public and not towards individuals; hence no one actively claims these measures.[26] This again disadvantages the already deprived as many public health programmes aim at population groups with high health risks. In addition, overall welfare diminishes because diseases that could have been prevented are not.

Individual rights lead to an unequal distribution of resources, thereby endangering 'the community–solidary–ethos upon which the NHS was founded' (Veitch 2012, p. 391). The NHS promises to provide equal access for all, according to medical need. If funds, which are raised by all members of society, were not sufficient to meet all needs, everyone had to queue. These basic principles are revoked by the exit option offered by the EU right to treatment abroad. Now, individuals can step out of the line and get their needs met, irrespective of the needs of others, and at the expense of all. If too many use the exit option, this inevitably challenges the legitimacy of the system: why should everyone contribute, if not the needy but an elite group gets a disproportional share?[27]

The individualisation of collective healthcare rights started 20 years ago with the Patient's Charter specifying for the first time the rights of patients under the NHS. Individualisation then intensified under Labour's consumerist approach to healthcare and was further driven by Europeanisation. I expect the process of individualisation to proceed in the future because the driving forces behind it continue to exist, and moreover, if once granted, individual rights can scarcely be withdrawn.

Notes

1 The causes of the universalisation of access in Germany are not considered here because this process just signifies a catching-up to the standards of other EU welfare states. The individualisation process, on the contrary, signifies a fundamental transformation of the collective right to healthcare and indicates profound alterations of social rights in Europe more generally.

2 If a reform did not clearly increase or decrease generosity or access, it was not considered for categorisation. This also applies to those reforms resulting from judicial judgements.

3 The classification was based exclusively on charges for drugs and medical aids.

4 Among the best known are Gallup Poll, National Opinion Poll (NOP), ICM Research, MORI and, since 2001, YouGov and Populus (Butler 2006, pp. 122ff.). MORI is the only polling institute providing data for the whole period under investigation. Data from Gallup is available only until 1999; NOP provided voting polls until 2005; and ICM has published its polling data since 1984. The decision regarding the existence of an electoral slack was based on data from MORI, ICM and Gallup. Thus, categorisation was always based on at least two data sources, which is important because results sometimes varied widely between institutes. Polling data was gathered from the British voting intention opinion poll database provided by Mark Pack, http://www.markpack. org.uk/opinion-polls/ (11.06.2014).

5 Only during September 2000 were the polls slightly negative for Labour.

6 Although negative recommendations of NICE are not binding for PCTs/CCGs, the respective treatments are usually not provided due to funding shortages.

7 For older poll data see Noelle-Neumann (1997), and for poll data since 1998 http://www. wahlrecht.de/umfragen/index.htm (16.05.2014).

8 In 1982, there was a special situation: the defection of the Liberals and the very strong position of the CDU/CSU in the polls allowed the new government to implement the Accompanying Budget Law 1983 with its far-reaching cuts. The 2.GKV NOG of 1997 is the result of a reform debate that had already begun in early 1995 (Wasem 1998). Negotiations, however, were prone to conflict, not only between the government and opposition, but also within the government coalition, and thus the passage of reform needed a long time.

9 Healthcare entitlement intentions of the Greens are not described here because their health policy did not widely differ from that of the Social Democrats. Furthermore, their influence on health policy was, despite a Green health minister during the first years, rather minor (Hartmann 2003, pp. 272f.).

10 This draft was abandoned in favour of a reform bill being supported by the opposition (GKV–Modernisierungsgesetz 2003).

11 In the past, the CDU has always formed a coalition with its Bavarian sister, the CSU. Although there are small differences between the two parties with regard to healthcare entitlement, the description treats both parties as having a single interest. References to the Christian Democrats in the following may be understood to mean both parties.

12 This background also helps to explain the restricted access to SHI for pensioners which resulted from the KVKG. With the cost-shifting between SPI and SHI, SHI membership of pensioners was no longer seen as a benefit of SPI, but as the task of SHI (Vincenti 2008, p. 530). In other words, automatic SHI membership of pensioners was abolished, and pensioners had to fulfil further criteria to be eligible for SHI membership.

13 The retrenchment reforms (e.g. charges for hospital treatment, exclusion of drugs for the treatment of minor diseases) had already been decided by the SPD/FDP government, but due to the abrupt change of government they were passed by the new CDU/CSU/FDP government in 1982 (Webber 1989, p. 266).

14 The Liberals were part of the federal government throughout the 1980s and 1990s until 1998, and again between 2010 and 2013. They often had a strong influence on healthcare

entitlement reforms despite being the smaller coalition partner (see above). Only during their last term in office did they depart from their liberal stance: from a very weak position, and with the fear of being voted out of the *Bundestag*, they abolished the unpopular practice fee.

15 For a detailed description of these processes, see Chapters 2.3 to 2.7.

16 Important is also differentiation. The differentiation narrative requires a more active consumer who is able to make informed choices and to engage with producers. There is a third strand in New Labour's public services discourse that is not related to consumerism but to the co-production of service users. This narrative is associated with concepts such as empowerment, opportunity and responsibility (Needham 2007, p. 5).

17 The fundamental decision about how much of the state budget to devote to healthcare and public health, and hence the weighting up between the interest of patients and the healthcare sector on the one hand and other interest groups (e.g. taxpayers, other social programmes, other state expenditure) on the other, remained within the hands of the Parliament.

18 The fact that differences between the NHS England and the other healthcare systems of Great Britain (NHS Wales, NHS Scotland, Health and Social Care in Northern Ireland) evoke far less outcry than variations within England supports this statement.

19 I exclusively refer to healthcare here. The case for public health and occupational health, where the EU possesses at least some competencies, is different.

20 For a detailed discussion of cases and concrete rules established by the ECJ with regard to patient mobility, see Chapter 2.7.

21 The NHS Act determined that the SoS has the duty to provide a 'comprehensive health service' (s. 1 NHS Act 1977). According to the NHS Act, treatment outside the UK was only possible for people suffering from respiratory tuberculosis (s. 5 (2)(b)). In addition, the DH could make a good will decision for patients fulfilling several strict criteria to seek treatment in another country (Obermaier 2009, p. 122).

22 For a detailed description of the content of the Patients' Rights Directive, see Chapter 2.7.

23 Some of the new rights can also be read as 'traditional patient rights' which are derived from the 'individual right to personal integrity and self-determination' (Palm and Baeten 2011, p. 272). However, with their clear purpose of enabling patients to (safely) participate in the European healthcare market, the new rights clearly differ from traditional patient rights.

24 The exclusive focus of the Patients' Rights Directive on market integration is also demonstrated by its legal foundation, which is Art. 114 TFEU. This regulation is concerned with the 'harmonisation of laws in pursuit of the development of the internal market' (Veitch 2012, p. 383). A similar argument is made by Sauter (2011).

25 Similarly, Newdick (2006, p. 1646).

26 This is well exemplified by the German case: SHI spent only 269 million Euro in 2001 on primary prevention, which is extremely low compared to the 1.4 billion Euro disbursed for secondary prevention alone the same year (Rosenbrock and Gerlinger 2014, p. 82).

27 A similar argument can be found by Newdick (2006, p. 1646).

Conclusion

All Western welfare states grant their members a social right to healthcare in cases of illness. The specific content of that right, however, varies between countries and over time. So far, very little is known about these historical and local variations since social rights research has almost exclusively covered reforms of cash benefits while widely neglecting social services. Addressing this research gap, this book has analysed how healthcare entitlement has been altered in the course of general welfare state transformation in England and Germany. The results confirm the findings of social rights studies for other social areas: generosity of legal healthcare entitlement was reduced during the late 1970s until the1990s, but has not been further cut since the beginning of the new millennium. Moreover, retrenchment, i.e. limitations to generosity, was primarily restricted to non-core areas of public healthcare (e.g. dental and optical appliances, OTC drugs), and the most vulnerable patients were largely exempted from cuts in cost coverage. More interesting, however, are the qualitative transformations of the social right to healthcare revealed by this study. Germany broadened access to healthcare and now provides a universal right. In England, the collective social right was partially transformed into an individual right.

This study not only presented empirical evidence of healthcare entitlement reforms, but also investigated the causes of welfare state change. Testing Pierson's 'new politics' thesis, it assessed whether the 'old' welfare state theories – in particular, the power resource approach – are still able to explain welfare reforms in times of austerity. Both case studies confirm the continued relevance of party politics. In Germany, however, the relationship between governing party and retrenchment is not as direct as in England because various institutional characteristics of the German political system impede on a direct transfer of party interests into legislation. The German case thus also demonstrates the importance of institutionalist theories for explaining welfare state reforms.

In *Chapter 1*, a framework for the assessment of alterations to healthcare rights was developed. The various features distinguishing healthcare from cash benefits made an adaptation of the classical categories of social rights research – access and generosity – necessary. In contrast to generosity of cash benefits, generosity of healthcare is two-dimensional: it involves the services to which beneficiaries are entitled (*service coverage*) and the amount of costs borne by the public healthcare system (*cost coverage*). The complexity of healthcare entitlement may explain why it has so far not been investigated by quantitative social rights researchers. To analyse generosity of and access to public healthcare, an in-depth study of individual countries is necessary. The analytical framework developed for this study has proven to be appropriate for exploring modifications to healthcare entitlement regulation. Although healthcare is unique amongst all welfare benefits, I suggest that this framework could also be applied to other social services such as long-term care or child care, which share many of the characteristics of healthcare.

Chapter 2 described, in detail, healthcare entitlement reforms in England over the last 35 years, and revealed a concentration of retrenchment under the Conservatives, as well as a fundamental transformation of the collective social right into a more individual one. Chapter 2 also illustrated the EU's substantial impact on national health policies, despite its lack of regulatory powers regarding the organisation of the healthcare systems of its Member States. The English case is particularly poignant because the rulings of the European Court of Justice concerning patient mobility fundamentally contradict the English social right to healthcare. The rulings established an individual and absolute right to treatment that had not formerly existed in the English NHS, and that endangers the collectivistic notion of the English social right.

Chapter 3 set out in detail the healthcare entitlement reforms conducted in Germany over the last 37 years and highlighted the special role of the joint self-administration in defining healthcare entitlement. The most striking development during this period was the universalisation of the social right to healthcare. German SHI traditionally gave access only to defined population groups. Access was restricted for particular groups during the 1970s, 1980s and 1990s. At the beginning of the new millennium, almost 200,000 people were without health insurance because they could not afford private insurance. In order to relieve the situation, Germany established universal access to healthcare by introducing the general obligation to insure in 2009. However, unconditional access to SHI would have contradicted the principle of reciprocal solidarity on which SHI is based and thus had to be realised by employing the private insurance sector to grant coverage to persons not eligible for SHI membership. Yet, as I argued in Chapter 4, this solution possesses an inherent contradiction: universality requires unconditional access; full access to healthcare, however, remains conditional upon the payment of contributions or premiums.

Chapter 4 summed up the findings from the case studies to answer the first research question. As written above, retrenchment of healthcare entitlement in both countries was restricted to the 1970s, 1980s and 1990s, and mainly affected non-core service areas. The two countries maintained the core values of their social rights: the English NHS kept universality and continues to guarantee access, irrespective of one's ability to pay; and the German SHI preserved its principle of providing all medically necessary treatments. Regarding the governance of healthcare entitlement, a similar development could be witnessed in both countries: England, as well as Germany, delegated coverage decisions to non-state actors. The delegation of complex and controversial decision-making to non-democratic actors possesses several advantages such as an increased efficiency of the decision-making process, higher credibility of decisions, and for politicians, the avoidance of blame. At the same time, however, the delegation of such important and contested decisions to non-democratic actors calls the legitimacy of these decisions into question. I argued in Chapter 4 that this is particularly problematic for the area of healthcare, where the distribution of vital resources is decided.

In addition, Chapter 4 analysed the individualisation of the collective social right to healthcare in England more thoroughly. The comparison of the English and German social rights to healthcare revealed fundamental conceptual differences: healthcare rights in the two countries differ with regard to their conceptual bases, population coverage, reference point, equality, absoluteness and enforceability, as well as in their levels of specification. In other words, England and Germany possess completely different types of social healthcare rights; namely, Germany grants an individual right to healthcare, while England provides a collective social right. These categorical differences are crucial because they influence the distribution of resources, as I argued in Chapter 5. The study covered only two cases, and thus we do not know if the distinction between individual and collective rights fully describes the family of social healthcare rights, and if it is also applicable to other welfare areas. The framework on which the categorisation was based includes very general characteristics and thus could also be applied to other social rights as well.

Chapter 5 investigated the causes of healthcare entitlement retrenchment in England and Germany. In addressing the scholarly debate about the transformation of the welfare state, Chapter 5 tested several hypotheses that strive to explain welfare state retrenchment. The analysis showed that in both countries, a budgetary crisis was a necessary but not sufficient condition for retrenchment. The occurrence of an electoral slack, on the contrary, had no impact on healthcare entitlement retrenchment. Moreover, Chapter 5 proved that the power resource approach very well explains retrenchment policies of the last 35 years: in England, significant healthcare entitlement retrenchment took place under the Conservatives only, and never under a Labour government. In Germany, the correlation between party rule and retrenchment policies is less evident because the influence of party politics was mediated through particular features of the political system. In particular, multi-party governments and the strong veto power of the *Bundesrat* (the federal council) increased the necessity for compromise. Thus, retrenchment reforms that, at first glance, contradict power resource theory (e.g. the extensive retrenchment under the Red–Green government in 2003, or limited retrenchment during the Kohl era) turn out to support its theses when reform processes are analysed more intensely.

Furthermore, Chapter 5 traced the roots of the individualisation of the collective social right to healthcare in England. It identified Europeanisation and marketisation on the national level as driving forces. Both processes involve a changing role for citizens: citizens are increasingly treated as consumers, and as such, are granted consumer rights. These rights, however, are individual rights aimed at strengthening consumer power. As such, they are directed towards the wellbeing of the individual and not towards the welfare of society. Hence, these processes signify a shift in the relationship balance between the individual and the collective, in favour of the individual. The individualisation of the collective social right to healthcare also implies the changing role of the state. The state is no longer directly responsible for the fulfilment of the right to healthcare; rather, it has assigned this task to a variety of actors. State provision and hierarchical control of health actors were superseded by a plurality of providers and market-like governance forms in England. This process mirrors the more general transformation of the state towards a 'regulatory state' (Majone 1997). Furthermore, it reflects the altered relationship between the state and its citizens. The state is no longer perceived as a strong and paternalistic power charged with the wellbeing of its subjects; instead, its role is to empower citizens to actively take part in the (quasi-)market. Nonetheless, despite the modified role of the state, it remains the ultimate guarantor of the right to healthcare.

In investigating entitlement to healthcare, this study filled the gap in social rights research for social services. Yet some notes about the limitation of this study are necessary. First, compared to cash benefits, the study of legal entitlement to healthcare has one major shortcoming: in healthcare, the disparity between legal and actual rights is usually quite significant as generosity of benefits are influenced by various factors including the design and availability of medical infrastructure, the financial incentives for providers or the actual needs of the population. These factors render a full account of actual access to and generosity of healthcare impossible. Second, the complexity of healthcare entitlement regulation limited the number of case studies feasible in the course of this research. Based on only two cases, it is not possible to generalise about the transformation of the social right to healthcare. However, as the study investigated two prime examples of healthcare system types, we can expect to find similar developments in other countries. With regard to the individualisation of the collective social right to healthcare, two studies already confirm my findings for Canada (Bhatia 2010; Redden 2002),[1] and I suppose this development to also be the case for other countries with collective social rights to healthcare (see below). This, however, must be proven by additional studies. Further investigation and comparison of individual social rights to healthcare would also provide interesting insights. Such an analysis could disclose detailed differences in generosity between countries, and over time, also offer a base of evidence for more general statements about healthcare entitlement retrenchment in advanced welfare states. The analytical framework developed by this study has proven practicable and could be used for these further inquiries.

I expect individualisation processes to take place in further countries with collective social rights to healthcare because collective social rights no longer meet the requirements of modern, capitalist, European welfare societies. Processes such as the individualisation and pluralisation of society, Europeanisation and the marketisation of social services, challenge the foundations of the collectivistic social rights approach. The reference point of collective social rights is the national society. This reference point, however, is becoming increasingly porous. Pluralisation and differentiation processes have weakened the sense of community, while at the same time, devolution and Europeanisation have created new groupings. Furthermore, collective social rights serve the public and not the individual interest. With advancing individualisation, however, the primacy of the collective is increasingly challenged. In my view, the greatest challenge to collective social rights is their incompatibility with welfare markets. A model of collective social rights presupposes a legitimate decision-making authority to determine the distribution of resources and, hence, concrete entitlement. If public allocation of resources is (at least partly) replaced by market allocation, or more specifically, if public provision is substituted by private provision, legitimacy is lost. Private providers cannot be charged with decisions about the distribution of resources because their choices are likely to be in their own interest instead of that of the common welfare. Lacking defined entitlement, patients have no means of countering provider power. With individual social rights, this problem does not arise. Entitlement is decided a priori by a legitimate public body (e.g. parliament, joint self-administration), and private providers are bound to these decisions. Armed with individual, enforceable entitlements, beneficiaries have the power to invoke their rights vis-à-vis providers.[2] Given these challenges, I see no future for collective social rights to healthcare; in the long run they will be transformed into individual rights.

However, some aspects of individual social rights are problematic. First, individual rights tend to favour the stronger members of society because they are able to claim their rights, a task much more difficult for the socially deprived or weaker individuals. Second, the focus of individual rights is on curative treatment because public health and group preventive measures are not claimed by individuals. Third, predetermined entitlements lead to increased expenditures should need or demand rise. Fourth, preoccupation with individual wellbeing diminishes societal welfare: within a system of finite resources, the allocation of the majority of resources towards individual curative treatment inevitably means fewer resources for other policies with a potentially greater impact on people's health such as education, housing or prevention, for example. On the other hand, individual social rights require explicit decision-making, and thus provide opportunity for societal negotiations and compromise. Given the vital and social importance of healthcare as well as the (re-)distributive effects of entitlements, entitlement decisions should be based on a broad societal compromise. In neither of the two countries studied is this still the case today. In England, entitlement decisions are implicit, resulting from resource allocation.[3] In Germany, entitlement decisions emanate from negotiations between payers and providers, thus reflecting payer and provider interests rather than societal compromise. It is unfeasible for the broad public to decide on the coverage of each single technology or service because such decision-making requires a high degree of expertise and knowledge. Decision-making is thus best delegated to a legitimate democratic institution with transparent decision-making procedures that allow for broad participation in order to facilitate public debate and societal compromise.

A public debate is necessary not only for decisions regarding concrete entitlement, but also for the overarching decision of the amount of resources to be devoted to healthcare. Given the importance attributed to health and healthcare in contemporary societies, as well as the expensive medical progress, it is to be expected that Western welfare societies will continue to spend an ever greater share of their resources on healthcare, despite the fact that often, funds dedicated to other public policies may actually improve health and wellbeing more than funds spent for curative care do. The debate about the generosity of healthcare entitlement is thus too narrow and should be complemented by a debate about requirements for healthy living in general.

Notes

1 Bhatia (2010) and Redden (2002) have studied the development of the social right to healthcare in Canada where public healthcare is an important symbol of national identity. Redden observed an individualisation of healthcare rights as a result of health reforms. Formerly, people had perceived healthcare as a citizenship right and a state's duty to publicly provide modern medical care to all citizens. After the 'individualistic turn', however, citizens have increasingly come to be regarded as consumers and the right to healthcare has increasingly been understood as an individual right that is purchased by paying taxes and is thus a legitimate claim against the state (Redden 2002, p. 41). Bhatia confirms this paradigm shift and describes the development of the social right to healthcare in Canada as a transformation from a moral obligation of the society to an 'individual civil right'.
2 Håkan and Bjørn (2013) make a similar argument.
3 Notable exceptions are the entitlement decisions taken by NICE, which result from transparent and inclusive deliberative processes.

Appendix

Table A.1 Full list of codes with description

Code Family	Code Name	Deductive/ Inductive	Code Description
Conditions of Conduct Criteria (CCCr)	CCCr Attendance	I	Service or cost coverage are contingent upon attendance at a hospital or other health service institution.
	CCCr Compliance	I	Service or cost coverage are contingent upon compliance of the patient.
	CCCr Healthy Behaviour	I	Service or cost coverage are contingent upon healthy behaviour/lifestyle of the insured person.
	CCCr Medical Examination	I	Service or cost coverage are contingent upon undergoing medical examinations.
	CCCr Other	I	Residual category: conditions of conduct criteria not belonging to any of the other codes in this family.
	CCCr Personal Negligence	I	Service or cost coverage are reduced in the case of personal negligence.
Change	Change Charge Decrease	D	Increase of cost coverage.
	Change Charge Increase	D	Decrease of cost coverage.
	Change DA	D	Change of defining authority (the person or body in charge of defining cost or service coverage).
	Change Definition	D	Cost or service coverage formerly having not been explicitly specified becomes defined by law.
	Change Easing of EligCr	D	Easing of eligibility criteria: more people become eligible for services or for exemption from paying charges.
	Change PopCovExclusion	D	Particular groups of persons are excluded from SHI membership or NHS coverage.
	Change PopCovInclusion	D	Particular groups of persons become eligible for SHI membership or NHS coverage.
	Change ServCr	I	Service criteria are changed.
	Change ServExclusion	D	Service coverage is reduced.
	Change ServInclusion	D	Service coverage is expanded.
	Change Tightening EligCr	D	Tightening of eligibility criteria: less people are eligible for receiving a particular service or for being exempted from paying charges.
	Change Tightening ServCr	I	Tightening of service criteria: fewer services are covered because service criteria became more restrictive.
Cost coverage		D	Main analytical category: concerns all relevant aspects that influence the direct cost burden of patients (co-payments, charges, remission and exemption from paying charges)

Defining Authority (DA)	DA Health Authorities	I	Coverage decisions are taken by a health authority (e.g. AHA, PCTs).
	DA Parliament	I	Coverage decisions are taken by the parliament.
	DA Provider	I	Coverage decisions are taken by the providers or the providers' association(s).
	DA Self-Administration	I	Coverage decisions are taken by the joint self-administration of the public healthcare system.
	DA SHI Fund	I	Coverage decisions are taken by the statutory health insurance funds or their association(s).
	DA SoS/Ministry	I	Coverage decisions are taken by the Secretary of State or the health ministry.
Eligibility Criteria (EligCr)	EligCr Benefit Receipt	I	Service or cost coverage are contingent upon the drawing of other social benefits (e.g. pension).
	EligCr Certain Age	I	Service or cost coverage are contingent upon a certain age of the beneficiary.
	EligCr Certain Disease	I	Service or cost coverage are contingent upon that the patient suffers from a particular disease.
	EligCr Emergency	I	Service or cost coverage only in emergency or urgent cases.
	EligCr Family	I	Service or cost coverage is conferred to family members.
	EligCr Hardship	I	Service or cost coverage in hardship or exceptional cases only.
	EligCr High Risk	I	Service or cost coverage for high risk groups/persons only.
Eligibility Criteria (EligCr)	EligCr Hospital Treatment	I	Service or cost coverage are contingent upon the treatment in a hospital.
	EligCr Low Income	I	Cost coverage is contingent upon low income or insufficient capital resources of the beneficiary.
	EligCr Medical Expenses	I	Cost coverage is contingent upon the amount of money already paid for charges and co-payments.
	EligCr Medical Need	I	Service coverage in the case of prevailing medical need only.
	EligCr Motherhood	I	Service or cost coverage for mothers only.
	EligCr Necessary	I	Service coverage only if treatment or diagnoses are medically necessary.
	EligCr Old Age	I	Service or cost coverage for old beneficiaries.
	EligCr Other	I	Residual category: eligibility criteria not belonging to any of the other defined codes of this family.
	EligCr Prior Approval	I	Service or cost coverage are contingent upon prior approval by the health fund or health authority.
	EligCr Residence	I	Service or cost coverage are contingent upon the residence of the beneficiary.
	EligCr Severity	I	Service or cost coverage are contingent upon the severity of the disease.

(Continued)

Table A.1 (Continued)

Code Family	Code Name	Deductive/ Inductive	Code Description
	EligCr Sex	I	Service or cost coverage are contingent upon the sex of the beneficiary.
	EligCr Subsidiarity	I	Service or cost coverage only if family members cannot provide support or if other social insurances do not cover costs.
	EligCr Sufficient Resources	I	Service coverage only if sufficient resources are available at the health facility.
	EligCr Treatment Possible	I	Service coverage only if treatment of the disease is possible or has sufficient chances of success.
	EligCr Undergoing Education	I	Service or cost coverage only for persons who are attending school or who are undergoing other education.
	EligCr Young Age	I	Service or cost coverage only for children and young adults.
Population Coverage Criteria (PCCr)	Population Coverage	D	Main analytical category: concerns the definition of population groups covered by the public healthcare system.
	PCCr Age	I	Population coverage is contingent upon the age of the person.
	PCCr Citizenship	I	Population coverage is contingent upon citizenship.
	PCCr Contribution Payment	I	Population coverage is contingent upon contribution payment.
	PCCr Disability	I	Population coverage is contingent upon disability.
	PCCr Employment	I	Population coverage is contingent upon employment.
	PCCr Family	I	Population coverage is conferred to family members.
	PCCr Income	I	Population coverage is contingent upon a particular height of income.
	PCCr Job-Promotion Progr.	I	Population coverage of people in job-promotion programmes.
	PCCr Other	I	Residual category: population coverage criteria not belonging to any of the other codes of this family.
	PCCr Private Insurance	I	Population coverage is contingent upon the insurance with a private health fund.
	PCCr Profession	I	Population coverage is contingent upon the profession of the insured.
	PCCr Public Pension	I	Population coverage is contingent upon the receipt of public pension.
	PCCr Qualifying Period	I	Population coverage is contingent upon a previous SHI membership of a defined period.
	PCCr Residence	I	Population coverage is contingent upon residence.
	PCCr SHI Membership	I	Population coverage is contingent upon previous SHI membership.
	PCCr Social Benefits	I	Population coverage is contingent upon the drawing of other social benefits.
	PCCr Student	I	Population coverage of students.
	PCCr Time Restriction	I	Accession to SHI is possible only within a given timeframe.

Service Area (SA)	SA Childcare	I	Regulations refer to childcare.
	SA Contraception	I	Regulations refer to contraception measures.
	SA Dental Appliances	I	Regulations refer to dental appliances.
	SA Dental Care	I	Regulations refer to dental care.
	SA Emergency	I	Regulations refer to emergency treatment.
	SA General	I	Regulations refer to medical services and goods in general.
	SA Hospital Care	I	Regulations refer to hospital care.
	SA Maternity Care	I	Regulations refer to maternity care.
	SA Medical Aids & Appl.	I	Regulations refer to medical aids and appliances.
	SA Medical Care	I	Regulations refer to medical care.
	SA Mental Health	I	Regulations refer to mental healthcare.
	SA Optical Care & Appl.	I	Regulations refer to optical care and appliances.
	SA Other	I	Residual category: regulations refer to service areas not belonging to any of the other codes in this family.
	SA Pharmaceuticals	I	Regulations refer to pharmaceuticals.
	SA Prevention	I	Regulations refer to preventive measures and treatments.
	SA Primary Care	I	Regulations refer to primary care.
Service Criteria (ServCr)	ServCr Appropriateness	I	Service coverage is restricted to appropriate services (synonyms: proper, adequate, zweckmäßig).
	ServCr Costs	I	Service coverage is restricted to services and goods that are cheaper than comparators.
	ServCr Effectiveness	I	Service coverage is restricted to effective services and goods.
	ServCr Efficiency	I	Service coverage is restricted to efficient services and goods.
	ServCr Evaluated/Standard	I	Service coverage is restricted to standard services and goods or to treatments that have been evaluated.
	ServCr Low Costs	I	Service coverage is restricted to services with a low price.
	ServCr Medical Need	I	Service coverage is restricted to services not being used to treat conditions with minor medical need.

(*Continued*)

Table A.1 (Continued)

Code Family	Code Name	Deductive/ Inductive	Code Description
	ServCr Necessary	I	Service coverage is restricted to services and goods that are 'necessary'.
	ServCr Other	I	Residual category: service criteria not belonging to any of the other codes in this family.
	ServCr Quality	I	Service coverage is restricted to quality services and goods.
	ServCr Sufficient	I	Service coverage comprises services and goods that are 'sufficient'.
	ServCr Timeframe	I	Service coverage is restricted within a particular timeframe (e.g. new glasses every three years only).
	Service Coverage	D	Main analytical category: concerns all regulations that determine the range of services and goods provided by the public healthcare system.

Table A.2 Charges for pharmaceuticals and medical appliances, England 1976–1997

Year	1976	1979	1980	1981	1982	1983	1984	1985	1986	1987	1988	1989	1990	1991	1992	1993	1994	1995	1996	1997
Statutory instr. (No.)	681	264	1503		289	306	298	326	432	368	427	419	537	579	365	420	690	643	583	559
Charge (£, per item)	0.20	0.45	0.70	1.00	1.30	1.40	1.60	2.00	2.20	2.40	2.60	2.80	3.05	3.40	3.75	4.25	4.75	5.25	5.50	5.65
Pre-payment certificates																				
4 months (£)	/	/	4.50	5.50	7.00	7.50	8.50	11.00	12.00	12.50	13.50	14.50	15.80	17.60	19.40	22.00	24.60	27.20	28.50	29.30
6 months (£)	2.00	4.50	/	/	/	/	/	/	/	/	/	/	/	/	/	/	/	/	/	/
12 months (£)	3.50	8.00	12.00	15.00	20.00	21.50	24.00	30.50	33.50	35.00	37.50	40.00	43.50	48.50	53.50	60.60	67.70	74.80	78.40	80.50

Table A.3 Charges for pharmaceuticals and medical appliances, England 1998–2013

Year	1998	1999	2000	2001	2002	2003	2004	2005	2006	2007
Statutory instr. (No.)	491	767	620	746	548	585	663	578	675	543
Charge (£, per item)	5.80	5.90	6.00	6.10	6.20	6.30	6.40	6.50	6.65	6.85
Pre-payment certificates										
4 months (£)	30.10	30.80	31.40	31.90	32.40	32.90	33.40	33.90	34.65	35.85
12 months (£)	82.70	84.60	86.20	87.60	89.00	90.40	91.80	93.20	95.30	98.70

Year	2007	2008	2009	2010	2011	2012	2013
Statutory instr. (No.)	543	1510	571	/	518	470	475
Charge (£, per item)	6.85	7.10	7.20	n.a.	7.40	7.65	7.85
Pre-payment certificates							
3 months (£)	26.85	27.85	28.25	n.a.	29.10	29.10	29.10
12 months (£)	98.70	102.50	104.00	n.a.	104.00	104.00	104.00

n.a.: no amendments

Table A.4 Charges for dental appliances, England 1979–1988

Year	1979	1979	1980	1981	1982	1983	1984	1985	1988
Statutory instrument (No.)		677	352	307	284	309	299	352	473
1. A metal based* denture									
having 1 to 3 teeth	£15	£18	£25	£29	£37	£40	£47	£50	£64
having 4 to 8 teeth	£16	£19	£27	£31	£39	£42	£49	£52	£69
having more than 8 teeth	£17	£20	£29	£33	£41	£44	£51	£55	£71
2. More than 1 metal or porcelain based denture	£30	£36	£50	£58	£74	£80	£92	£98	/
3. A denture based in materials other than metal*									
having 1 to 3 teeth	£10	£12	£17	£19	£20	£22	£24	£26	£26
having 4 to 8 teeth	£11	£13	£18	£20	£21	£23	£26	£28	£34
having more than 8 teeth	£12	£14	£19	£21	£22	£24	£28	£30	£40
4. More than 1 denture based in materials other than metal*	£20	£24	£30	£33	£35	£38	£44	£47	£62
Maximum charge	£30	£36	£54	£60	£90	£95	£110	£115	£150

* Until 1988: or porcelain based.

Table A.5 Charges for dental appliances, England 1989–2005

Year	1989	1991	1992	1993	1994	1995	1996	1997	1998	1999	2000	2001	2002	2003	2004	2005
Statutory instr.(No.)	394	581	369	419	530	444	389	558	490	544	596	707	544	586	1091	576
Charges	0.75 x fees	n.a.	n.a.	0.80 x fees	n.a.	n.a.	n.a.	n.a.	n.a.	n.a.	n.a.	n.a.	n.a.	n.a.	n.a.	n.a.
Maximum charge	£150	£200	£225	£250	£275	£300	£325	£330	£340	£348	£354	£360	£366	£372	£378	£384

n.a.: no amendment

Table A.6 Charges for dental appliances, England 2005–2013

Year	2005	2007	2008	2009	2011	2012	2013
Statutory instrument (No.)	3477	544	547	407	519	502	475
Band 1: Diagnosis, treatment planning and maintenance and urgent treatment	£15.50	£15.90	£16.20	£16.50	£17.00	£17.50	£18.00
Band 2: Treatment	£42.40	£43.60	£44.60	£45.60	£47.00	£48.00	£49.00
Band 3: Provision of appliances	£189	£194.00	£198.00	£198.00	£204.00	£209.00	£214.00

Table A.7 Charges for medical appliances, England 1979–1980

Year	1979	1979	1980	1980
Statutory instrument (No.)	/	681	264	1503
All (per item)	20p	45p	70p	£1.00
Elastic hosiery				
Anklet, kneecap or legging	25p	50p	80p	n.a.
Above-knee stocking, below-knee stocking or thigh stocking (each)	50p	£1	£1.60	n.a.
Fabric support and wigs				
Fabric support (other than elastic hosiery)	£2.00	£4.50	£7.00	n.a.
Bespoke wig	£7.50	£17.00	£26.50	n.a.
Stock wig	£2.50	£6.00	£9.50	n.a.

n.a.: no amendment

Table A.8 Charges for medical appliances, England 1981–2013

Year	1981	1982	1983	1984	1985	1986	1987	1988	1989	1990	1991	1992	1993	1994	1995	1996	1997
Statutory instr. (No.)	501	289	306	298	326	432	368	427	419	537	579	365	420	690	643	583	559
All (per item)	n.a.	£1.30	£1.40	£1.60	£2.00	£2.20	£2.40	£2.60	£2.80	£3.05	£3.40	£3.75	£4.25	£4.75	£5.25	£5.50	£5.65
Elastic hosiery																	
Above-knee stocking, below-knee stocking or thigh stocking (each)	n.a.	n.a.	n.a.	£1.70	£2.00	£2.20	£2.40	£2.60	£2.80	£3.05	£3.40	£3.75	£4.25	£4.75	£5.25	£5.50	£5.65
Fabric support and wigs																	
Surgical brassiere	£7.00	n.a.	n.a.	£7.35	£10.00	n.a.	£11.00	n.a.	£12.00	£13.00	£14.50	£16.00	£18.00	£18.50	£19.00	£19.25	£19.75
Abdominal or spinal support	£9.50	£11.00	n.a.	£11.55	£14.00	n.a.	£15.00	n.a.	£16.00	£17.00	£19.00	£21.00	£24.00	£24.50	£27.00	£28.30	£29.05
Stock modacrylic wig	£11.50	£14.00	£15.00	£16.00	£21.00	n.a.	£22.00	n.a.	£24.00	£26.00	£29.00	£32.00	£36.00	£40.00	£44.00	£46.00	£47.00
Partial human hair wig	£28.00	n.a.	£30.50	£32.00	£40.00	£55.00	£58.00	n.a.	£62.00	£67.00	£74.50	£82.00	£93.00	£104.00	£115.00	£120.00	£123.00
Full bespoke human hair wig	£45	n.a.	£49.00	£51.00	£64.00	£86.00	£90.00	n.a.	£97.00	n.a.	£108.00	£119.00	£135.00	£151.00	£167.00	£175.00	£179.50
Tights	/	/	/	£3.40	£4.00	£4.40	£4.80	£5.20	£5.60	£6.10	£6.80	£7.50	£8.50	£9.50	£10.50	£11.00	£11.30

Year	1998	1999	2000	2001	2002	2003	2004	2005	2006	2007	2008	2009	2011	2012	2013
Statutory instrument (No.)	491	767	620	746	548	585	663	578	675	543	571	411	518	470	475
All (per item)	£5.80	£5.90	£6.00	£6.10	£6.20	£6.30	£6.40	£6.50	£6.65	£6.85	£7.10	£7.20	£7.40	£7.65	£7.85
Elastic hosiery															
Anklet, kneecap or legging	/	£5.90	£12.00	£12.20	£12.40	£12.60	£12.80	£13.00	£13.30	£13.70	£14.20	£14.40	£14.80	£15.30	£15.70
Fabric support															
Surgical brassiere	£19.75	£19.95	£20.30	£20.60	£20.90	£21.20	£21.50	£21.80	£22.30	£23.10	£24.00	£24.35	£25.10	£25.70	£26.35
Abdominal or spinal support	£29.50	£29.95	£30.50	£31.00	£31.50	£32.00	£32.50	£33.00	£33.75	£34.95	£36.30	£36.80	£37.90	£38.80	£39.75
Stock modacrylic wig	£48.00	£49.00	£49.90	£50.70	£51.50	£52.30	£53.10	£53.90	£55.10	£57.00	£59.20	£60.00	£61.85	£63.35	£64.95
Partial human hair wig	£126.00	£129.00	£131.50	£133.70	£135.90	£138.00	£140.15	£142.30	£145.55	£150.75	£156.60	£158.90	£163.80	£167.85	£172.00
Full bespoke human hair wig	£184.50	£188.50	£192.20	£195.40	£198.60	£201.70	£204.90	£208.10	£212.85	£220.50	£229.50	£232.45	£239.45	£245.40	£251.55
Tights	£11.60	£11.80	£12.00	£12.20	£12.40	£12.60	£12.80	£13.00	£13.30	£13.70	£14.20	£14.40	£14.80	£15.30	£15.70

Table A.9 Categorisation of healthcare entitlement retrenchment, England

Year	1979	1980	1981	1982	1983	1984	1985	1986
Retrenchment grade[a]	XXXX	XXXX	–	XX	X	XX	XXX	X
Reason for classification	Charge increase > 5 x inflation	Charge increase > 5 x inflation	–	Charge increase ≥ 3 x inflation	Charge increase ≥ 1.5 x inflation	Charge increase ≥ 1.5 x inflation and 1 relevant exclusion	Charge increase ≥ 3 x inflation and 1 relevant exclusion	Charge increase ≥ 1,5x inflation
Service coverage	–	–	–	–	–	Exclusions: Glasses*	Drug limited lists*	–
Charge increase / inflation rate[b]	9.0	6.7	0	3.4	1.7	2.8	4.1	2.9

Year	1987	1988	1989	1990	1991	1992	1993	1994
Retrenchment grade[a]	X	X	X	–	X	XX	XXX	XXX
Reason for classification	Charge increase ≥ 1.5 x inflation	Charge increase ≥ 1.5 x inflation	Charge increase ≥ 1.5 x inflation	–	Charge increase ≥ 1.5 x inflation	Charge increase ≥ 1.5 x inflation and 1 relevant exclusion	Charge increase > 5 x inflation	Charge increase > 5 x inflation
Service coverage	–	–	–	–	–	Expansion of limited list*	–	–
Charge increase / inflation rate[b]	2.2	2.0	1.5	1.3	1.5	2.3	5.2	6.0

Year	1995	1996	1997	1998	1999	2000	2001	2002
Retrenchment grade[a]	XX	X	X	X	–	X	–	–
Reason for classification	Charge increase ≥ 3 x inflation	Charge increase ≥ 1.5 x inflation	Charge increase ≥ 1.5 x inflation	Charge increase ≥ 1.5 x inflation	–	Charge increase ≥ 1.5 x inflation	–	–
Service coverage	–	–	–	–	–	–	Exclusions: nicotine substitutes	Grey list: medical appl. for erectile dysfunction
Charge increase / inflation rate[b]	4.2	2.0	1.7	1.7	1.3	2.1	1.4	1.2

Year	2003	2004	2005	2006	2007	2008	2009	2010	2011	2012	2013
Retrenchment grade[a]	–	X	–	–	–	–	–	–	–	–	–
Reason for classification	–	Charge increase ≥ 1.5 x inflation	–	–	–	–	–	–	–	–	–
Service coverage	–	–	–	–	–	–	–	–	–	–	–
Charge increase / inflation rate[b]	1.1	2.0	0.3	1.0	1.3	1.0	0.6	0	0.6	1.2	1.3

Sources: OECD (2014a), for charges see Table 2.3 and Table 2.5.

a XXX: charge increase ≥ 5 x inflation rate; or charge increase ≥ 3 x inflation rate and one or more relevant service exclusions; or more than one relevant service exclusion; XX: charge increase ≥ 3 x inflation rate; or charge increase ≥ 1.5 x inflation rate; or several smaller exclusions. Relevant service exclusion: a service that is needed by a large group of patients is excluded from NHS coverage. Only charges for drugs and medical aids were considered.

b The relative annual charge increase for drugs and medical aids divided by the inflation rate for the particular year.

Table A.10 Categorisation of healthcare entitlement retrenchment, Germany

Year	1977	1978	1979	1980	1981	1982	1983	1984	1985	1986	1987	1988
Retrenchment grade[a]	XXX	–	–	–	X	XX	–	–	–	–	–	XXX
Service coverage	(Negative list drugs)*	–	–	–	Introduction of a timeframe for glasses	Exclusions: • drugs for the treatment of minor diseases*	–	–	–	–	–	Restrictions for new diagnosis and treatment methods in ambulatory medical and dental care* Exclusions: • medical aids • (negative list)* • caring products for contact lenses Tightening eligibility: – orthod. treatment – spectacles
Cost coverage	New charges: • spectacles* Charge increase: • dental appl. • drugs & med. aids Tightening eligibility: • dental appl. • drugs & med. aids*	–	–	–	Charge increase: • dental appliances • drugs	New charges: • hospital treatment* Charge increase: • drugs	–	–	–	–	–	Introduction of a reference pricing system for drugs, med. aids & appl., spectacles* Charge increase: • drugs • hospital treatment
Restriction of SHI membership	for pensioners* for family members*	–	–	–	for disabled	/	–	–	–	–	–	for voluntarily insured* for students

Year	1989	1990	1991	1992	1993	1994	1995	1996	1997	1998	1999
Retrenchment grade [a]	–	–	–	XX	–	–	–	XX	X(X)	–	XX
Service coverage	–	Drug negative list*	–	(Drug positive list)* Exclusions: • bridges that substitute more than 4 teeth • orthod. treatment for adults* • vaccinations for holidays Tightening eligibility: • dental appl. for non-residents	–	–	–	Exclusions: • artificial dentition based on implants • dental appl. for people born after 1978* • glasses frames* • health promotion	–	–	Exclusion of hospital services became possible*; (Drug positive list)* Exclusions: • individual prophylactic dental services for adults
Cost coverage	–	–	–	Charge increase: • drugs • hospital treatment	–	–	–	New charges: • ambulatory psychotherapy by psychotherapists Charge increase: • drugs	(Automatic increase of charges) (charges rise with contribution rate)* New charges: • bandages, foot orthotics, med. aids for compression therapy Charge increase: • drugs • hospital treatment • remedies	–	–
Restriction of SHI membership	–	–	–	–	–	–	–	–	–	–	for people over 54 who want to return to SHI* for particular family members

(Continued)

Table A.10 (Continued)

Year	2000	2001	2002	2003	2004	2005	2006	2007	2008	2009	2010	2011	2012	2013
Retrenchment grade [a]	–	–	–	XXX	–	–	–	X	–	–	–	–	–	–
Service coverage	Expansion of drug negative list	–	–	Exclusions: • sterilisation • OTC drugs* • lifestyle-drugs • visual aids* • (dental appliances) Tightening eligibility: – artificial insemination	–	–	–	No choice amongst different drug brands	–	–	–	–	–	–
Cost coverage	–	–	–	New charges: • artificial insemination • med. aids & appl.* • practice charge* • supportive social care Charge increase: • drugs • hospital treatment	–	–	–	Charge increase for people who have not attended preventive examinations; Cost-sharing if treatment became necessary as a 'result of a medically not indicated procedure'	–	–	–	–	–	–
Restriction of SHI membership	–	–	–	/	–	–	–	for unemployed not compulsorily insured with SHI	–	–	–	–	–	–

a X minor retrenchment: one relevant cut and/or several smaller cuts; XX medium retrenchment: more than one relevant cut or several smaller cuts in each of the three categories; XXX extensive retrenchment: more than three relevant cuts in at least two categories and smaller cuts; Relevant cut: introduction of a new charge in one of the core service areas; exclusion of a larger group of services or a service that is needed by a larger group of patients; tightening of eligibility for a larger group of patients; increase of conditionality of SHI membership for a larger group of SHI members.

Note: Reforms in parenthesis were decided but not realised.

References

Abel-Smith, B and Mossialos, E 1994, 'Cost Containment and Healthcare Reform: A Study of the European Union', *Health Policy*, vol. 28, no. 2, pp. 89–132.

Altenstetter, C 1997, 'Health Policy-Making in Germany: Stability and Dynamics', in C Altenstetter and JW Bjorkman (eds), *Health Policy Reform, National Variations, and Globalization*, Macmillan, Basingstoke, pp. 136–61.

Appleby, J 2013, *What Happened to the Extra NHS Billions?*, The King's Fund, viewed 26 August 2014, http://www.kingsfund.org.uk/blog/2013/06/what-happened-extra-nhs-billions.

Bandelow, NC 1998, *Gesundheitspolitik: Der Staat in der Hand einzelner Interessengruppen? Probleme, Erklärungen, Reformen*, Leske + Budrich, Opladen.

Bandelow, NC and Hartmann, A 2007, 'Weder rot noch grün. Machterosion und Interessenfragmentierung bei Staat und Verbänden in der Gesundheitspolitik', in C Egle and R Zohlnhöfer (eds), *Ende des rot-grünen Projektes: Eine Bilanz der Regierung Schröder 2002–2005*, VS Verl. für Sozialwissenschaften, Wiesbaden, pp. 334–54.

Bandelow, NC and Schubert, K 1998, 'Wechselnde Strategien und kontinuierlicher Abbau solidarischen Ausgleichs: Eine gesundheitspolitische Bilanz der Ära Kohl', in G Wewer and NC Bandelow (eds), *Bilanz der Ära Kohl: Christlich-liberale Politik in Deutschland 1982–1998*, Leske + Budrich, Opladen, pp. 113–27.

Beck, U and Beck-Gernsheim, E 2002, *Individualization: Institutionalized Individualism and Its Social and Political Consequences*, SAGE Publ., London.

Beckmann, J and Kuhn, H 1989, *Gesundheitsreform: Ein kritischer Ratgeber*, Lamuv, Göttingen.

Bhatia, V 2010, 'Social Rights, Civil Rights, and Health Reform in Canada', *Governance*, vol. 23, no. 1, pp. 37–58.

Blair, T 1998, *The Third Way: New Politics for the New Century*, Fabian Society, London.

Blank, F 2007, *Analyzing Social Rights in Different Contexts: A Qualitative Multi-dimensional Approach: Paper Presented at the ESPAnet Conference 2007*, Vienna.

——— 2011, *Soziale Rechte 1998–2005: Die Wohlfahrtsstaatsreformen der rot-grünen Bundesregierung*, VS Verl. für Sozialwissenschaften, Wiesbaden.

Bloor, K and Maynard, A 1993, *Expenditure on the NHS during and after the Thatcher Years: Its Growth and Utilisation*, Discussion Paper no. 113, Centre for Health Economics, University of York, York.

BMG 1995, *Daten des Gesundheitswesens*, Schriftenreihe des Bundesministeriums für Gesundheit, vol. 51, Nomos, Baden-Baden.

——— 2001, *Daten des Gesundheitswesens*, Schriftenreihe des Bundesministeriums für Gesundheit, vol. 137, Nomos, Baden-Baden.

────── 2013, *Daten des Gesundheitswesens*, viewed 7 May 2014, <http://www.bundes gesundheitsministerium.de/fileadmin/dateien/Publikationen/Gesundheit/Broschueren/ Daten_des_Gesundheitswesens_2013.pdf>.

BMJFG 1980, *Daten des Gesundheitswesens*, Schriftenreihe des Bundesministers für Jugend, Familie und Gesundheit, vol. 151, Kohlhammer, Stuttgart.

────── 1983, *Daten des Gesundheitswesens*, Schriftenreihe des Bundesministers für Jugend, Familie und Gesundheit, vol. 152, Kohlhammer, Stuttgart.

Böhm, K 2008, *Politische Steuerung des Gesundheitswesens: Die Rolle von Korporatismus und Wettbewerb im Krankenhaus*, Diskussionspapier 01–2008, Institut für Medizinsoziologie, Frankfurt.

Böhm, K and Landwehr, C 2014, 'The Europeanization of Healthcare Coverage Decisions: EU-Regulation, Policy Learning and Cooperation in Decision-Making', *Journal of European Integration*, vol. 36, no. 1, pp. 17–35.

Böhm, K, Landwehr, C and Steiner, N 2014, 'What Explains "Generosity" in the Public Financing of High-Tech Drugs? An Empirical Investigation of 25 OECD Countries and 11 Controversial Drugs', *Journal of European Social Policy*, vol. 24, no. 1, pp. 39–55.

Böhm, K, Schmid, A, Götze, R, Landwehr, C and Rothgang, H 2012, *Classifying OECD Healthcare Systems: A Deductive Approach*, TranState Working Papers no. 165, SfB "Transformations of the State", Bremen.

────── 2013, 'Five Types of OECD Healthcare Systems: Empirical Results of a Deductive Classification', *Health Policy*, vol. 113, no. 3, pp. 258–69.

Bölt, U and Graf, T 2012, '20 Jahre Krankenhausstatistik', in *Wirtschaft und Statistik*, no. 02/2012, pp. 112–38., viewed 28 August 2013, <https://www.destatis.de/DE/Pub likationen/WirtschaftStatistik/Gesundheitswesen/20JahreKrankenhausstatistik. pdf?__blob=publicationFile>.

Bonoli, G 2012, 'Blame Avoidance and Credit Claiming Revisited', in G Bonoli and D Natali (eds), *The Politics of the New Welfare State*, Oxford University Press, Oxford, pp. 93–107.

Bonoli, G and Natali, D 2012, 'Multidimensional Transformations in the Early 21st Century Welfare States', in G Bonoli and D Natali (eds), *The Politics of the New Welfare State*, Oxford University Press, Oxford, pp. 287–304.

Bosanquet, N 2007, 'The Health and Welfare Legacy', in A Seldon (ed.), *Blair's Britain: 1997–2007*, Cambridge University Press, Cambridge, pp. 385–407.

Boyle, S 2011, *United Kingdom (England): Health System Review*, Health Systems in Transition 13–1, European Observatory on Health Systems and Policies, Copenhagen, viewed 26 August 2014, <http://www.euro.who.int/__data/assets/pdf_file/0004/135148/e94836.pdf>.

Brandhorst, A 2003, 'Gesundheitspolitik zwischen 1998 und 2003: Nach der Reform ist vor der Reform', in A Gohr and M Seeleib-Kaiser (eds), *Sozial- und Wirtschaftspolitik unter Rot-Grün*, Westdt. Verl., Wiesbaden, pp. 211–28.

Braun, B 1998, *Das Märchen von der Kostenexplosion: Populäre Irrtümer zur Gesundheitspolitik*, 2nd edn, Fischer-Taschenbuch-Verl., Frankfurt.

Breyer, F and Haufler, A 2000, 'Healthcare Reform: Separating Insurance from Income Redistribution', *International Tax and Public Finance*, vol. 7, nos. 4–5, pp. 445–61.

British Medical Association 2010, *General Practitioners: Briefing Paper*, British Medical Association, viewed 12 August 2013, <http://bma.org.uk/-/media/Files/Word%20files/ News%20views%20analysis/pressbriefing_GPs.doc>.

Busse, R and Riesberg, A 2004, *Germany: Health System Review*, Health Systems in Transition 6–9, WHO Regional Office for Europe on behalf of the European Observatory on Health Systems and Policies, Copenhagen, viewed 26 August 2014, <http://www.euro. who.int/__data/assets/pdf_file/0018/80703/E85472.pdf>.

Busse, R, Schreyögg, J and Gericke, C 2007, *Analyzing Changes in Health Financing Arrangements in High-Income Countries: A Comprehensive Framework Approach*, Health, Nutrition and Population (HNP) Discussion Paper, The International Bank for Reconstruction and Development/The World Bank, Washington, viewed 2 July 2009, <http://www.mig.tu-berlin.de/fileadmin/a38331600/2007.publications/dp.2007.busse_ BusseAnalyzingChangesinHealthFinancingFinal.pdf>.

Butler, D 2006, *British Political Facts Since 1979*, Palgrave Macmillan, Basingstoke.

Butler, D and Kavanagh, D 1997, *The British General Election of 1997*, Macmillan, Basingstoke.

Butterwegge, C 2001, *Wohlfahrtsstaat im Wandel: Probleme und Perspektiven der Sozialpolitik*, 3rd edn, Leske + Budrich, Opladen.

Carpenter, D 2012, 'Is Health Politics Different?', *Annual Review of Political Science*, vol. 15, no. 1, pp. 287–311.

Carroll, E 1999, *Emergence and Structuring of Social Insurance Institutions: Comparative Studies on Social Policy and Unemployment Insurance*, Swedish Institute for Social Research, Stockholm.

Castles, FG 2001, 'On the Political Economy of Recent Public Sector Development', *Journal of European Social Policy*, vol. 11, no. 3, pp. 195–211.

―――― 2004, *The Future of the Welfare State: Crisis Myths and Crisis Realities*, Oxford University Press, Oxford.

Chadwick, A and Heffernan, R 2003, 'Introduction', in A Chadwick and R Heffernan (eds), *The New Labour Reader*, Polity Press, Cambridge, pp. 1–25.

Christensen, T and Lægreid, P 2011, 'Introduction', in T Christensen and P Lægreid (eds), *The Ashgate Research Companion to New Public Management*, Ashgate, Farnham, pp. 1–13.

Clarke, J and Newman, J 1997, *The Managerial State: Power, Politics and Ideology in the Remaking of Social Welfare*, SAGE Publ., London.

Clarke, J, Newman, JE, Smith, N, Vidler, E and Westmarland, L 2007, *Creating Citizen-Consumers: Changing Publics and Changing Public Services*, SAGE Publ., London.

Clasen, J and Clegg, D 2007, 'Levels and Levers of Conditionality: Measuring Change within Welfare States', in J Clasen and NA Siegel (eds), *Investigating Welfare State Change: The 'Dependent Variable Problem' in Comparative Analysis*, Edward Elgar, Cheltenham, pp. 166–91.

Clasen, J and Daniel, C 2006, 'New Labour Market Risks and the Revision of Unemployment Protection Systems in Europe', in K Armingeon and G Bonoli (eds), *The Politics of Post-Industrial Welfare States: Adapting Post-war Social Policies to New Social Risks*, Routledge, London, pp. 192–210.

Clasen, J and Siegel, NA (eds) 2007, *Investigating Welfare State Change: The 'Dependent Variable Problem' in Comparative Analysis*, Edward Elgar, Cheltenham.

Clayton, R and Pontusson, J 1998, 'Welfare State Retrenchment Revisited: Entitlement Cuts, Public Sector Restructuring, and Inegalitarian Trends in Advanced Capitalist Societies', *World Politics*, vol. 51, no. 1, pp. 67–98.

Collier, J 1985, 'Licensing and Provision of Medicines in the United Kingdom: An Appraisal', *Lancet*, 17 August, pp. 377–81.

Conrad, P 2007, *The Medicalization of Society: On the Transformation of Human Conditions into Treatable Disorders*, Johns Hopkins University Press, Baltimore.

Davis, G 2007, 'The Effect of Mrs Watts' Trip to France on the National Health Service', *King's Law Journal*, vol. 18, no. 1, pp. 158–67.

Dean, H 2002, *Welfare Rights and Social Policy*, Prentice Hall, Harlow.

Department of Health 1992, *The Health of the Nation. A Strategy for Health in England*, Cm 1986, HMSO, London.

—————— 1998, *A First Class Service: Quality in the New NHS,*, Department of Health, London.

—————— 2007, *Patient Mobility. Advice to Local Healthcare Commissioners on Handling Requests for Hospital Care in Other European Countries Following the ECJ's Judgment in the Watts Case*, Gateway Reference no. 8010, London, viewed 12 December 2013, <http://webarchive.nationalarchives.gov.uk/20130107105354/http://www.dh.gov.uk/prod_consum_dh/groups/dh_digitalassets/@dh/@en/documents/digitalasset/dh_073851.pdf>.

—————— 2009a, *Defining Guiding Principles for Processes Supporting Local Decision Making about Medicines*, London, viewed 8 November 2013, <http://webarchive.nationalarchives.gov.uk/20130107105354/http://www.dh.gov.uk/prod_consum_dh/groups/dh_digitalassets/documents/digitalasset/dh_093433.pdf>.

—————— 2009b, *Guidance on NHS Patients Who Wish to Pay for Additional Private Care*, London, viewed 12 November 2013, <http://webarchive.nationalarchives.gov.uk/20130107105354/http://www.dh.gov.uk/prod_consum_dh/groups/dh_digitalassets/documents/digitalasset/dh_096576.pdf>.

—————— 2011a, *Guidance on Implementing the Overseas Visitors Hospital Charging Regulations*, London, viewed 16 August 2013, <http://webarchive.nationalarchives.gov.uk/20130513204013/https://www.gov.uk/government/uploads/system/uploads/attachment_data/file/152376/dh_134418.pdf.pdf>.

—————— 2011b, *Resource Accounts 2010–11*, HC no. 1011, Stationery Office, London, viewed 12 August 2013, <https://www.gov.uk/government/uploads/system/uploads/attachment_data/file/215448/dh_130154.pdf>.

Deppe, H 2000, *Zur sozialen Anatomie des Gesundheitssystems: Neoliberalismus und Gesundheitspolitik in Deutschland*, VSA-Verl., Frankfurt.

—————— 2005, *Zur sozialen Anatomie des Gesundheitssystems: Neoliberalismus und Gesundheitspolitik in Deutschland*, 3rd edn, VSA-Verl., Frankfurt.

Die Ersatzkasse 1978, 'Hilfsmittelkatalog verabschiedet', *Die Ersatzkasse*, no. 10, pp. 425–30.

Dobbs-Smith, I 1999, 'The Supply and Reimbursement of Medicines under the NHS', in J O'Grady, I Dobbs-Smith, N Walsh and M Spencer (eds), *Medicines, Medical Devices and the Law*, Greenwich Medical Media, London, pp. 71–98.

Döhler, M 1990, *Gesundheitspolitik nach der "Wende": Policy-Netzwerke und ordnungspolitischer Strategiewechsel in Grossbritannien, den USA und der Bundesrepublik Deutschland*, Edition Sigma, Berlin.

Döhler, M and Manow-Borgwardt, P 1992a, 'Gesundheitspolitische Steuerung zwischen Hierarchie und Verhandlung', *Politische Vierteljahresschrift*, vol. 33, no. 4, pp. 571–96.

—————— 1992b, 'Korporatisierung als gesundheitspolitische Strategie', *Staatswissenschaften und Staatspraxis*, vol. 3, no. 1, pp. 64–106.

Dormont, B, Oliveira-Martins, J, Pelgrin, F and Suhrcke, M 2010, 'The Growth of Health Expenditures: Ageing vs. Technological Progress', in P Garibaldi, J Oliveira-Martins and JC van Ours (eds), *Ageing, Health, and Productivity: The Economics of Increased Life Expectancy*, Oxford University Press, Oxford, pp. 16–38.

Driver, S and Martell, L 2002, *New Labour: Politics after Thatcherism*, Polity Press, Cambridge.

Dworkin, R 1977, *Taking Rights Seriously*, Harvard University Press, Cambridge, MA.

Ebbinghaus, B and Schulze, I 2008, 'Krise und Reform der Alterssicherung in Europa', in F Boll (ed.), *Der Sozialstaat in der Krise: Deutschland im internationalen Vergleich*, Archiv für Sozialgeschichte/Einzelveröffentlichungen, Dietz, Bonn, pp. 269–96.

Eekhoff, J 2008, *Beschäftigung und soziale Sicherung*, 4th edn, Mohr Siebeck, Tübingen.

Egle, C, Ostheim, T and Zohlnhöfer, R 2003, 'Einführung: Eine Topographie des rot-grünen Projekts', in C Egle, T Ostheim and R Zohlnhöfer (eds), *Das rot-grüne Projekt: Eine Bilanz der Regierung Schröder 1998–2002*, Westdt. Verl., Wiesbaden, pp. 9–25.

Egle, C and Zohlnhöfer, R 2010, 'Die Große Koalition – eine "Koalition der neuen Möglichkeiten"?', in C Egle and R Zohlnhöfer (eds), *Die zweite Große Koalition: Eine Bilanz der Regierung Merkel 2005–2009*, VS Verl. für Sozialwissenschaften, Wiesbaden, pp. 11–25.

Elmelund-Praestkaer, C and Baggesen, M 2012, 'Policy or Institution? The Political Choice of Retrenchment Strategy', *Journal of European Public Policy*, vol. 19, no. 7, pp. 1089–107.

Engelhard, W 2012, '§ 12', in K Engelmann and R Schlegel (eds), *Juris Praxis Kommentar SGB V – Gesetzliche Krankenversicherung*, 2nd edn, Juris, Saarbrücken.

Esping-Andersen, G 1990, *The Three Worlds of Welfare Capitalism*, Princeton University Press, Princeton.

——— 1996, 'After the Golden Age? Welfare State Dilemmas in a Global Economy', in G Esping-Andersen (ed.), *Welfare States in Transition: National Adaptations in Global Economies*, SAGE Publ., London, pp. 1–31.

——— 1999, *Social Foundations of Postindustrial Economies*, Oxford University Press, Oxford.

Evans, B 1999, *Thatcherism and British Politics 1975–1999*, Sutton, Phoenix Mill.

Evans, EJ 2004, *Thatcher and Thatcherism*, 2nd edn, Routledge, London.

Evers, A and Guillemard, A 2013, 'Introduction: Marshall's Concept of Citizenship and Contemporary Welfare Reconfiguration', in A Evers and A Guillemard (eds), *Social Policy and Citizenship: The Changing Landscape*, Oxford University Press, New York, pp. 3–34.

Evers, A and Olk, T 1996, *Wohlfahrtspluralismus: Vom Wohlfahrtsstaat zur Wohlfahrtsge-sellschaft*, Westdt. Verl., Opladen.

Faist, T 2007, 'Die transnationale soziale Frage. Soziale Rechte und Bürgerschaften im globalen Kontext', in J Mackert (ed.), *Moderne (Staats)Bürgerschaft: Nationale Staats-bürgerschaft und die Debatten der Citizenship Studies*, VS Verl. für Sozialwissen-schaften, Wiesbaden, pp. 285–307.

Ferrera, M 2008, 'The European Welfare State: Golden Achievements, Silver Prospects', *West European Politics*, vol. 31, nos. 1–2, pp. 82–107.

Fisher, J and Wlezien, C 2012, 'Introduction: The General Election of 2010', in J Fisher and C Wlezien (eds), *The UK General Election of 2010: Explaining the Outcome*, Routledge, London, pp. 1–4.

Ford, A 2012, 'The Concept of Exceptionality: A Legal Farce?', *Medical Law Review*, vol. 20, no. 3, pp. 304–36.

Freeman, R and Moran, M 2000, 'Reforming Healthcare in Europe', *West European Politics*, vol. 23, no. 2, pp. 35–58.

Fries, JF, Bruce, B and Chakravarty, E 2011, 'Compression of Morbidity 1980–2011: A Focused Review of Paradigms and Progress', *Journal of Aging Research*, vol. 2011, no. 3, pp. 1–10.

Ganßmann, H 1993, 'Sind soziale Rechte universalisierbar?', *Zeitschrift für Soziologie*, vol. 22, no. 5, pp. 385–94.

Gelijns, A and Rosenberg, N 1994, 'The Dynamics of Technological Change in Medicine', *Health Affairs*, vol. 13, no. 3, pp. 28–46.

George, AL and Bennett, A 2005, *Case Studies and Theory Development in the Social Sciences*, MIT Press, Cambridge, MA.

Gerlinger, T 2002, *Zwischen Korporatismus und Wettbewerb: Gesundheitspolitische Steuerung im Wandel*, Veröffentlichungsreihe der Arbeitsgruppe Public Health, P02–204, Wissenschaftszentrum Berlin für Sozialforschung, Berlin.

——— 2004, 'Privatisierung – Liberalisierung – Re-Regulierung. Konturen des Umbaus des Gesundheitssystems', *WSI-Mitteilungen*, vol. 57, no. 9, pp. 501–6.

——— 2009, 'Competitive Transformation and the State Regulation of Health Insurance Systems: Germany, Switzerland and the Netherlands Compared', in I Dingeldey and H Rothgang (eds), *Governance of Welfare State Reform: A Cross National and Cross Sectoral Comparison of Policy and Politics*, Edward Elgar, Cheltenham, pp. 145–75.

Gerlinger, T, Mosebach, K and Schmucker, R (eds) 2010, *Gesundheitsdienstleistungen im europäischen Binnenmarkt*, Frankfurter Schriften zur Gesundheitspolitik und zum Gesundheitsrecht, vol. 11, Lang, Frankfurt.

Gerring, J 2007, *Case Study Research: Principles and Practices*, Cambridge University Press, Cambridge.

Giaimo, S 2001, 'Who Pays for Healthcare Reform', in P Pierson (ed.), *The New Politics of the Welfare State*, Oxford University Press, Oxford, pp. 334–67.

Giaimo, S and Manow, P 1999, 'Adapting the Welfare State: The Case of Healthcare Reform in Britain, Germany, and the United States', *Comparative Political Studies*, vol. 32, no. 8, pp. 967–1000.

Gibis, B, Koch-Wulkan, PW and Bultman, J 2004, 'Shifting Criteria for Benefit Decisions in Social Health Insurance Systems', in RB Saltman, R Busse and J Figueras (eds), *Social Health Insurance Systems in Western Europe*, European Observatory on Health Systems and Policies Series, Open University Press, Maidenhead, pp. 189–206.

Gilbert, N 2002, *Transformation of the Welfare State: The Silent Surrender of Public Responsibility*, Oxford University Press, Oxford.

Goodin, RE and Rein, M 2001, 'Regimes on Pillars: Alternaitve Welfare State Logics and Dynamics', *Public Administration*, vol. 79, no. 4, pp. 769–801.

gpk 2011a, 'Gespräch mit Rainer Hess: Unparteiischer Vorsitzender des Gemeinsamen Bundesausschusses', *Gesellschaftspolitische Kommentare*, vol. 52, special ed. no. 1, pp. 3–13.

——— 2011b, 'Gespräch mt Johann-Magnus von Stackelberg: Stellvertretender Vorsitzender des GKV-Spitzenverbandes', *Gesellschaftspolitische Kommentare*, vol. 52, special ed. no. 1, pp. 14–21.

Greer, SL 2006, 'Uninvited Europeanization: Neofuctionalism and the EU in Health Policy', *Journal of European Public Policy*, vol. 13, no. 1, pp. 134–52.

Griffiths, R 1983, *NHS Management Inquiry: Report to the Secretary of State for Social Services*, Mimeo, London.

Grimshaw, D and Rubery, J 2012, 'The End of the UK's Liberal Collectivist Social Model? The Implications of the Coalition Government's Policy during the Austerity Crisis', *Cambridge Journal of Economics*, vol. 36, no. 1, pp. 105–26.

The Guardian 2013, *DATABLOG: Deficit, National Debt and Government Borrowing – How Has It Changed Since 1946?*, 22 May, The Guardian, viewed 25 November 2013, <http://www.theguardian.com/news/datablog/2010/oct/18/deficit-debt-government-borrowing-data#zoomed-picture>.

Hacker, JS 2004, 'Dismantling the Healthcare State?: Political Institutions, Public Policies and the Comparative Politics of Health Reform', *British Journal of Political Science*, vol. 34, no. 4, pp. 693–724.

Haggett, E 2001, *The Human Rights Act 1998 and Access to NHS Treatments and Services: A Practical Guide*, SoPPUCL, The Constitution Unit, London, viewed 4 April 2013, <http://www.ucl.ac.uk/spp/publications/unit-publications/78.pdf>.

Håkan, J and Bjørn, H 2013, 'Towards a Post-Marshallian Framework for the Analysis of Social Citizenship', in A Evers and A Guillemard (eds), *Social Policy and Citizenship: The Changing Landscape*, Oxford University Press, New York, pp. 35–79.

Ham, C 2009, *Health Policy in Britain*, 6th edn, Palgrave Macmillan, Basingstoke.

Harcker, R 2012, *NHS Funding and Expenditure*, House of Commons Library SN/SG/724, House of Commons, viewed 25 October 2013, <http://www.nhshistory.net/parlymoney.pdf>.

Hartley, BH 1981, 'Clinical Pharmacology: Prescription Writing', *BMJ*, vol. 282, no. 6265, pp. 711–4.

Hartmann, A 2003, 'Patientennah, leistungsstark, finanzbewusst? Die Gesundheitspolitik der rot-grünen Bundesregierung', in C Egle, T Ostheim and R Zohlnhöfer (eds), *Das rot-grüne Projekt: Eine Bilanz der Regierung Schröder 1998–2002*, Westdt. Verl., Wiesbaden, pp. 259–81.

———— 2010, 'Die Gesundheitsreform der Großen Koalition: Kleinster gemeinsamer Nenner oder offenes Hintertürchen?', in C Egle and R Zohlnhöfer (eds), *Die zweite Große Koalition: Eine Bilanz der Regierung Merkel 2005–2009*, VS Verl. für Sozialwissenschaften, Wiesbaden, pp. 327–49.

Hassenteufel, P and Palier, B 2008, 'Towards Neo Bismarckian Healthcare States? Comparing Health Insurance Reforms in Bismarckian Welfare Systems', in B Palier and C Martin (eds), *Reforming the Bismarckian Welfare Systems*, Blackwell Publ., Malden, MA, pp. 40–61.

Hayek, FA 1976, *The Mirage of Social Justice*, Law, Legislation and Liberty, vol. 2, Routledge and Kegan Paul, London.

Hegelich, S, Knollmann, D and Kuhlmann, J 2011, *Agenda 2010: Strategien, Entscheidungen, Konsequenzen*, VS Verl. für Sozialwissenschaften, Wiesbaden.

Heinze, H 1976, '§§165-, 376d', in H Bley (ed.), *RVO-, SGB-Gesamtkommentar: Sozialgesetzbuch, Sozialversicherung: Kommentar zum gesamten Recht der Reichsversicherungsordnung einschließlich zwischenstaatlicher Abkommen und internationaler Übereinkommen*, Chmielorz, Wiesbaden.

Heppell, T 2013, *How Labour Governments Fall: From Ramsay Macdonald to Gordon Brown*, Palgrave Macmillan, New York.

Hermann, C 2007, 'Die Privatisierung von Gesundheit in Europa', in H Ivansits (ed.), *Privatisierung von Gesundheit: Blick über die Grenzen*, Sozialpolitik in Diskussion, Dokumentation der gleichnamigen Tagung vom November 2007 AK-Bildungszentrum Wien, vol. 5, Wien, pp. 5–21, viewed 11 March 2014, <http://media.arbeiterkammer.at/PDF/Sozialpolitik_in_Diskussion_5.pdf>.

Hervey, TK and McHale, JV 2004, *Health Law and the European Union*, Cambridge University Press, Cambridge.

HM Government 2010, *The Coalition: Our Programme for Government*, Cabinet Office, London, viewed 2 December 2013, <https://www.gov.uk/government/uploads/system/uploads/attachment_data/file/78977/coalition_programme_for_government.pdf>.

HMSO 1991, *The Citizen's Charter: Raising the Standard: Presented to Parliament by the Prime Minister by Command of Her Majesty, July 1991*, Cm. no. 1599, London.

HM Treasury 2010, *Budget 2010*, HC 61, The Stationery Office, London, viewed 6 January 2014, <http://www.direct.gov.uk/prod_consum_dg/groups/dg_digitalassets/@dg/@en/documents/digitalasset/dg_188581.pdf>.

Hockley, T 2012, 'A Giant Leap by Small Steps: The Conservative Party and National Health Service Reform', PHD thesis, London School of Economics and Political Science, London.

Huber, E and Stephens, JD 2001, *Development and Crisis of the Welfare State: Parties and Policies in Global Markets*, University of Chicago Press, Chicago.

Hughes, D 1993, 'General Practitioners and the New Contract: Promoting Better Health through Financial Incentives', *Health Policy*, vol. 25, pp. 39–50.

Hunter, DJ 1982, 'Organising for Health: The National Health Service in the United Kingdom', *Journal of Public Policy*, vol. 2, no. 3, p. 263.

Huster, E 1982, 'Krankenversorgung und Gesundheitssicherung', *Gewerkschaftliche Monatshefte*, vol. 33, no. 11, pp. 697–713.

Immergut, EM 1992, *Health Politics: Interests and Institutions in Western Europe*, Cambridge University Press, Cambridge.

Iversen, T and Soskice, D 2006, 'Electoral Institutions and the Politics of Coalitions: Why Some Democracies Redistribute More Than Others', *American Political Science Review*, vol. 100, no. 2, pp. 165–81.

Jensen, C 2008, 'Worlds of Welfare Services and Transfers', *Journal of European Social Policy*, vol. 18, no. 2, pp. 151–62.

―――― 2011a, 'Marketization via Compensation: Healthcare and the Politics of the Right in Advanced Industrialized Nations', *British Journal of Political Science*, vol. 41, no. 4, pp. 907–26.

―――― 2011b, 'The Forgotten Half: Analysing the Politics of Welfare Services', *International Journal of Social Welfare*, vol. 20, no. 4, pp. 404–12.

Jochem, S 1999, *Sozialpolitik in der Ära Kohl: Die Politik des Sozialversicherungsstaates*, ZeS-Arbeitspapier, 12/99, Zentrum für Sozialpolitik, Universität Bremen, Bremen.

Jordan, J 2011, 'Healthcare Politics in the Age of Retrenchment', *Journal of Social Policy*, vol. 40, no. 1, pp. 113–34.

Jost, TS 2003, *Disentitlement?: The Threats Facing Our Public Health-Care Programs and a Rights-Based Response*, Oxford University Press, Oxford.

Kamps, N 2009, *Grundlagen der Hilfsmittel- und Pflegehilfsmittelversorgung: Arbeitshilfe zum SGB V und SGB XI; Einführung in das Hilfsmittelverzeichnis*, Walhalla-Fachverl., Regensburg.

Kangas, O and Palme, J 2007, 'Social Rights, Structural Needs and Social Expenditure: A Comparative Study of 18 OECD Countries 1960–2000', in J Clasen and NA Siegel (eds), *Investigating Welfare State Change: The 'Dependent Variable Problem' in Comparative Analysis*, Edward Elgar, Cheltenham, pp. 106–29.

Kaufmann, F 2003a, *Die Entstehung sozialer Grundrechte und die wohlfahrtsstaatliche Entwicklung*, Schöningh, Paderborn.

―――― 2003b, *Varianten des Wohlfahrtsstaats: Der deutsche Sozialstaat im internationalen Vergleich*, Suhrkamp, Frankfurt.

The King's Fund 2013, *An Alternative Guide to the New NHS in England*, viewed 2 December 2013, <http://www.kingsfund.org.uk/projects/nhs-65/alternative-guide-new-nhs-england>.

Klein, R 2007, 'The New Model NHS: Performance, Perceptions and Expectations', *British Medical Bulletin*, vol. 81–82, no. 1, pp. 39–50.

―――― 2010, *The New Politics of the NHS: From Creation to Reinvention*, 6th edn, Radcliffe Publ., Oxford.

Klein, R, Day, P and Redmayne, S 1996, *Managing Scarcity: Priority Setting and Rationing in the National Health Service*, Open University Press, Buckingham.

Kornelius, B and Roth, D 2007, 'Bundestagswahl 2005: Rot-Grün abgewählt. Verlierer bilden die Regierung', in C Egle and R Zohlnhöfer (eds), *Ende des rot-grünen Projektes: Eine Bilanz der Regierung Schröder 2002–2005*, VS Verl. für Sozialwissenschaften, Wiesbaden, pp. 29–59.

Korpi, W 1989, 'Power, Politics and State Autonomy in the Development of Social Citizenship', *American Sociological Review*, vol. 54, no. 3, pp. 309–29.

——— 2003, 'Welfare State Regress in Western-Europe: Politics, Institutions, Globalization, and Europeanization', *Annual Review of Sociology*, vol. 29, pp. 589–609.

Korpi, W and Palme, J 2003, 'New Politics and Class Politics in the Context of Austerity and Globalization: Welfare State Regress in 18 Countries, 1975–95', *American Political Science Review*, vol. 97, no. 3, pp. 425–46.

Krauskopf, D 1997, '§ 33', in D Krauskopf (ed.), *Soziale Krankenversicherung*, C.H. Beck, München, pp. 1–24.

Kruse, J and Hänlein, A 2004, *Das neue Krankenversicherungsrecht*, Nomos, Baden Baden.

Kvist, J 2007, 'Exploring Diversity: Measuring Welfare State Change with Fuzzy-Set Methodology', in J Clasen and NA Siegel (eds), *Investigating Welfare State Change: The 'Dependent Variable Problem' in Comparative Analysis*, Edward Elgar, Cheltenham, pp. 198–214.

Labour Party 1997, *New Labour: Because Britain Deserves Better*, Labour Party, London.

Landwehr, C 2013, 'Procedural Justice and Democratic Institutional Design in Health-Care Priority-Setting', *Contemporary Political Theory*, vol. 12, no. 4, pp. 296–317.

Landwehr, C and Böhm, K 2011a, 'Delegation and Institutional Design in Health-Care Rationing', *Governance*, vol. 24, no. 4, pp. 665–88.

——— 2011b, 'Prioritätensetzung und explizite Rationierung in der Gesundheitspolitik: Entscheidungsverfahren und Leistungskataloge im internationalen Vergleich', in S Schüttemeyer (ed.), *Politik im Klimawandel: Keine Macht für gerechte Lösungen?*, Nomos, Baden-Baden, pp. 341–54.

——— 2014, 'Strategic Institutional Design: Two Case Studies of Non-Majoritarian Agencies in Healthcare Priority Setting', *Government and Opposition*, forthcoming.

Le Grand, J, Winter, D and Wooley, F 1991, 'The National Health Service: Safe in Whose Hands?', in N Barr and J Hills (eds), *The State of Welfare: The Welfare State in Britain Since 1974*, Clarendon Press, Oxford, pp. 88–134.

Lister, R 2003, *Citizenship: Feminist Perspectives*, 2nd edn, New York University Press, New York.

——— 2007, 'Staatsbürgerschaft und Differenz. Plädoyer für einen differenzierten Universalismus', in J Mackert (ed.), *Moderne (Staats)Bürgerschaft: Nationale Staatsbürgerschaft und die Debatten der Citizenship Studies*, VS Verl. für Sozialwissenschaften, Wiesbaden, pp. 395–413.

Littlejohns, P, Weale, A, Chalkidou, K, Faden, R and Teerawattananon, Y 2012, 'Social Values and Health Policy: A New International Research Programme', *Journal of Health Organization and Management*, vol. 26, no. 3, pp. 285–92.

Maarse, H 2006, 'The Privatization of Healthcare in Europe: An Eight-Country Analysis', *Journal of Health Politics, Policy and Law*, vol. 31, no. 5, pp. 981–1014.

Majone, G 1997, 'From the Positive to the Regulatory State: Causes and Consequences of Changes in the Mode of Governance', *Journal of Public Policy*, vol. 17, no. 2, pp. 139–67.

——— 1999, 'The Regulatory State and Its Legitimacy Problems', *West European Politics*, vol. 22, no. 1, pp. 1–24.

Mann, M 1987, 'Ruling Class Strategies and Citizenship', *Sociology*, vol. 21, no. 3, pp. 339–54.

Marshall, TH 1950, *Citizenship and Social Class and Other Essays*, Cambridge University Press, London.

Mau, S 2007, 'Mitgliedschaftsräume, wohlfahrtsstaatliche Solidarität und Migration', in J Mackert (ed.), *Moderne (Staats)Bürgerschaft: Nationale Staatsbürgerschaft und die Debatten der Citizenship Studies*, VS Verl. für Sozialwissenschaften, Wiesbaden, pp. 215–33.

McCarvill, P 2010, *Equality, Entitlements and Localism*, Institute for Public Policy Research, London, viewed 19 December 2013, <http://www.onenorthwest.org.uk/documents/Equality_Entitlements_and_Localism%5B1%5D.pdf>.

McHale, JV 2007, 'Rights to Medical Treatment in EU Law', *Medical Law Review*, vol. 15, no. 1, pp. 99–108.

―――― 2011, 'Healthcare, the United Kingdom and the Draft Patients' Rights Directive: One Small Step for Patient Mobility But a Huge Leap for a Reformed NHS?', in JW van de Gronden, E Szyszczak, U Neergard and M Krajewski (eds), *Healthcare and EU Law*, T.M.C. Asser Press, The Hague, pp. 241–62.

―――― 2012, 'Exploring Patients' Rights: What Does the NHS Constitution Tell Us?', *British Journal of Nursing*, vol. 21, no. 9, pp. 552–3.

Mills, A, Gilson, L, Hanson, K and Palmer, N 2008, 'What Do We Mean by Rigorous Health-Systems Research?', *The Lancet*, vol. 372, pp. 1527–9.

Montanari, I and Nelson, K 2013, 'Social Service Decline and Convergence: How Does Healthcare Fare?', *Journal of European Social Policy*, vol. 23, no. 1, pp. 102–16.

Montgomery, J 2002, *Healthcare Law*, 2nd edn, Oxford University Press, Oxford.

Moran, M 2000, 'Understanding the Welfare State: The Case of Healthcare', *British Journal of Politics and International Relations*, vol. 2, no. 2, pp. 135–60.

Mossialos, E and Palm, W 2003, 'The European Court of Justice and the Free Movement of Patients in the European Union', *International Social Security Review*, vol. 56, no. 2, pp. 3–29.

Mossialos, E, Permanand, G, Baeten, R and Hervey, T 2010a, 'Health System Governance in Europe: The Role of European Union Law and Policy', in E Mossialos, G Permanand, R Baeten and T Hervey (eds), *Health Systems Governance in Europe: The Role of European Union Law and Policy*, Cambridge University Press, Cambridge, pp. 1–83.

―――― (eds) 2010b, *Health Systems Governance in Europe: The Role of European Union Law and Policy*, Cambridge University Press, Cambridge.

Needham, C 2007, *The Reform of Public Services under New Labour: Narratives of Consumerism*, Palgrave Macmillan, Basingstoke.

Newdick, C 2005, *Who Should We Treat? Rights, Rationing, and Resources in the NHS*, 2nd edn, Oxford University Press, Oxford.

―――― 2006, 'Citizenship, Free Movement and Healthcare: Cementing Individual Rights by Corroding Social Solidarity', *Common Market Law Review*, vol. 43, no. 6, pp. 1645–68.

―――― 2007, 'Judicial Supervision of Health Resource Allocation: English Experience', in TS Jost (ed.), *Readings in Comparative Health Law and Bioethics*, 2nd edn, Carolina Academic Press, Durham, NC, pp. 59–70.

―――― 2009, 'The European Court of Justice, Transnational Healthcare, and Social Citizenship – Accidental Death of a Concept?', *Wisconsin International Law Journal*, vol. 26, no. 3, pp. 844–67.

Newhouse, JP 1993, *Free for All?: Lessons from the RAND Health Insurance Experiment*, Harvard University Press, Cambridge, MA.

NICE 2005, *Social Value Judgements: Principles for the Development of NICE Guidance*, National Institute for Health and Clinical Excellence, London, viewed 6 January 2014, <http://www.nice.org.uk/media/873/2F/SocialValueJudgementsDec05.pdf>.

———— 2008, *Social Value Judgements: Principles for the Development of NICE Guidance*, 2nd edn, National Institute for Health and Clinical Excellence, London, viewed 11 November 2013, <http://www.nice.org.uk/media/C18/30/SVJ2PUBLICATION2008. pdf>.

———— 2009, *Appraising Life-Extending, End of Life Treatments*, National Institute for Health and Clinical Excellence, London, viewed 11 November 2013, <http://www.nice. org.uk/media/E4A/79/SupplementaryAdviceTACEoL.pdf>.

Niedermayer, O 2011, 'Das deutsche Parteiensystem nach der Bundestagswahl 2009', in O Niedermayer (ed.), *Die Parteien nach der Bundestagswahl 2009*, VS Verl. für Sozial-wissenschaften, Wiesbaden, pp. 7–35.

Noelle-Neumann, E 1997, *Allensbacher Jahrbuch der Demoskopie 1993–1997*, vol. 10, Saur, München.

Noweski, M 2004, *Der unvollendete Korporatismus: Staatliche Steuerungsfähigkeit im ambulanten Sektor des deutschen Gesundheitswesens*, Wissenschaftszentrum Berlin für Sozialforschung, Berlin.

Nussbaum, MC 2011, *Creating Capabilities: The Human Development Approach*, Belknap Press, Cambridge.

Obermaier, AJ 2009, *The End of Territoriality?: The Impact of ECJ Rulings on British, German, and French Social Policy*, Ashgate, Burlington.

OECD 2012a, *OECD Health Data: Expenditure and Financing*, Organization for Eco-nomic Co-operation and Development, Paris, viewed 04 June 2013, <http://stats.oecd. org/Index.aspx?DataSetCode=SHA>.

———— 2012b, *OECD Health Data: Health Status*, Organization for Economic Co-operation and Development, Paris.

———— 2012c, *Social Spending during the Crisis: Social Expenditure (SOCX) Data Update 2012*, Organization for Economic Co-operation and Development, Paris, viewed 4 June 2013, <http://www.oecd.org/els/soc/OECD2012SocialSpendingDuringThe Crisis8pages.pdf>.

———— 2014a, *Key Short Term Indicators*, Main Economic Indicators (database), Organi-zation for Economic Co-operation and Development, Paris, viewed 26 August 2014, <http://stats.oecd.org/viewhtml.aspx?datasetcode=KEI&lang=en>.

———— 2014b, *Labour Force Statistics: Summary Tables*, OECD Employment and Labour Market Statistics (database), Organization for Economic Co-operation and Develop-ment, Paris, viewed 26 August 2014, <http://stats.oecd.org/viewhtml.aspx?datasetcode= ALFS_SUMTAB&lang=en>.

———— 2014c, *OECD Health Data: Expenditure and Financing: Main Indicators*, OECD Health Statistics (database), Organization for Economic Co-operation and Development, Paris, viewed 20 August 2014, <http://stats.oecd.org/Index.aspx?DataSetCode=SHA>.

Office of Health Economics 2013, *GDP and NHS Expenditure, and Per Capita, UK, 1949/50–2011/12*, viewed 5 May 2014, <www.ohe.org/page/health-statistics/access-the-data/expenditure/data.cfm>.

Office for National Statistics 2014, *Public Sector Finances: April 2014*, London, viewed 13 June 2014, <http://www.ons.gov.uk/ons/rel/psa/public-sector-finances/april-2014/ stb-april-2014.html>.

Official Election Statistics 2014, 5 June, viewed 21 August 2014, <http://www.bundeswahl leiter.de/de/bundestagswahlen/fruehere_bundestagswahlen/>.

Orloff, AS 1993, 'Gender and the Social Rights of Citizenship: The Comparative Analysis of Gender Relations and Welfare States', *American Sociological Review*, vol. 58, no. 3, pp. 303–28.

Orlowski, U and Wasem, J 2003, *Gesundheitsreform 2004: GKV-Modernisierungsgesetz (GMG)*, Economica-Verl., Heidelberg.

———— 2007, *Gesundheitsreform 2007 (GKV-WSG): Änderungen und Auswirkungen auf einen Blick*, C.F. Müller, Heidelberg.

Palm, W and Baeten, R 2011, 'The Quality and Safety Paradox in the Patients' Rights Directive', *The European Journal of Public Health*, vol. 21, no. 3, pp. 272–4.

Palm, W and Glinos, IA 2010, 'Enabling Patient Mobility in the EU: Between Free Movement and Coordination', in E Mossialos, G Permanand, R Baeten and T Hervey (eds), *Health Systems Governance in Europe: The Role of European Union Law and Policy*, Cambridge University Press, Cambridge, pp. 509–60.

Paquet, R and Schroeder, W 2009, 'Gesundheitsreform 2007: Akteure, Interessen und Prozesse', in R Paquet and W Schroeder (eds), *Gesundheitsreform 2007: Nach der Reform ist vor der Reform*, VS Verl. für Sozialwissenschaften, Wiesbaden, pp. 11–29.

Perschke-Hartmann, C 1994, *Die doppelte Reform: Gesundheitspolitik von Blüm zu Seehofer*, Leske + Budrich, Opladen.

Pierson, P 1994, *Dismantling the Welfare State?: Reagan, Thatcher, and the Politics of Retrenchment*, Cambridge University Press, Cambridge.

———— 1996, 'The New Politics of the Welfare State', *World Politics*, vol. 48, no. 2, pp. 143–79.

———— 2001, 'Coping with Permanent Austerity: Welfare State Restructuring in Affluent Democracies', in P Pierson (ed.), *The New Politics of the Welfare State*, Oxford University Press, Oxford, pp. 410–56.

Plant, R 1998, 'Citizenship, Rights, Welfare', in J Franklin (ed.), *Social Policy and Social Justice: The IPPR Reader*, Polity Press, Cambridge, pp. 57–72.

Pollock, AM, Price, D, Viebrock, E, Miller, E and Watt, G 2007, 'The Market in Primary Care', *BMJ*, vol. 335, no. 7618, pp. 475–7.

Quinn, T, Bara, J and Bartle, J 2012, 'The UK Coalition Agreement of 2010: Who Won?', in J Fisher and C Wlezien (eds), *The UK General Election of 2010: Explaining the Outcome*, Routledge, London, pp. 175–92.

Rankin, J, Allen, J and Brooks, R 2007, *Great Expectations: Achieving a Sustainable Health System*, Institute for Public Policy Research, London.

Redden, CJ 2002, *Healthcare, Entitlement and Citizenship*, University of Toronto Press, Toronto.

Reiners, H 2009, *Mythen der Gesundheitspolitik*, Huber, Bern.

Reiners, H and Müller, O 2012, *Die Reformfibel: Gesundheitsgesetze von Blüm bis Bahr*, KomPart, Berlin.

Reiners, H, Volkholz, V, Botschafter, P, Preisler, K and Thiele, W 1977, *Gesundheitssystem in der Bundes Republik Deutschland*, VSA-Verl., Hamburg.

Rhodes, M 1996, 'Globalization and West European Welfare States: A Critical Review of Recent Debates', *Journal of European Social Policy*, vol. 6, no. 4, pp. 305–27.

Richards, M 2008, *Improving Access to Medicines for NHS Patients: A Report for the Secretary of State for Health by Professor Mike Richards CBE*, viewed 12 November 2013, <http://webarchive.nationalarchives.gov.uk/20130107105354/http://www.dh.gov.uk/prod_consum_dh/groups/dh_digitalassets/@dh/@en/documents/digitalasset/dh_089952.pdf>.

Ritter, GA 1991, *Wahlen in Deutschland 1946–1991: Ein Handbuch*, Beck, München.

———— 2007, 'Rahmenbedingungen der innerdeutschen Einigung', in GA Ritter and HG Hockerts (eds), *1989–1994, Bundesrepublik Deutschland: Sozialpolitik im Zeichen der Vereinigung*, Nomos, Baden-Baden, pp. 1–106.

Rivett, G 1998, *From Cradle to Grave: Fifty Years of the NHS*, King's Fund, London.

Robinson, S, Dickinson, H, Williams, I, Freeman, T, Rumbold, B and Spence, K 2011, *Setting Priorities in Health: A Study of English Primary Care Trusts*, Nuffield Trust, London, viewed 15 August 2013, <http://www.nuffieldtrust.org.uk/sites/files/nuffield/setting-priorities-in-health-research-report-sep11.pdf>.

Rosenberg, P 1969, *Die soziale Krankenversicherung. Pflichtversicherung oder freiwillige Vorsorge?*, Bund-Verlag, Köln.

Rosenbrock, R and Gerlinger, T 2014, *Gesundheitspolitik: Eine systematische Einführung*, 3rd edn, Huber, Bern.

Rosewitz, B and Webber, D 1990, *Reformversuche und Reformblockaden im deutschen Gesundheitswesen*, Schriften des Max-Planck-Instituts für Gesellschaftsforschung, Köln, vol. 5, Campus, Frankfurt.

Ross, F 2000, ' "Beyond Left and Right": The New Partisan Politics of Welfare', *Governance*, vol. 13, no. 2, pp. 155–83.

Rothgang, H 2009, 'Converging Governance in Healthcare Systems', in I Dingeldey and H Rothgang (eds), *Governance of Welfare State Reform: A Cross National and Cross Sectoral Comparison of Policy and Politics*, Edward Elgar, Cheltenham, pp. 21–42.

——— 2010, 'Introduction to the Book', in H Rothgang, M Cacace, F Lorraine, S Grimmeisen, A Schmid and C Wendt (eds), *The State and Healthcare: Comparing OECD Countries*, Palgrave Macmillan, Basingstoke, pp. 3–9.

Rothgang, H, Cacace, M, Lorraine, F, Grimmeisen, S, Schmid, A and Wendt, C (eds) 2010, *The State and Healthcare: Comparing OECD Countries*, Palgrave Macmillan, Basingstoke.

Sachverständigenrat für die Konzertierte Aktion im Gesundheitswesen 1994, *Gesundheitsversorgung und Krankenversicherung 2000: Eigenverantwortung, Subsidiarität und Solidarität bei sich ändernden Rahmenbedingungen*, Sachstandsbericht Sachverständigenrat für die Konzertierte Aktion im Gesundheitswesen, vol. 1994, Nomos, Baden-Baden.

Saltman, RB and Figueras, J 1997, *European Healthcare Reform: Analysis of Current Strategies*, World Health Organization Regional Office for Europe, Copenhagen.

Sauter, W 2011, *Harmonisation in Healthcare: The EU Patients' Rights Directive*, TILEC Discussion Paper 2011–030, Tilburg University, Tilburg, viewed 9 December 2013, <http://ssrn.com/abstract=1859251>.

Scharpf, FW 2002, 'The European Social Model: Coping with the Challenges of Diversity', *Journal of Common Market Studies*, vol. 40, no. 4, pp. 645–70.

Schmid, A, Cacace, M and Rothgang, H 2010, 'The Changing Role of the State in Healthcare Financing', in H Rothgang, M Cacace, F Lorraine, S Grimmeisen, A Schmid and C Wendt (eds), *The State and Healthcare: Comparing OECD Countries*, Palgrave Macmillan, Basingstoke, pp. 25–52.

Schmid, A and Wendt, C 2010, 'The Changing Role of the State in Healthcare Service Provision', in H Rothgang, M Cacace, F Lorraine, S Grimmeisen, A Schmid and C Wendt (eds), *The State and Healthcare: Comparing OECD Countries*, Palgrave Macmillan, Basingstoke, pp. 53–71.

Schmidt, MG 2003, 'Rot-grüne Sozialpolitik (1998–2002)', in C Egle, T Ostheim and R Zohlnhöfer (eds), *Das rot-grüne Projekt: Eine Bilanz der Regierung Schröder 1998–2002*, Westdt. Verl., Wiesbaden, pp. 239–58.

——— 2005a, 'Rahmenbedingungen', in MG Schmidt (ed.), *1982–1989, Bundesrepublik Deutschland: Finanzielle Konsolidierung und institutionelle Reform*, Geschichte der Sozialpolitik in Deutschland seit 1945, vol. 7, Nomos, Baden-Baden, pp. 1–30.

———— 2005b, *Sozialpolitik in Deutschland: Historische Entwicklung und internationaler Vergleich*, Lehrbuch, 3rd edn, vol. 2, VS Verl. für Sozialwissenschaften, Wiesbaden.

———— 2010, 'Die Sozialpolitik der zweiten Großen Koalition (2005 bis 2009)', in C Egle and R Zohlnhöfer (eds), *Die zweite Große Koalition: Eine Bilanz der Regierung Merkel 2005–2009*, VS Verl. für Sozialwissenschaften, Wiesbaden, pp. 302–26.

Schulten, T and Böhlke, N 2009, 'Die Privatisierung von Krankenhäusern in Deutschland und ihre Auswirkungen auf Beschäftigte und Patienten', in N Böhlke, T Gerlinger, K Mosebach, R Schmucker and T Schulten (eds), *Privatisierung von Krankenhäusern: Erfahrungen und Perspektiven aus Sicht der Beschäftigten*, VSA-Verl., Hamburg, pp. 97–123.

Scruggs, L 2006, 'The Generosity of Social Insurance, 1971–2002', *Oxford Review of Economic Policy*, vol. 22, no. 3, pp. 349–64.

Secretary of State for Health 1999, *Directions to the National Institute for Clinical Excellence*, London.

———— 2001, *Directions to Health Authorities, Primary Care Trusts and NHS Trusts in England*, London.

———— 2005, *Directions and Consolidating Directions to the National Institute for Health and Clinical Excellence*, London.

———— 2009, *Directions to Primary Care Trusts and NHS Trusts Concerning Decisions about Drugs and Other Treatments*, Department of Health, London, viewed 13 August 2014, <http://webarchive.nationalarchives.gov.uk/20130107105354/http://www. dh.gov.uk/prod_consum_dh/groups/dh_digitalassets/@dh/@en/documents/digitalasset/ dh_096065.pdf>.

Seeleib-Kaiser, M 2003, 'Rot-Grün am Ende?', in A Gohr and M Seeleib-Kaiser (eds), *Sozial- und Wirtschaftspolitik unter Rot-Grün*, Westdt. Verl., Wiesbaden, pp. 347–61.

Sheldrick, BM 2003, 'Judicial Review and the Allocation of Healthcare Resources in Canada and the United Kingdom', *Journal of Comparative Policy Analysis*, vol. 5, no. 2, pp. 149–66.

Siegel, NA 2007, 'When (Only) Money Matters: The Pros and Cons of Expenditure Analysis', in J Clasen and NA Siegel (eds), *Investigating Welfare State Change: The 'Dependent Variable Problem' in Comparative Analysis*, Edward Elgar, Cheltenham, pp. 43–71.

Starke, P and Obinger, H 2009, 'Are Welfare States Converging? Recent Social Policy Developments in Advanced OECD Countries', in I Dingeldey and H Rothgang (eds), *Governance of Welfare State Reform: A Cross National and Cross Sectoral Comparison of Policy and Politics*, Edward Elgar, Cheltenham, pp. 113–41.

Statistisches Bundesamt 2014, *Statistik der Bundesagentur für Arbeit, Arbeitslosigkeit im Zeitverlauf*, Statistisches Bundesamt, Wiesbaden, viewed 28 January 2014, <https:// www.destatis.de/DE/ZahlenFakten/Indikatoren/LangeReihen/Arbeitsmarkt/lrarb003. html#Fussnote1a>.

Steffen, M (ed.) 2005, *Health Governance in Europe: Issues, Challenges and Theories*, Routledge, London.

Stolt, E 1973, *Die Ersatzkassen der Krankenversicherung: Geschichte, Gestalt, Recht*, 7th edn, Asgard, Bonn.

Syrett, K 2004, 'Impotence or Importance? Judicial Review in an Era of Explicit NHS Rationing', *Modern Law Review*, vol. 67, no. 2, pp. 289–304.

———— 2011, 'Health Technology Appraisal and the Courts: Accountability for Reasonableness and the Judicial Model of Procedural Justice', *Health Economics, Policy and Law*, vol. 6, no. 4, pp. 469–88.

Talbot-Smith, A and Pollock, AM 2006, *The New NHS: A Guide*, Routledge, London.

Taylor, I 1999, 'Raising the Expectation Interest: New Labour and the Citizen's Charter', *Public Policy and Administration*, vol. 14, no. 4, pp. 29–38.

Taylor-Gooby, P 2005, 'New Risks and Social Change', in P Taylor-Gooby (ed.), *New Risks, New Welfare: The Transformation of the European Welfare State*, Oxford University Press, Oxford, pp. 1–28.

——— 2012, 'Root and Branch Restructuring to Achieve Major Cuts: The Social Policy Programme of the 2010 UK Coalition Government', *Social Policy and Administration*, vol. 46, no. 1, pp. 61–82.

Thorpe, A 2008, *A History of the British Labour Party*, 3rd edn, Palgrave Macmillan, Basingstoke.

Thränhardt, D 1996, *Geschichte der Bundesrepublik Deutschland 1949–1990*, Wissenschaftliche Buchgesellschaft, Darmstadt.

Timmins, N 2012, *Newer Again? The Story of the Health and Social Care Act 2012*, The King's Fund, Institute for Government, London.

Trägårdh, L and Svedberg, L 2013, 'The Iron Law of Rights: Citizenship and Individual Empowerment in Modern Sweden', in A Evers and A Guillemard (eds), *Social Policy and Citizenship: The Changing Landscape*, Oxford University Press, New York, pp. 222–56.

Turner, B 1990, 'Outline of a Theory of Citizenship', *Sociology*, vol. 24, no. 2, pp. 189–217.

Urban, H 2001, *Wettbewerbskorporatistische Regulierung im Politikfeld Gesundheit: Der Bundesausschuss der Ärtzte und Krankenkassen und die gesundheitspolitische Wende*, Arbeitsgruppe Public Health, Berlin.

Veitch, K 2012, 'Juridification, Medicalisation, and the Impact of EU Law: Patient Mobility and the Allocation of Scarce NHS Resources', *Medical Law Review*, vol. 20, no. 3, pp. 362–98.

Velasco-Garrido, M and Busse, R 2010, *Health Systems Research in Europe: Draft Report, Prepared for the Working Conference 'Health Services Research in Europe', 8–9 April 2010*, Berlin, viewed 22 April 2013, <http://www.nivel.nl/sites/default/files/bestanden/Report_Parallel%20Session_I_Health_Systems.pdf>.

Vincenti, A 2008, 'Gesundheitswesen und Sicherung bei Krankheit', in MH Geyer (ed.), *1974–1982, Bundesrepublik Deutschland: Neue Herausforderungen, wachsende Unsicherheiten*, Geschichte der Sozialpolitik in Deutschland seit 1945, vol. 6, Nomos, Baden-Baden, pp. 517–56.

Waller, P and Yong, B 2012, 'Case Studies II: Tuition Fees, NHS Reform, and Nuclear Policy', in R Hazell and B Yong (eds), *The Politics of Coalition: How the Conservative-Liberal Democrat Government Works*, Hart Pub., Oxford, pp. 172–89.

Wasem, J 1998, 'Im Schatten des GSG: Gesundheitspolitik in der 13. Wahlperiode des Deutschen Bundestages – eine (vorläufige) Bilanz', *Arbeit und Sozialpolitik*, vol. 52, nos. 7–8, pp. 18–30.

Wasem, J and Greß, S 2005, 'Gesundheitswesen und Sicherung bei Krankheit', in MG Schmidt (ed.), *1982–1989, Bundesrepublik Deutschland: Finanzielle Konsolidierung und institutionelle Reform*, Geschichte der Sozialpolitik in Deutschland seit 1945, vol. 7, Nomos, Baden-Baden, pp. 392–412.

Wasem, J, Greß, S and Hessel, F 2007, 'Gesundheitswesen und soziale Sicherung bei Krankheit', in GA Ritter and HG Hockerts (eds), *1989–1994, Bundesrepublik Deutschland: Sozialpolitik im Zeichen der Vereinigung*, Nomos, Baden-Baden, pp. 652–79.

Weaver, RK 1986, 'The Politics of Blame Avoidance', *Journal of Public Policy*, vol. 6, no. 4, pp. 371–98.

Webber, D 1988, 'Krankheit, Geld und Politik. Zur Geschichte der Gesundheitsreformen in Deutschland', *Leviathan*, vol. 16, no. 2, pp. 156–203.

——— 1989, 'Zur Geschichte der Gesundheitsreformen in Deutschland (II. Teil): Norbert Blüms Gesundheitsreform und die Lobby', *Leviathan*, vol. 17, no. 2, pp. 262–300.

Wennemo, I 1994, *Sharing the Costs of Children: Studies on the Development of Family Support in the OECD Countries*, Swedish Institute for Social Research, Stockholm.

Whitney, R 1988, *National Health Crisis: A Modern Solution*, Shepheard-Walwyn, London.

WHO 2009, *Scaling Up Research and Learning for Health Systems: Now Is the Time: Report of a High Level Task Force, Presented and Endorsed at the Global Ministerial Forum on Research for Health 2008, Bamako, Mali*, World Health Organization, Geneva.

Wille, M and Koch, E 2007, *Die Gesundheitsreform 2007: Grundriss*, Beck, München.

Wood, M 2013, *Holding Back the Tide: Hyper-Politicization and Ministerial Reactions to the Herceptin Postcode Lottery Crisis: Paper Presented at the PSA Annual General Conference, 25–27 March 2013*, Cardiff.

World Bank 1994, *Averting the Old Age Crisis: Policies to Protect the Old and Promote Growth; Summary*, World Bank, Washington, DC.

Yule, B 1993, 'Dental Care in the NHS: Reforms with Teeth?', *Health Policy*, vol. 25, nos. 1–2, pp. 63–80.

Zanon, E 2011, 'Healthcare across Borders: Implications of the EU Directive on Cross-border Healthcare for the English NHS', *Eurohealth*, vol. 17, nos. 1–2, pp. 34–6.

Zimmermann, C 2012, *Der gemeinsame Bundesausschuss: Normsetzung durch Richtlinien sowie Integration neuer Untersuchungs- und Behandlungsmethoden in den Leistungs-katalog der GKV*, Springer, Berlin.

Zipperer, M 1978, 'Die Auswirkungen des KVKG', *Die Ortskrankenkasse*, vol. 60, no. 1, pp. 11–29.

Zohlnhöfer, R and Egle, C 2007, 'Der Episode zweiter Teil – ein Überblick über die 15. Legislaturperiode', in C Egle and R Zohlnhöfer (eds), *Ende des rot-grünen Projektes: Eine Bilanz der Regierung Schröder 2002–2005*, VS Verl. für Sozialwissenschaften, Wiesbaden, pp. 11–25.

Index